New Advances in Palliative Care

New Advances in Palliative Care

Guest Editors

Georg Bollig
Erika Zelko

MDPI

Basel • Beijing • Wuhan • Barcelona • Belgrade • Novi Sad • Cluj • Manchester

Guest Editors
Georg Bollig
Department of Anesthesiology, Intensive Care, Palliative Medicine and Pain Therapy
HELIOS Klinikum Schleswig
Schleswig
Germany

Erika Zelko
Institute for General Medicine
Johannes Keppler University Linz
Linz
Austria

Editorial Office
MDPI AG
Grosspeteranlage 5
4052 Basel, Switzerland

This is a reprint of the Special Issue, published open access by the journal *Healthcare* (ISSN 2227-9032), freely accessible at: https://www.mdpi.com/journal/healthcare/special_issues/advance_palliative_care.

For citation purposes, cite each article independently as indicated on the article page online and as indicated below:

Lastname, A.A.; Lastname, B.B. Article Title. *Journal Name* **Year**, *Volume Number*, Page Range.

ISBN 978-3-7258-6936-7 (Hbk)
ISBN 978-3-7258-6937-4 (PDF)
https://doi.org/10.3390/books978-3-7258-6937-4

Contents

About the Editors

Georg Bollig

Georg Bollig, Associate Professor PD Dr. med., PhD, MAS (Palliative Care), DEAA, is a physician, researcher, and social entrepreneur.

After completing his medical studies at the universities of Cologne, Vienna, and Seattle, he became a specialist in anesthesiology, pain therapy, and palliative care. He received a Master's Degree in Palliative Care and Organisational Ethics from the University of Klagenfurt/IFF Vienna. His PhD at the University of Bergen, Norway, focused on palliative care, ethical challenges, and end-of-life decision-making in nursing homes. From 2016 to 2022, he worked as a senior consultant in Palliative Medicine at the University Hospital of Southern Jutland and as a Clinical Associate Professor in Palliative Care at the University of Southern Denmark. Currently, he works as a senior consultant in Palliative Medicine and is the head of Palliative Medicine at the academic teaching hospital Helios Klinikum Schleswig in Germany. In addition to his clinical work, Bollig is an Associate Professor in Palliative Medicine at the Department of Palliative Medicine, University of Cologne, Faculty of Medicine and University Hospital, Cologne, Germany. Bollig was the first scholar to introduce the idea of a Last Aid Course, and he is the leader of the International Last Aid working group and the Last Aid Research Group International (LARGI). His current research interests include public palliative care education (PPCE), Last Aid Courses, and telepalliative care. He has received a number of recognitions and awards for his work with Last Aid Courses, including awards from the German Association for Palliative Medicine and the Order of Merit of Schleswig-Holstein.

Erika Zelko

Erika Zelko, PhD, is a university professor at Johannes Kepler University in Linz and practices as a family physician in an outpatient clinical setting. She is an active collaborator at the University of Maribor's Institute for Palliative Care and serves as the head of the Institute of General Practice at Johannes Kepler University, Linz. Her research interests focus on palliative and end-of-life care, primary healthcare, the early identification of palliative needs, caregiver support, and community-based approaches to palliative care. She is a co-founder of the LARGI Research Group, a group dedicated to community palliative care, and is an instructor of the Last Aid program. Her work includes participation in national and international research projects, peer-reviewed publications, and contributions to educational and policy initiatives aimed at strengthening patient-centered and ethically grounded palliative care across healthcare settings.

Preface

Today, palliative care is seen as an essential part of healthcare. According to the World Health Organization's (WHO) definition, "Palliative care is an approach that improves the quality of life of patients and their families facing the problems associated with life-threatening illness, through the prevention and relief of suffering by means of early identification and impeccable assessment and treatment of pain and other problems, physical, psychosocial and spiritual." Nevertheless, palliative care is often associated with cancer and oncology patients, and both professionals and the public are lacking an awareness that patients with other chronic life-limiting diseases, including patients of different ethnicities and those from diverse backgrounds, may benefit from the provision of palliative care by community health services and/or specialized palliative care teams. New, inclusive approaches for all patients in need are paramount. During the COVID-19 pandemic, palliative care provision was hampered, and new methods for providing palliative care during a pandemic were developed, including telemedicine and telepalliative care. There are many questions that have been raised concerning the inclusion of individuals other than cancer patients in palliative care. These include how to provide palliative care in a pandemic setting or alongside curative intended therapy in intensive care and emergency medicine contexts. This reprint, "New Advances in Palliative Care", highlights recent advances and challenges in palliative care, addressing the inclusion of diverse patient groups in palliative care, palliative care in pandemic times, telepalliative care, and the use of modern technology in the field of palliative care. These articles will help guide researchers and clinicians from various fields, as well as the policymakers, officials, and politicians who are responsible for public health decisions and policies for the future.

Georg Bollig and Erika Zelko
Guest Editors

healthcare

MDPI

Editorial

New Advances in Palliative Care—State of the Field, Its Challenges and Advances at the End of the Year 2025

Georg Bollig [1,2,3,4,*] **and Erika Zelko** [3,5,6]

1 Department of Anesthesiology, Intensive Care, Palliative Medicine and Pain Therapy, Helios Klinikum Schleswig, St. Jürgener Str. 1-3, 24837 Schleswig, Germany
2 Department of Palliative Medicine, Faculty of Medicine and University Hospital, University of Cologne, Kerpener Str. 62, 50937 Köln, Germany
3 Last Aid Research Group International (LARGI), 24837 Schleswig, Germany; erika.zelko@jku.at
4 Letzte Hilfe Deutschland gGmbH, 24837 Schleswig, Germany
5 Institute for Palliative Medicine, Medical Faculty, University of Maribor, Taborska cesta 9, 2000 Maribor, Slovenia
6 Institute for General Medicine, Medical Faculty, Johannes Keppler University, Altenberger Str. 69, 4040 Linz, Austria
* Correspondence: georg.bollig@helios-gesundheit.de

1. Introduction

In recent decades, palliative care has become an essential component of modern healthcare systems. According to the World Health Organization (WHO), "Palliative care is an approach that improves the quality of life of patients and their families facing problems associated with life-threatening illness, through the prevention and relief of suffering by means of early identification and impeccable assessment and treatment of pain and other problems, physical, psychosocial and spiritual" [1]. Despite its recognized importance, an estimated 56.8 million people worldwide require palliative care each year, while only approximately 14% of those in need actually receive it [1]. This underlines the urgent need to strengthen and expand palliative care services around the world. Today we know that the need for palliative care is high, not only in cancer patients but also in patients with chronic non-oncologic conditions [2]. Unfortunately, palliative care is still frequently associated solely with imminent death or limited to oncology patients. Awareness remains insufficient among both healthcare professionals and the general public that individuals with other chronic, life-limiting conditions—as well as people from diverse ethnic, cultural, and social backgrounds—may also significantly benefit from palliative care delivered by community health services and specialized palliative care teams. To address these gaps, new approaches that promote inclusivity and foster collaboration among communities, informal carers, and healthcare professionals are essential. The Lancet Commission on the Value of Death and a number of other experts have stated that there is a need to improve death literacy, knowledge, and skills in palliative care and end-of-life care for everyone [3–6]. The COVID-19 pandemic further highlighted vulnerabilities in palliative care provision, as established services were disrupted and innovative methods of care delivery had to be developed. Digital solutions are often not fully implemented in palliative care and there is a need for development of digital infrastructures in the field of palliative care [7]. Telehealth and telepalliative care emerged as important tools to maintain communication and support patients and families during this unprecedented period [8–10]. Other new ways of including technology in palliative care provision are in the pilot phase, as, for example, the drone-based delivery of medication [11]. By the end of 2025, palliative care has continued to evolve globally. When Cicely Saunders started the palliative care and hospice movement in the 1960s, the first advances were the recognition of the needs of seriously ill and dying people by healthcare professionals, establishing hospices as places for both short-term and long-term palliative care, end-of-life care for those in need and of course the efforts to provide symptom relief for distressing symptoms, first of all providing access to opioids as morphine to treat pain and dyspnea. Later on, the focus broadened to a number of diseases other than cancer and to an increased availability of palliative care in the communities. Palliative Care and Palliative Medicine became in the course of this recognized fields for nurses, physicians and other healthcare professionals. Today, palliative medicine is recognized as a distinct medical specialty in some countries as Great Britain and Australia, while in others like Germany and the USA remains a subspecialty. In 2025, Dr. Balfour Mount—widely regarded as the father of palliative care in Canada and the physician who coined the term "palliative care"—passed away [12], marking a significant moment in the history of the field. His death reminds us to look back and acknowledge the achievements already made in palliative care but also to focus on the challenges that lie ahead. Looking back at the relatively short history of palliative care, the most important recent developments in the field from our point of view have been the early integration of palliative care in oncology, the expansion of the role of palliative care for patients with other chronic life-limiting diseases than cancer and telepalliative care in order to reach more people with specialized palliative care in rural areas or despite other hindrances to personal treatment at home or in an outpatient clinic. The most important gaps that should be addressed in the future include the knowledge about palliative care provision for all in need, taking into account the increasing need for palliative care and the demographic change, the broad implementation of early palliative care, how to improve public awareness and inclusion of informal carers in palliative care provision at home, the cooperation of professionals with lay people in compassionate communities and how to include new technologies as telepalliative care in the best interest of patients, relatives and healthcare professionals.

2. An Overview of Published Articles in This Special Issue

The aim of this Special Issue, "New Advances in Palliative Care", is to highlight recent developments and ongoing challenges related to the inclusion of diverse patient groups, palliative care during pandemics, telepalliative care, and the integration of modern technologies into palliative practice. The articles included in this Special Issue address a broad spectrum of topics within this framework and reflect perspectives from patients, relatives, volunteers, and healthcare professionals. Grimm et al. (contribution 1) present an approach to improve end-of-life outcomes through a minimal invasive intervention (MINI), which shows potential for enhancing patient-centered care and palliative care delivery in acute hospital settings (contribution 2). In the context of primary palliative care in the community, the role of primary healthcare professionals is crucial for identifying patient needs and ensuring timely referral to specialist services when required (contribution 3). Düzgün et al. highlight the potential contribution of university students as volunteers within caring communities (contribution 4), emphasizing the value of civic engagement in end-of-life care. Informal caregivers play a vital role in providing palliative and end-of-life care at home and should be adequately supported by specialized palliative care teams and through education for the public (contribution 5, contribution 12). Telehealth can serve as an additional modality to support informal caregivers in the home setting (contribution 5). However, caregivers' needs are often insufficiently addressed, leaving them vulnerable to emotional strain and financial burden (contribution 6). Hagen and Zelko demonstrate that the likelihood of dying at home is strongly associated with the availability of home-based healthcare services. Their registry-based study showed that patients with breast cancer and

https://doi.org/10.3390/healthcare14020206

heart failure were more likely to die at home than patients with dementia (contribution 7). This finding underscores the urgent need for broad implementation of caring communities and equitable access to palliative care irrespective of diagnosis. MacAden and Muirhead introduce the Dementia Education for Workforce Excellence (DEWE) program, an innovative educational resource that promotes person- and relationship-centered dementia care across all stages of the disease trajectory (contribution 8). Furthermore, a systematic review by Farrukh et al. suggests that re-irradiation may prolong survival in patients with progressive diffuse intrinsic pontine glioma as part of palliative treatment strategies (contribution 9). Public awareness remains a cornerstone of effective palliative care delivery. Spary-Kainz et al. demonstrate that public information campaigns can positively influence the home care of seriously ill individuals (contribution 10). Herrera-Gomez et al. describe the challenges connected to identifying palliative care needs and the referral to specialized palliative care (contribution 11). Bollig et al. report on ten years of practical and scientific experience with Last Aid Courses as means for Public Palliative Care Education. Educational measures like the LAC can contribute to raise public awareness for the topics of death, dying, and grief and may encourage lay people to participate in end-of-life care provision in the community.

3. Conclusions

Collectively, the contributions in this Special Issue enrich the growing body of palliative care knowledge grounded in practice, theory, and research from diverse global contexts. They show that the cooperation between healthcare professionals, patients, relatives, and lay people in a compassionate community approach can be a solution to provide palliative care for more patients in need. Together, we have to strive to make palliative care available for more people in need. As part of this collaboration and joint effort to improve palliative care provision around the world, further research and sustained implementation efforts are required to translate the scientific evidence into equitable, worldwide palliative care provision. With the contributions in this issue, some knowledge gaps could be addressed, as described above. Nevertheless, the field of palliative care practice and research has to be developed further. Future directions for improvement in practice and research are as follows:

- ○ Early integration of Palliative Care;
- ○ Make Palliative Care available everywhere for all in need;
- ○ Public awareness and participation of lay persons in Palliative Care provision in compassionate communities;
- ○ New technologies to support Palliative Care (e.g., telepalliative care);
- ○ Encourage an open public debate on assisted dying.

Although we know that early integration of palliative care in the course of different diseases is meaningful, early integration is still lacking in many clinical situations. Up to 10% of patient visits in the Emergency Department are due to palliative care needs [13]. Early recognition of these needs can help to reduce symptom burden. More efforts are needed to make early integration of palliative care a standard throughout healthcare, including all emergency departments. As shown above, the overall need for palliative care worldwide is much higher than the actual numbers of palliative care provision [1]. Therefore, we need a combination of different measures in order to be able to address the future palliative care needs worldwide. Based on the findings presented in this Special Issue and our broader perspective, future challenges in palliative care include ensuring access for all individuals in need and developing innovative models to support informal caregivers both financially and through practical and psychological assistance. As articulated by Kellehear, palliative and end-of-life care are "everybody's business" [14]. His "95% rule" emphasizes that seriously ill and dying individuals spend only about 5% of their final

https://doi.org/10.3390/healthcare14020206

year of life in direct contact with healthcare services, while the remaining 95% depends on informal caregivers—family members, friends, and community members—to provide care [14]. Public awareness and contribution of lay people is urgently needed. One measure to improve public knowledge is public palliative care education throughout society starting already in school. The example of Last Aid Courses for the public is shown in contribution 12. These LACs can improve palliative care knowledge and encourage people to participate in end-of-life provision in the model of compassionate communities (contribution 12) [14]. The integration of digitalization and new technologies as telepalliative care and other technical innovations may help to provide palliative care for more people living in rural areas without direct access to specialist palliative care [7–11]. Another important challenge for the future is an open public debate about assisted suicide and the connection to palliative care. In many countries, a number of people are for or against it. This is also true for palliative care practitioners [15]. Therefore, an open debate of all people, including healthcare professionals, ethicists, and politicians, is needed in order to find practical ways to support people at the end of life. The availability of palliative care for everyone in need, adequate funding of palliative care services [16], and the best possible symptom relief for suffering patients are from our point of view the most important measures to address the wish for assisted death.

To meet the increasing demand for palliative care within communities, enhanced collaboration between lay people and healthcare professionals, supported by a caring community approach, is essential. Telepalliative care holds significant promise, but further research and practice-based models are needed to integrate this approach effectively into routine care and community structures. When everyone contributes, we can collectively strive to ensure compassionate care for all those in need.

Author Contributions: G.B. and E.Z. contributed equally to the conceptualization, curation, and writing of this editorial. All authors have read and agreed to the published version of the manuscript.

Conflicts of Interest: The authors declare no conflicts of interest.

List of Contributions:

1. Grimm, J.S.; Kasdorf, A.; Voltz, R.; Strupp, J. From MINI to Meaningful Change—A German Pilot Study to Improve Patient Outcomes in End-of-Life Care. *Healthcare* **2025**, *13*, 2024. https://doi.org/10.3390/healthcare13162024.
2. Kasdorf, A.; Werner, B.; Grimm, J.S.; Dust, G.; Simon, S.T.; Voltz, R.; Strupp, J., on behalf of the Cologne Research and Development Network (CoRe-Net) Study Group. Promising Concept, Challenging Implementation of a Minimally Invasive Intervention (MINI) to Identify Patients in Their Last Year of Life—A Multi-Methods Feasibility Study at a German University Hospital. *Healthcare* **2025**, *13*, 2784. https://doi.org/10.3390/healthcare13212784.
3. Barreto, C.; Silva, M.M.d.; Fernandes, A.F.C.; Yanez, R.J.V.; Laranjeira, C. The Practices of Portuguese Primary Health Care Professionals in Palliative Care Access and Referral: A Focus Group Study. *Healthcare* **2025**, *13*, 1576. https://doi.org/10.3390/healthcare13131576.
4. Düzgün, G.; Kılıç Öztürk, Y.; Polat, G.; Şahin, S. Volunteer Services in Palliative Care by Third Age University Students. *Healthcare* **2024**, *12*, 2591. https://doi.org/10.3390/healthcare12242591.
5. Caetano, P.; Querido, A.; Laranjeira, C. Preparedness for Caregiving Role and Telehealth Use to Provide Informal Palliative Home Care in Portugal: A Qualitative Study. *Healthcare* **2024**, *12*, 1915. https://doi.org/10.3390/healthcare12191915.
6. Pieper, S.; Kasdorf, A.; Voltz, R.; Strupp, J. "What Do You Get? Nothing": A Qualitative Analysis of the Financial Impact of Family Caregiving for a Dying Relative at Home in Germany. *Healthcare* **2025**, *13*, 810. https://doi.org/10.3390/healthcare13070810.
7. Hagen, T.P.; Zelko, E. Exploring End-of-Life Care for Patients with Breast Cancer, Dementia or Heart Failure: A Register-Based Study of Individual and Institutional Factors. *Healthcare* **2024**, *12*, 943. https://doi.org/10.3390/healthcare12090943.

8. Macaden, L.; Muirhead, K. Dementia Education for Workforce Excellence: Evaluation of a Novel Bichronous Approach. *Healthcare* **2024**, *12*, 590. https://doi.org/10.3390/healthcare12050590.
9. Farrukh, S.; Habib, S.; Rafaqat, A.; Sarfraz, Z.; Sarfraz, A.; Sarfraz, M.; Robles-Velasco, K.; Felix, M.; Cherrez-Ojeda, I. Emerging Therapeutic Strategies for Diffuse Intrinsic Pontine Glioma: A Systematic Review. *Healthcare* **2023**, *11*, 559. https://doi.org/10.3390/healthcare11040559.
10. Spary-Kainz, U.; Posch, N.; Paier-Abuzahra, M.; Lieb, M.; Avian, A.; Zelko, E.; Siebenhofer, A. Palliative Care Survey: Awareness, Knowledge and Views of the Styrian Population in Austria. *Healthcare* **2023**, *11*, 2611. https://doi.org/10.3390/healthcare11192611.
11. Herrera-Gomez, M.I.; Iribarne-Duran, M.L.; Carcia-Caro, M.P.; López-Morales, M.; Esteban-Burgos, A.A.; Montoya-Juárez, R. Experiences of Primary Care Nurse Case Managers in Palliative Care Needs Identification and Complex Chronic Patients' Referral to Advanced Palliative Care Resources. *Healthcare* **2026**, *14*, 85. https://doi.org/10.3390/healthcare14010085.
12. Bollig, G.; Mills, J.; Müller-Koch, S.; Pani, P.; Neumann, B.; Zelko, E. Last Aid Courses as a Means for Public Palliative Care Education—A Narrative Review of the Literature and 10 Years of Experience Around the World with Implications for Future Research. *Healthcare* **2026**, *14*, 96. https://doi.org/10.3390/healthcare14010096.

References

1. World Health Organization. Palliative Care. Available online: https://www.who.int/news-room/fact-sheets/detail/palliative-care (accessed on 19 December 2025).
2. Villanueva-Quispe, A.; Rivarola-Hidalgo, M.; Fuentes-Yufra, A.; Ale-Sánchez, M.; Copaja-Corzo, C.; Flores-Cohaila, J.A.; Miranda-Chavez, B. Need for palliative care in patients with chronic diseases in a hospital in a developing country. *Palliat. Care Soc. Pract.* **2025**, *19*, 1–8. [CrossRef] [PubMed]
3. Sallnow, L.; Smith, R.; Ahmedzai, S.H.; Bhadelia, A.; Chamberlain, C.; Cong, Y.; Doble, B.; Dullie, L.; Durie, R.; Finkelstein, E.A.; et al. Report of the Lancet Commission on the Value of Death: Bringing death back into life. *Lancet* **2022**, *399*, 837–884. [CrossRef] [PubMed]
4. Bollig, G.; Hayes Bauer, E. Last Aid Courses as measure for public palliative care education—A narrative review. *Ann. Palliat. Med.* **2021**, *10*, 8242–8253. [CrossRef] [PubMed]
5. McIlfatrick, S.; Hasson, F.; McLaughlin, D.; Johnston, G.; Roulston, A.; Rutherford, L.; Noble, H.; Kelly, S.; Craig, A.; Kernohan, W.G. Public awareness and attitudes toward palliative care in Northern Ireland. *BMC Palliat. Care* **2013**, *12*, 34. [CrossRef] [PubMed]
6. Bollig, G.; Brandt Kristensen, F.; Wolff, D.L. Citizens appreciate talking about death and learning end-of-life care—A mixedmethods study on views and experiences of 5469 Last aid Course participants. *Prog. Palliat. Care* **2021**, *29*, 140–148. [CrossRef]
7. Hodiamont, F.; Jansky, M.; Golic, L.; Bausewein, C.; Hriskova, K. Is digitalization still an uncharted territory for palliative care? Use of electronic patient records and assessment instruments in German specialist palliative care: Results of an online survey. *BMC Health Serv. Res.* **2025**, *Online ahead of print.* [CrossRef] [PubMed]
8. Sigaard, J.A.V.; Joensen, E.D.R.; Birgisdottir, U.R.; Spindler, H.; Dinesen, B. Telepalliation creates a sense of security: A qualitative study of patients with cancer receiving palliative care. *Palliat. Med.* **2025**, *Online ahead of print.* [CrossRef] [PubMed]
9. Bandini, J.; Tsuei, J.; Kavalieratos, D.; Ahluwalia, S.C.; Vazquez, E.; Curseen, K.; Harrison, J.M. "Telehealth Allows for Flexibility and More Equity": Provider Perspectives on Telehealth for Outpatient Palliative Care for Underserved Patients. *J. Palliat. Med.* **2025**, *28*, 655–660. [CrossRef] [PubMed]
10. Haydon, H.M.; Lotfaliany, M.; Broadbent, A.; Snoswell, C.L.; Smith, A.C.; Brydon, J.-A.; Caffery, L.J.; Thomas, E.E. Telehealth-facilitated palliative care enables more people to die at home: An analysis of clinical outcomes and service activity data. *BMC Palliat. Care* **2025**, *24*, 22. [CrossRef] [PubMed]
11. Fink, F.; Otto, S.C.; Grünthal, M.; Lehmann, A.; Jahn, P. Family Caregivers' Perspectives on the Potential of Drone-Based Medication Delivery in Palliative Home Care: Qualitative Focus Group Study. *JMIR Hum. Factors* **2025**, *12*, e80320. [CrossRef] [PubMed]
12. McGill. Balfour Mount. Available online: https://www.mcgill.ca/palliativecare/about/portraits/balfour-mount (accessed on 19 December 2025).
13. Munsch, C.; Bergrath, S.; Kreß, J.S.; Graeven, U.; Rödler, J.V. Patient Characteristics and Different Decision Paths for Establishing Palliative Care for Patients Admitted via the Emergency Department. *J. Clin. Med.* **2025**, *14*, 8935. [CrossRef] [PubMed]
14. Kellehear, A. The social nature of dying and the social model of health. In *Oxford Textbook of Public Health Palliative Care*; Oxford University Press: Oxford, UK, 2022; pp. 22–29.

https://doi.org/10.3390/healthcare14020206

15. Grove, G.L.; Lovell, M.R.; Butow, P.; Hughes, I.; Best, M. Shaping a knowable event or embracing a mysterious journey: A mixed methods study on palliative care clinician views on voluntary assisted dying. *Palliat. Support. Care* **2025**, *23*, e153. [CrossRef] [PubMed]
16. Finlay, I.G. Pain, palliative care, and the politics of dying: Rethinking suffering in the assisted suicide debate. *Br. J. Pain* **2025**, *Online ahead of print*. [CrossRef] [PubMed]

https://doi.org/10.3390/healthcare14020206

healthcare

MDPI

Article

From MINI to Meaningful Change—A German Pilot Study to Improve Patient Outcomes in End-of-Life Care

Jana Sophie Grimm [1,*], Alina Kasdorf [1], Raymond Voltz [1,2,3] and Julia Strupp [1]

[1] Department of Palliative Medicine, Faculty of Medicine and University Hospital, University of Cologne, 50937 Cologne, Germany; alina.kasdorf@uk-koeln.de (A.K.); raymond.voltz@uk-koeln.de (R.V.); julia.strupp@uk-koeln.de (J.S.)

[2] Center for Health Services Research, Faculty of Medicine and University Hospital, University of Cologne, 50937 Cologne, Germany

[3] Center for Integrated Oncology Aachen Bonn Cologne Dusseldorf (CIO ABCD), Faculty of Medicine and University Hospital, University of Cologne, 50937 Cologne, Germany

* Correspondence: jana.s.grimm@protonmail.com

Abstract: Background/Objectives: Early identification of terminally ill patients is crucial for enhancing care, patient and care partner satisfaction, and healthcare staff confidence in discussing disease trajectories. Yet, timely recognition remains challenging. To address this, we developed a minimally invasive intervention (MINI) for general hospital wards. We aimed to evaluate the MINI's feasibility in facilitating an earlier identification of terminally ill patients and improving patient reported outcomes in a hospital setting. **Methods**: This prospective, two-arm pre-post intervention study at a university hospital evaluated the MINI alongside usual care. Patient-reported outcomes, including quality of life (SF-12), palliative care needs (IPOS), and functional status (ECOG), were collected at baseline and every three months over 12 months. Participants were allocated to a control or intervention group. **Results**: Of 188 patients identified using the Surprise Question, 58 completed the baseline assessment. While physical functioning (SF-12 PCS) remained comparable, the intervention group experienced clinically meaningful improvements in mental health (SF-12 MCS) at three months, with positive trends at six months. This group also showed a decline in palliative care needs, reduced emotional symptoms, and improved performance status, evidenced by significant differences in non-parametric analyses. These findings underscore the MINI's potential to significantly improve patient well-being. **Conclusions**: This pilot study demonstrated the feasibility of the MINI and suggests it may foster meaningful system-wide change in patient-centred care within acute hospital settings, leading to improved patient outcomes and more confident healthcare staff in identifying terminally ill patients. However, given the small sample size, these findings should be interpreted with caution. Future research with larger cohorts and extended intervention periods is warranted to fully elucidate the MINI's impact and refine strategies for improving care for terminally ill patients.

Keywords: terminal care; quality of life; patient care; hospitals; feasibility studies

1. Introduction

Palliative care is often only associated with the dying phase, but its scope is broader than that [1–3]. It involves early planning and the consideration of the wishes and needs of patients and their family and friends regarding care options and their preferred place of death in their last year of life. It emphasizes enabling patients and their families to maintain the highest possible quality of life until the end of their lives [2].

On a global scale, the increasing prevalence of chronic, life-limiting conditions, including cancer, cardiovascular diseases, respiratory diseases, and renal diseases, as well as ageing populations, underscores the growing need for comprehensive palliative care interventions within healthcare systems [4]. Terminally ill patients in their last year of life face various imponderables [5]. Owing to the advanced and incurable nature of the disease, care provision creates multidimensional treatment and delivery requirements, all of which influence health-related quality of life and contribute to perceived suffering [6,7]. Although evidence supports the need for palliative care in both cancer and non-cancer patients, inequalities in communication and access to specialist palliative care persist [8]. Moreover, late and non-empathetic communication about the prospect of death is associated with distress, whereas empathic discussions are linked to fewer transitions in the last year of life [9]. Data suggest that 40.7% to 96.1% of patients who die would benefit from palliative care [10]. Early communication about the disease and care planning can improve quality of life, increase patient autonomy, and enhance satisfaction [11].

Nevertheless, identifying patients in their last year of life, particularly those with conditions other than cancer, remains challenging, leading to delays in palliative care referral, unmet palliative care needs, and difficulties in shared decision making about care options [12,13]. Consequently, patients' wishes often remain unclear for too long [11]. Beyond patient outcomes, the quality of end-of-life care is profoundly influenced by the well-being and engagement of family and friend caregivers. Understanding and supporting caregivers by addressing aspects such as their quality of life [14], burden [15], self-efficacy, confidence, and preparedness [16,17] is an integral part of comprehensive palliative care.

General hospital wards serve as critical checkpoints in the last year of life. In a preceding study by our research team [5], 91% of terminally ill patients were hospitalized at least once during their last year of life. This setting thus provides an ideal opportunity to determine whether a patient is terminally ill and in need of palliative care and to initiate appropriate care accordingly. Unfortunately, this opportunity is rarely seized. In addition, satisfaction with general hospital services is the lowest among all healthcare settings, particularly compared with nursing homes and home care [6,13]. Although 68% of patients would have preferred to die at home, between 42% and 47% of deaths in Germany occur in hospitals [5]. In most cases, deaths in the last year of life are not unexpected, but result from previously diagnosed progressive diseases, the interaction of risk factors or diseases (multimorbidity), or the end of a natural ageing process. Particularly for non-cancer diseases, integration into palliative care structures may be delayed or absent [8]. Transitions from curative to palliative care are fluid. However, there is no consensus on the optimal timing of palliative care integration, although earlier involvement is thought to be most beneficial. Additional barriers include the life-sustaining culture of hospitals, where preventing death is the norm, combined with budgetary and time constraints and the absence of established standards for patients likely to die in the foreseeable future [18].

To improve care and satisfaction for terminally ill patients and their families while enhancing healthcare professionals' (HCPs) confidence and competence, we developed a minimally invasive intervention (MINI) that incorporates simple yet effective clinical tools. This intervention employs a two-sided, trigger-question-based approach involving HCPs, patients, and family carers [6]. We aimed to evaluate the MINI's feasibility in facilitating an earlier identification of terminally ill patients and improving patient-reported outcomes in a hospital setting. Specifically, using patient-reported outcome measures (PROMS), we investigated key healthcare outcomes, including quality of life, palliative care needs, and functional status in terminally ill patients. By promoting the early identification of palliative care needs and fostering communication through collaborative decision making, the MINI may address critical gaps in end-of-life care [2,12,19].

2. Materials and Methods

2.1. Study Design

This phase II pilot study is part of the broader project "Last Year of Life Study Cologne—Part 2 (LYOL-C-II)". The study employs a prospective interventional design using a mixed-methods approach in a pre-post structure divided into two phases, as detailed in the study protocol [6]. This paper reports data collected from terminally ill patients during the second phase. The effects of the intervention on hospital staff (Kasdorf et al., in preparation [20]) and care partner data, including the Zarit Burden Interview [15] (Grimm et al., in preparation [21]), are reported separately. Patient data were used to assess the feasibility and potential of the minimally invasive intervention (MINI), alongside usual care, to enhance patient-reported outcomes, including quality of life (SF-12 [22]), palliative care needs (IPOS [23]), and functional status (ECOG [24,25]). The study was conducted in accordance with the Declaration of Helsinki and received ethical approval from the Ethics Commission of the Faculty of Medicine of Cologne University (20-1431). The trial is registered in the German Clinical Trials Register (DRKS00022378, registration date: 10 February 2021). This study was reported in accordance with the STROBE Statement for observational studies [26]. The STROBE checklist can be found in the Supplementary Material.

2.2. Intervention and Study Procedure

The intervention was developed to facilitate the early identification of patients in their last year of life and to prompt HCPs to revisit and revise the existing care plan. To this end, it integrates the *12-month Surprise Question (SQ)* ("Would I be surprised if this patient died in the next 12 months?") [27] and the *Supportive and Palliative Care Indicators Tool* (SPICT-DE™) [28], both of which are concise, validated screening instruments designed to flag individuals who may benefit for palliative services and guide advanced care planning discussions. In addition, patients and their care partners received a *"Conversation Guide for Your Healthcare,"* a question prompt sheet (QPS) intended to structure and enable dialogues about prognosis, preferences, and care priorities for patients and their care partners [6].

Patients were allocated to either a control arm—receiving usual care and assessed prior to implementation of the MINI—or an intervention arm, in which usual care was supplemented by the MINI. In the control arm, a small team of senior physicians applied the 12-month SQ, either individually or collaboratively to identify eligible patients. In the intervention arm, all ward staff (physicians, nurses, and case managers) underwent a single comprehensive 60–90 min training session that addressed core palliative care principles, the rationale for early integration, and empathic communication techniques for discussing terminal illness. After the training, staff used the SQ in conjunction with SPICT-DE™ to screen all patients and encourage patients (and their care partners) to use the QPS during discussions about care preferences and trajectories. A schematic overview of the MINI is shown in Figure 1 (inspired by Afshar et al. [29]).

2.3. Recruitment Procedure

Recruitment for this prospective, two-arm pre-post intervention study followed a four-step procedure:

1. **Initial Screening**: HCPs (medical and nursing staff) on participating wards (Ward 1, primarily treating non-cancer patients; Ward 2, cancer inpatients/outpatients) identified eligible patients. This occurred during regular contact (visits and team meetings) or with study personnel (researchers (JG, BW) or study nurse (LW)) present at least twice weekly. **Inclusion criteria were** (a) patients who were identified via the Surprise Question ("Would you be surprised if this patient died within 12 months?" to which the answer was recorded as "no") and the SPICT-DE™ tool; (b) aware of their

incurable disease and limited prognosis; (c) aged ≥ 18 years; (d) capable of providing informed consent; (e) cognitively able to participate; and (f) fluent in German;

2. **Recruitment Log Completion**: For each flagged patient, HCPs completed a standardized recruitment log and confirmed all inclusion criteria, especially the patient's awareness of their condition's incurability;
3. **Patient Contact Form**: HCPs provided identified patients with a contact form to indicate their willingness to be contacted by the study team. These forms were securely collected by study personnel from the physician's office. Study personnel regularly contacted wards to ensure ongoing screening;
4. **Informed Consent and Baseline**: Study personnel retrieved forms, contacted interested patients, and provided detailed study information. If patients were interested, the conversation guide (QPS) was distributed and their written informed consent was obtained. Care partner contact details were also collected for burden assessment, with this data to be published separately (Grimm et al., in preparation [21]). A baseline assessment (T0) was scheduled only after consent was secured.

HCPs ask themselves or as a team (not in front of the patient) during visits, team meetings, or other moments of patient contact:

"Would I be surprised if this patient died in the next 12 months?"

- If no, the patient is eligible for the study;
- If unsure, use the SPICT-DE™; identification occurs if two or more indicators are present (combined from general and specific indicators);
- If yes, the patient is not yet considered in their last year of life. In consequence, the SQ should be asked regularly due to dynamic disease progression.

Eligible **patients** (identified as "No" with SQ or with at least two SPICT indicators) received the conversation guide. Its use was encouraged for their contact with HCPs or when organizing their own care.

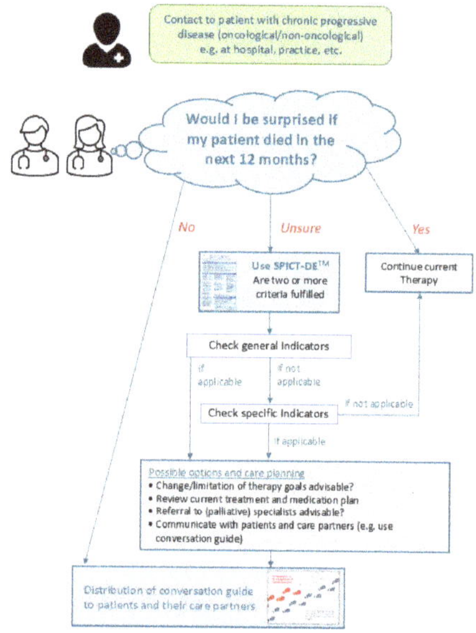

Figure 1. Illustration of the minimally invasive intervention (MINI).

2.4. Data Collection

The study, initially planned for 36 months starting May 2020, aimed to recruit 36 patients per group, totaling 72 participants [6]. Overall data collection spanned from February 2021 to August 2023. Recruitment for the control group (CG) in Ward 1 (non-cancer patients) started in February 2021, followed by the intervention group (IG) in April 2022. In Ward 2 (cancer inpatients/outpatients), CG recruitment began in June 2021, with IG recruitment in September 2022. Both concluded in August 2023.

Quantitative data were collected over 12 months for both CG and IG at five time points: baseline (T0) at enrolment, and at 3 (T1), 6 (T2), 9 (T3), and 12 months (T4) post-enrolment. Data were gathered through face-to-face interviews at the University Hospital, patients' homes, or via telephone. Researchers read instructions and questions aloud, and participants responded verbally. Interviews typically lasted 40–90 min, varying with patient health and mood. In addition to quantitative data, field notes from HCPs, patients, and relatives, as well as interview comments, provided qualitative insights. Due to various implementation delays (discussed elsewhere), only T0 to T2 results will be compared for a clearer analysis of control and intervention phases.

2.5. Measurements

Participant Characteristics. We collected patients' sociodemographic and specific disease characteristics at baseline (T0) and their preferred final place of care at each time point (T0–T4). Reasons for non-participation were also assessed.

Potential effects. The primary patient outcome was self-reported quality of life (QoL) using the "*Short-Form Health Service (SF-12)*" [22,30–32]. The SF-12 is commonly used for measuring QoL using two norm-based summary scales (*Physical Component Score*, PCS-12; *Mental Component Score*, MCS-12) with a population mean of 50 and a standard deviation of 10. The possible range for each score domain is 0–100, with higher scores indicating better QoL. Further, we assessed palliative care needs using the "*Integrated Palliative care Outcome Scale (IPOS)*". It consists of a total sum scale (0–68) and three subscales (*physical symptoms* (0–40), *emotional problems* (0–16), and *communication and practical issues* (0–12)) [23]. The higher the score, the greater the need. Moreover, the functional status of the patients was assessed during the survey by the respective interviewers. For this purpose, the "*Eastern Cooperative Oncology Group Performance Status (ECOG)*" [24,25] was used with scores from 0 to 5, in which higher values indicate lower performance status.

2.6. Statistical Analysis

Data are presented as the mean $\pm$ standard deviation for continuous variables and as counts (percentages) for categorical variables. Group differences were assessed using independent samples t-tests for normally distributed data and Mann–Whitney U tests otherwise, with normality being assessed via the Shapiro–Wilk test. A significance threshold of $\alpha < 0.05$ was used. No a priori dichotomization ("high" vs. "low") was performed to preserve validity in this exploratory pilot study. The intervention effects were evaluated using linear mixed-effects models (LMMs) with restricted maximum likelihood (REML) estimation and Satterthwaite approximation for degrees of freedom. Time was modelled as a categorical factor with three levels (baseline, three months, and six months). Fixed effects included group, time, group $\times$ time interaction, gender, ward, and age (mean-centred), with categorical predictors being dummy-coded (reference: intervention group, six months, male, gynecology ward). Random intercepts were specified for each participant and an AR(1) residual covariance structure was applied. Random slopes and alternative structures were tested but were omitted due to convergence issues. Missing data in this pilot were documented at each time point and handled under the missing at random (MAR) assumption via likelihood-based REML to include participants with partial data. Due to the exploratory nature of the pilot study, formal multiplicity adjustment (e.g., Bonferroni corrections) was omitted to avoid obscuring potentially meaningful associations. To mitigate potential selection bias from screening, we used standardized screening logs. All analyses were conducted using SPSS version 28. Qualitative comments and field notes were analyzed following the approach outlined by Miles et al. [33].

3. Results

3.1. Allocation and Dropout

A total of 188 patients were identified using the Surprise Question within the control and intervention phase. Of these, 110 met the formal inclusion criteria, of whom 66 signed the informed consent form. However, only 58 started the baseline assessment. Among these, 33 (56.9%) were control participants and 25 (43.1%) were intervention participants. This corresponds to an overall participation rate of 50.9%, with rates of 55.2% for the control group and 42.86% for the intervention group. In the control phase, 88 patients were identified using the SQ, with 49 patients on the non-cancer ward and 39 patients on the cancer ward. Despite more non-cancer patients being initially identified, slightly more cancer patients eventually participated. In the intervention phase, the distribution was comparable: 47 of the 100 identified patients were on the non-cancer ward, and 50 were on the cancer ward. Despite this balance, a higher proportion of cancer patients participated in the study (18 vs. 6). The non-participation of patients was attributed to various reasons: a lack of interest (33.8%), emotional or physical exhaustion (28.4%), cognitive impairment (18.9%), death (6.8%), and other reasons (12.2%). Figure 2 provides allocation and dropout details.

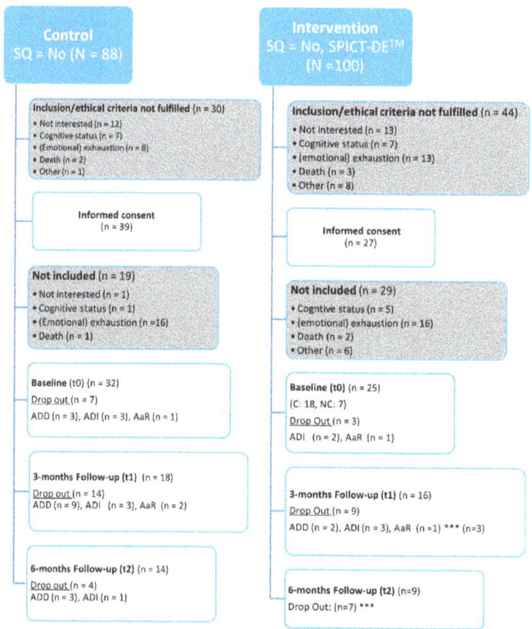

Figure 2. Flowchart with allocation and dropout details with classification of attrition based on Higginson et al. [34,35] (attrition due to death (ADD), attrition due to illness (ADI), attrition at random (AaR)); *** attrition due to end of study period.

3.2. General Sample Characteristics at Baseline

A total of 79.3% of the patients were female and 20.7% were male. The proportion of women outnumbered men in both the control and intervention groups (75.8% and 84%, respectively). At baseline, the mean age of the patients was 63.28 years ± 13.43, with the mean age of the control patients being marginally higher (64.76 years ± 13.63 years) than that of the intervention patients (61.32 years ± 13.17 years). Male patients were on average approximately 10 years older. Gender differences in age were greater in the intervention group, with a mean age of 48 years for female intervention participants compared to 72 years for male intervention participants. A total of 67% of patients in the control group and 56% in the intervention had a nursing care grade. If patients had a nursing care grade, they were more likely to have a higher care grade, i.e., care grades 2–4, and, thus, were more dependent on help (Spearman's $p = 0.636$, $p < 0.001$). The majority of patients stated that they had known about their underlying disease for at least one year or longer (82.5%). In the control group, 12.1% had known about their illness for at least one month but less than six months. In the intervention group, 8.3% stated that they had only learnt about their illness 24 h ago. Looking at the distribution of the underlying disease, more participants had cancer (60.3%). The patients consistently preferred their own home or a hospice as their final place of care. Approximately 21.4% of patients reported experiencing financial hardship due to their illness; however, a greater proportion of control patients reported this issue (31.3% vs. 8.3%). Details are shown in Table 1.

Table 1. Sample characteristics of both control and intervention patients ($n = 58$).

Characteristics	Control n (%) M (SD)	Intervention n (%) M (SD)	Total n (%) M (SD)
Care partner enrolled in study			
No	18 (52.9)	19 (73.1)	37 (61.7)
Yes	16 (47.1)	7 (26.9)	23 (38.3)
Care setting of recruitment			
Internal medicine unit	16 (48.5)	7 (28.0)	23 (39.7)
Gynecological inpatient unit	4 (12.1)	2 (8.0)	6 (10.3)
Gynecological outpatient unit	13 (39.4)	16 (64.0)	30 (50.0)
Highest school qualification *			
High school or lower	12 (36.4)	10 (43.5)	22 (39.3)
Vocational degree	14 (42.4)	7 (30.4)	21 (37.5)
University degree	7 (21.2)	6 (26.1)	13 (23.2)
Age	64.76 ± 13.63	61.32 ± 13.17	63.28 ± 13.43
Sex			
Female	25 (75.8)	21 (84.0)	46 (79.3)
Male	8 (24.2)	4 (16.0)	12 (20.7)
Relationship status			
Single	2 (6.1)	7 (29.2)	9 (15.8)
Married/civil partnership	19 (57.6)	12 (50.0)	31 (53.6)
Divorced	7 (21.2)	2 (8.3)	9 (15.8)
Widowed	5 (15.2)	3 (12.5)	8 (14.0)
Religion (NA 2)			
None	6 (18.8)	6 (25.0)	12 (21.4)
Christianity	24 (75.0)	18 (75.0)	42 (75.0)
Islam	2 (6.3)	0 (0.0)	2 (3.6)
Employment			
No	25 (78.1)	16 (80.7)	40 (71.4)
Currently on sick leave	3 (9.4)	4 (16.7)	7 (12.5)
Yes	4 (12.5)	4 (16.7)	8 (14.3)
Children (NA 1)			
No	4 (12.1)	8 (33.3)	12 (21.1)
Yes	29 (87.9)	16 (66.7)	45 (78.9)
1	10 (31.3)	4 (16.7)	14 (25.0)
2	10 (31.1)	9 (37.5)	19 (33.9)
3 or more	8 (25.0)	3 (12.5)	11 (19.6)
Living situation (NA 1)			
Living alone	6 (18.2)	9 (37.5)	15 (26.3)
Living with another person	27 (81.8.4)	15 (62.5)	42 (73.7)

Table 1. *Cont.*

Characteristics	Control n (%) M (SD)	Intervention n (%) M (SD)	Total n (%) M (SD)
Care Grade ** (NA 1)			
No	10 (30.3)	11 (45.8)	21 (36.8)
Yes	23 (69.7)	13 (54.2)	36 (63.2)
Care grade 1	1 (3.0)	1 (4.2)	2 (3.5)
Care grade 2	8 (24.2)	2 (8.3)	10 (17.5)
Care grade 3	11 (33.3)	5 (20.8)	16 (28.1)
Care grade 4	3 (9.1)	4 (16.7)	7 (12.3)
Unsure	0 (0.0)	1 (4.2)	1 (1.8)
Planned/applied for	2 (6.1)	0 (0.0)	2 (3.5)
Knowledge about incurability (NA 3)			
<24 h	0 (0.0)	2 (8.7)	2 (3.6)
1 week to <1 month	0 (0.0)	1 (4.3)	1 (1.8)
1 to <6 months	4 (12.5)	1 (4.3)	5 (9.1)
6 months to <1 year	1 (3.1)	0 (0.0)	1 (1.8)
≥1 year	27 (84.4)	19 (82.6)	47 (86.6)
Financial problems			
No	16 (50.0)	14 (58.3)	30 (51.7)
Rather not	2 (6.3)	4 (16.7)	6 (10.3)
Rather yes	4 (12.5)	3 (12.5)	7 (12.1)
Yes	10 (31.3)	2 (8.3)	12 (21.4)
Not sure	0 (0.0)	1 (4.2)	1 (1.8)

Note: NA = no data; M = mean; SD = standard deviation. * *School qualification* based on German system. ** Nursing *care grades* are used in the German care system to classify people's dependency on care as follows: 1. slight impairment of independence; 2. considerable impairment of independence; 3. severe impairment of independence; 4. most severe impairment of independence; 5. most severe impairment of independence with special requirements for nursing care.

3.3. *Self-Reported Health-Related Quality of Life with the Short-Form Health Service (SF-12)*

3.3.1. Physical Component Score

The mean physical quality of life of patients was found to be low (see Figure 3 and Table 2). Across both groups and at each time point, the data were found to be below the average German standard sample mean of 48.22 ± 8.77. At baseline (T0), the mean PCS for the intervention group was marginally higher (M = 33.40, SD = 5.50) in comparison to the control group (M = 31.34, SD = 5.53). However, these differences were not significant for the PCS between the intervention group and the control group ($t(56) = -1.246$, $p = 0.109$). Following a three-month period (T1), both groups demonstrated a slight increase in their scores, with the intervention group continuing to report higher scores (M = 35.14, SD = 7.20) in comparison to the control group (M = 32.54, SD = 6.51).

The differences were not significant ($t(28.621) = -1.081$, $p = 0.142$). At the six-month follow-up (T2), both groups demonstrated a decline in PCS, with the intervention group reporting an average score of M = 29.74 (SD = 4.93) and the control group exhibiting an average score of M = 29.24 (SD = 5.54). Comparable to the T0 and T1 results, these differences did not reach statistical significance ($t(18) = -0.590$, $p = 0.281$).

A linear mixed-effects model was used to compare the PCSs at baseline, three months, and six months between the control and intervention groups. The group × time interaction was not significant ($F(2, 49.06) = 0.02$, $p = 0.977$, see Table 2B), indicating no differential effects over time. There was a significant effect of time ($F(2, 47.70) = 4.00$, $p = 0.025$), with PCS being higher at baseline and three months than at six months. However, neither of these contrasts reached significance ($\beta_{T0 \text{ vs. } T2} = 2.64$, $p = 0.233$; $\beta_{T1 \text{ vs. } T2} = 3.48$, $p = 0.111$, see Table 2A). No significant main effect of group was found ($F(1, 60.78) = 0.44$, $p = 0.511$). Among the covariates, only ward was significant, with patients in the internal medicine ward scoring, on average, 4.45 points lower than those in the gynecology ward

(F(1, 54.69) = 5.04, $p = 0.029$; β = −4.45, $p = 0.029$). The random intercept variance was 11.20 and residual variance was 20.44 (ICC ≈ 0.35). The AR(1) autocorrelation was low (ρ = 0.17, $p = 0.692$, see Table 2C).

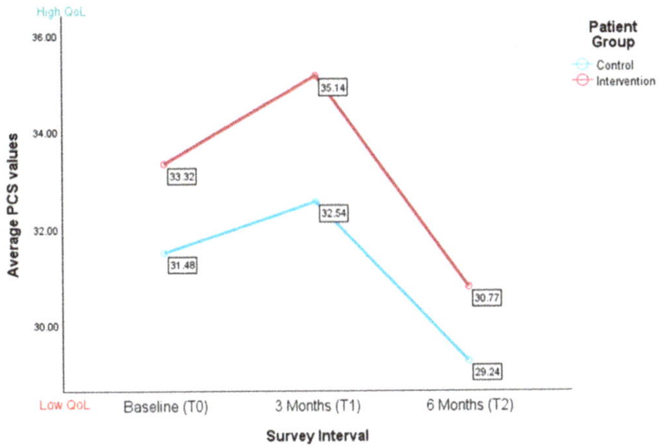

Figure 3. Average physical component scores for control and intervention groups ($n = 58$); the higher the score, the better the patient's physical quality of life.

Table 2. Mixed-effects model results for the SF-12 physical component score (PCS).

A. Fixed-Effect Estimates						
Parameter	**β**	**Std. Error**	**df**	**t-Value**	***p*-Value**	**95% CI**
Intercept	35.53	2.98	86.82	11.26	<0.001	[27.61, 39.44]
Group (control)	−1.16	2.55	79.50	−0.46	0.650	[−6.23, 3.91]
Time (T0 vs. T2)	2.64	2.17	30.96	1.22	0.233	[−1.79, 7.08]
Time (T1 vs. T2)	3.48	2.15	60.86	1.62	0.111	[−1.82, 7.79]
Group × Time (control × T0)	0.09	2.64	28.10	0.03	0.974	[−5.32, 5.49]
Group × Time (control × T1)	0.45	2.62	59.06	0.17	0.865	[−4.80, 5.69]
Gender (female)	−1.88	2.16	55.28	−0.87	0.387	[−6.20, 2.44]
Ward (internal medicine)	−4.45	1.98	54.69	−2.24	0.029 *	[−8.43, −0.48]
Age	−0.03	0.06	45.33	−0.42	0.675	[−0.15, 0.10]

B. Type III Tests of Fixed Effects				
Parameters	**Num df**	**Den df**	**F**	***p*-value**
Group	1	60.78	0.44	0.511
Time	2	47.70	4.00	0.025 *
Group × Time	2	49.06	0.02	0.977
Gender	1	55.28	0.76	0.387
Ward	1	54.69	5.04	0.029 *
Age	1	45.33	0.18	0.675

C. Variance Components and AR (1) Parameter			
Component	**Estimate**	**Std. Error**	**95% CI**
Random-intercept variance	11.20	11.70	[1.44, 86.85]
Residual variance	20.44	10.77	[7.28, 57.38]
AR(1)	0.17	0.44	[−0.61, 0.79]

Note CI = confidence interval; df = degrees of freedom; β = unstandardized coefficient. * $p < 0.05$. Reference categories: Group = intervention; Time = T2 6 months; Gender = male; Ward = gynecology.

3.3.2. Mental Component Score (MCS)

At baseline (T0), the control group (M = 38.63, SD = 7.53) and the intervention group (M = 38.09, SD = 7.25) showed no significant difference in MCS (t(56) = −0.287, p = 0.388). After three months (T1), the intervention group (M = 42.03, SD = 4.82) reported significantly higher MCSs than the control group, indicating a better QoL (M = 38.10, SD = 7.06, t(29.691) = −1.894, p = 0.034). At six months (T2), the intervention group continued to report higher MCSs (M = 44.67, SD = 6.24) compared to the control group (M = 39.68, SD = 7.27), although the difference was not statistically significant (t(18) = −1.525, p = 0.071). Both groups showed below-average MCSs compared to the German standard sample mean (for 1998) of 51.41 ± 8.55 (see Figure 4).

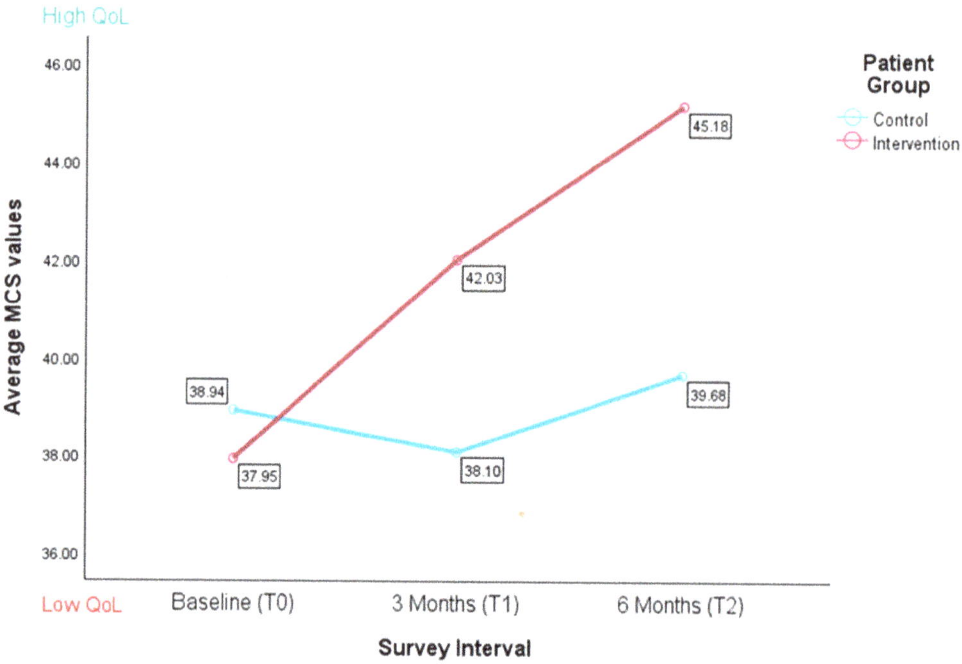

Figure 4. Average mental component scores for control and intervention groups (n = 58); the higher the score, the better the mental quality of life.

An LMM compared MCSs between the control and intervention groups at baseline, three months, and six months. The group × time interaction was not significant (F(2, 55.34) = 2.00, p = 0.146, see Table 3B), indicating no difference between the groups over time. The main effect of time was also not significant (F(2, 54.25) = 2.24, p = 0.116), although baseline scores were lower than 6-month scores ($\beta_{\text{T0 vs. T2}}$ = −6.21, p = 0.032, see Table 3A). There were also no significant main effects of group (F(1, 51.64) = 1.58, p = 0.215) and none of the covariates were significant (all $p > 0.05$). The random intercept variance was 19.04 and the residual variance was 31.88 (ICC ≈ 0.37). The AR(1) autocorrelation was non-significant (ρ = −0.20, p = 0.433, see Table 3C).

Table 3. Mixed-effects model results for the SF-12 mental component score (PCS).

A. Fixed-Effect Estimates						
Parameter	**β**	**Std. Error**	**df**	**t-Value**	**Sig.**	**95% CI**
Intercept	43.97	3.75	86.39	11.72	<0.001	[36.51, 51.42]
Group (control)	−4.49	3.28	79.41	−1.37	0.175	[−11.01, 2.04]
Time (T0 vs. T2)	−6.21	2.79	39.95	−2.23	0.032 *	[−11.85, 0.57]
Time (T1 vs. T2)	−2.45	3.04	56.84	−0.81	0.424	[−8.55, 3.64]
Group × Time (control × T0)	5.52	3.71	38.02	1.64	0.110	[−1.30, 12.34]
Group × Time (control × T1)	1.18	3.76	53.67	0.32	0.754	[−6.36, 8.72]
Gender (female)	0.47	2.64	53.38	0.18	0.859	[−4.82, 5.76]
Ward (internal medicine)	−0.52	2.41	51.50	−0.22	0.830	[−5.36, 4.32]
Age	0.037	0.07	39.47	0.51	0.611	[−0.12–0.18]
B. Type III Tests of Fixed Effects						
Parameters	**Num df**	**Den df**	**F**	***p*-value**		
Group	1	51.64	1.58	0.215		
Time	2	54.25	2.24	0.116		
Group × Time	2	55.34	2.00	0.146		
Gender	1	53.38	0.03	0.859		
Ward	1	51.50	0.05	0.830		
Age	1	39.47	0.26	0.611		
C. Variance Components and AR (1) Parameter						
Component	**Estimate**	**Std. Error**	**95% CI**			
Random-intercept variance	19.04	7.41	[7.71, 47.03]			
Residual variance	31.88	7.41	[20.21, 50.27]			
AR(1)	−0.20	0.26	[−0.62, 0.31]			

Note CI = confidence interval; df = degrees of freedom; β = unstandardized coefficient; * $p < 0.05$. Reference categories: Group = intervention; Time = T2 6 months; Gender = male; Ward = gynecology.

3.4. *Palliative Care Needs Using the Integrated Palliative Care Outcome Scale (IPOS)*

3.4.1. IPOS Number of Physical, Emotional, and Communication Problems

At baseline, both the control and intervention patients reported on average having 11 out of 17 possible problems, encompassing physical or emotional symptoms as well as communication or practical issues (control: SD = 2.59, range = 6–14; intervention: SD = 2.74, range = 5–15). Over time, the average number of reported problems decreased for both groups, although no significant differences were observed.

3.4.2. IPOS Total Scores

The IPOS scores for the control group initially demonstrated a decline, followed by an upward trajectory. In contrast, the intervention group exhibited a pronounced downward trend, indicating better symptom management, especially from the baseline to the three-month follow-up, as seen in Figure 5.

The Mann–Whitney U tests revealed that, at all three time points, the control patients had significantly higher total sum scores than the intervention patients, indicating greater palliative care needs in the control group (t0: U = 250.000, Z = −2.415, p = 0.008; t1: U = 83.500, Z = −1.865, p = 0.031, t2: U = 21.500, Z = −2.055, p = 0.020). In particular, the IPOS scores for the control group initially declined and subsequently increased, whereas the intervention group exhibited a pronounced downward trend—most notably from the baseline to the three-month follow-up (see Figure 5).

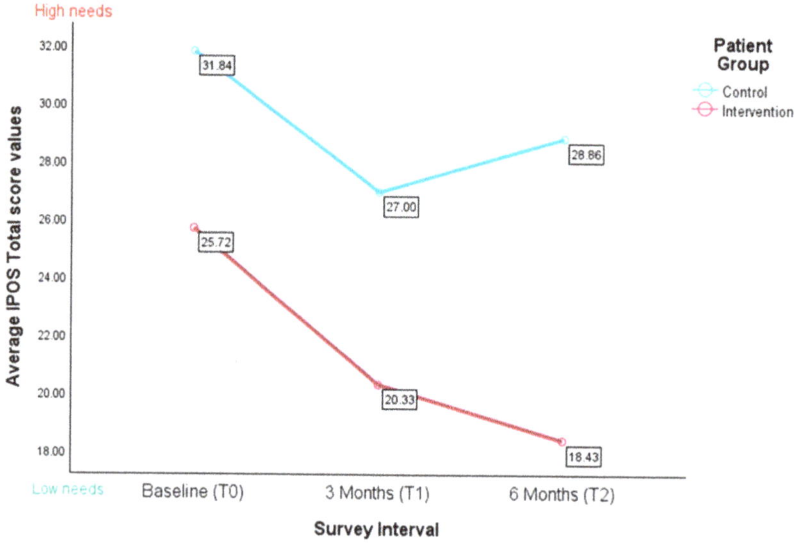

Figure 5. Average IPOS total scores for the control and intervention group (n = 58); the higher the score, the higher potential palliative care needs.

An LMM revealed no significant group × time interaction (F(2, 47.68) = 0.45, p = 0.638, see Table A2) or main effect of time (F(2, 46.74) = 1.91, p = 0.159). However, there was a significant main effect of group (F(1, 56.79) = 6.43, p = 0.014), with control patients scoring on average 8.8 points higher than the intervention group (β = 8.77, p = 0.030). None of the covariates were significant (all p > 0.05), though there was a positive trend for age (p = 0.068). Variance component estimates indicated modest between-subject variability (random intercept variance = 8.89, residual variance = 85.90, ICC ≈ 0.09) and non-significant AR(1) autocorrelation (ρ = 0.62, p = 0.113).

3.4.3. IPOS Subscale for Physical Symptoms

The Mann–Whitney U test revealed a significant difference at three months, with the control group reporting higher physical symptom scores (U = 83.000, Z = −1.886, p = 0.030; see Figure 6). A linear mixed-effect model showed a trend for the group × time interaction towards significance (F(2, 39.82) = 3.13, p = 0.055; see Table 4B). There was no main effect of time (F(2, 39.19) = 0.98, p = 0.384). Pairwise contrasts relative to the six months reference indicated higher scores at baseline (β = 3.75, p = 0.071) and at three months (β = 0.60, p = 0.747; see Table 4A), neither of which reached significance. The omnibus test for group was marginal (F(1, 55.48) = 3.43, p = 0.069), but the specific group contrast was significant, with control patients scoring 5.71 points higher on average than intervention patients (β = 5.71, p = 0.039). None of the covariates were significant (all p > 0.05), although age showed a trend towards significance (p = 0.085). Variance component estimates indicated substantial between-subject variability (random intercept variance = 29.31, residual variance = 21.62, ICC ≈ 0.58). The AR(1) autocorrelation was non-significant (ρ = 0.38, p = 0.381; see Table 4C).

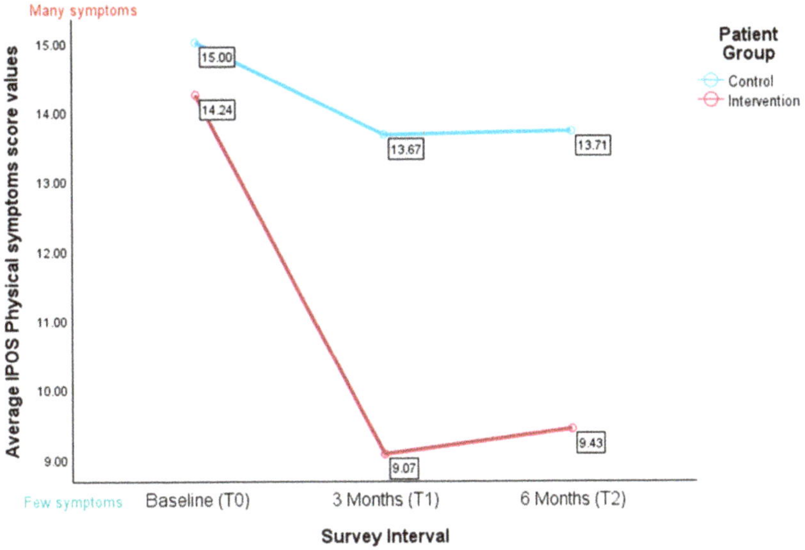

Figure 6. Average values for the IPOS subscale for physical symptoms (n = 58); the higher the score, the higher perceived physical symptom burden.

Table 4. Mixed-effects model results for the IPOS physical symptoms subscale.

Pannel A. Fixed-Effect Estimates						
Parameter	**β**	**Std. Error**	**df**	**t-Value**	**Sig.**	**95% CI**
Intercept	9.06	3.65	67.61	2.48	0.016 *	[−1.77, 16.34]
Group (control)	5.71	2.72	85.11	2.10	0.039 *	[0.31, 11.12]
Time (T0 vs. T2)	3.75	2.00	29.96	2.87	0.071	[−0.34, 7.84]
Time (T1 vs. T2)	0.60	1.86	50.69	0.32	0.747	[−3.14, 4.35]
Group × Time (control × T0)	−5.13	2.50	27.76	−2.05	0.050	[−10.25, −0.01]
Group × Time (control × T1)	−1.24	2.30	49.61	−0.54	0.594	[−5.86, 3.39]
Gender (female)	1.95	2.94	50.28	0.67	0.509	[−3.95, 7.85]
Ward (internal medicine)	0.05	2.69	49.74	0.02	0.984	[−5.34, 5.45]
Age	0.15	0.08	45.00	1.76	0.085	[−0.02, 0.31]
Panel B Type III Tests of Fixed Effects						
Parameters	**Num df**	**Den df**	**F**	***p*-value**		
Group	1	55.48	3.43	0.069		
Time	2	39.19	0.98	0.384		
Group × Time	2	39.82	3.13	0.055		
Gender	1	50.28	0.44	0.509		
Ward	1	49.74	0.00	0.984		
Age	1	45.00	3.11	0.085		
C. Variance Components and AR (1) Parameter						
Component	Estimate	Std. Error	95% CI			
Random-intercept variance	29.31	17.46	[9.12, 94.21]			
Residual variance	21.62	14.83	[5.63, 82.95]			
AR(1)	0.38	0.43	[−0.53, 0.88]			

Note CI = confidence interval; df = degrees of freedom; β = unstandardized coefficient; * $p < 0.05$. Reference categories: Group intervention; Time = T2 6 months; Gender = male; Ward = gynecology.

3.4.4. IPOS Subscale for Emotional Symptoms

The control group showed higher mean scores for the subscale for emotional symptoms compared to those in the intervention group. These differences were statistically significant at baseline (U = 182.000, z = −3.525, $p < 0.001$) and at six-month follow-up (U = 19.000, z = −2.257, $p = 0.023$) (see Figure 7).

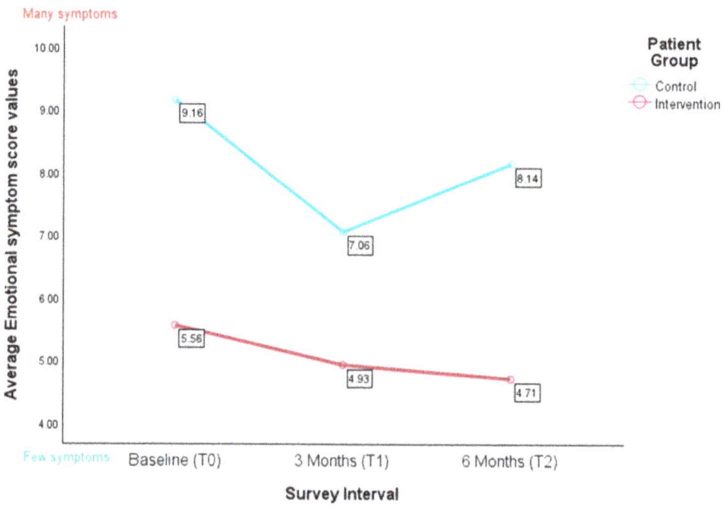

Figure 7. Average values for the IPOS subscale for emotional symptoms ($n = 58$); the higher the score, the higher perceived emotional symptom burden.

A linear mixed model revealed no significant group × time interaction (F(2, 55.92) = 0.78, $p = 0.466$, see Table 5B). There was also no main effect of time (F(2, 54.31) = 1.33, $p = 0.272$). The omnibus test revealed a significant main effect for group (F(1, 49.20) = 10.44, $p = 0.002$), though the specific contrast trended towards significance only (β = 2.76, $p = 0.075$, see Table 5A). None of the covariates were significant (all $p > 0.05$). Variance component estimates (Table 5C) showed a residual variance of 11.29 and a random-intercept variance of 0.37 (ICC ≈ 0.03). The AR(1) autocorrelation was non-significant (ρ = 0.37, $p = 0.387$).

Table 5. Mixed-effects model results for the IPOS subscale emotional symptoms.

A. Fixed-Effect Estimates						
Parameter	β	Std. Error	df	t-Value	Sig.	95% CI
Intercept	5.90	1.76	71.98	3.35	0.001	[2.39, 9.41]
Group (control)	2.76	1.54	99.25	1.80	0.075	[−0.29, 5.81]
Time (T0 vs. T2)	0.30	1.36	40.59	0.22	0.825	[−2.45, 3.05]
Time (T1 vs. T2)	0.06	1.30	64.24	0.05	0.963	[−2.53, 2.65]
Group × Time (control × T0)	0.84	1.70	36.50	0.49	0.625	[−2.60, 4.28]
Group × Time (control × T1)	−0.70	1.62	60.09	−0.43	0.668	[−3.93, 2.54]
Gender (female)	−0.51	1.30	49.04	−0.39	0.699	[−3.11, 2.10]
Ward (internal medicine)	−0.58	1.18	50.54	−0.49	0.625	[−3.00, 1.80]
Age	0.02	0.04	38.81	0.45	0.653	[−0.06, 0.09]

Table 5. *Cont.*

B. Type III Tests of Fixed Effects				
Parameters	**Num df**	**Den df**	**F**	***p*-value**
Group	1	49.20	10.44	0.002 *
Time	2	54.31	1.33	0.272
Group × Time	2	55.93	0.78	0.466
Gender	1	49.04	0.15	0.699
Ward	1	50.54	0.24	0.625
Age	1	38.81	0.21	0.653

C. Variance Components and AR (1) Parameter			
Component	**Estimate**	**Std. Error**	**95% CI**
Random-intercept variance	0.37	0.43	[−0.53, 0.88]
Residual variance	0.37	8.00	$[0, 5.73 \times 10^{15}]$ **
AR(1)	11.29	8.00	[2.83, 45.05]

Note CI = confidence interval; df = degrees of freedom; β = unstandardized coefficient; * $p < 0.05$. Reference categories: Group = intervention; Time = T2 6 months; Gender = male; Ward = gynecology. ** Variance CIs are Wald-type (estimate ± 1.96 × SE), truncated at zero, with large upper bounds shown in scientific notation.

The qualitative data (field notes) also revealed emotional concerns held by the patients. In particular, some patients expressed the wish to not think about their illness all the time. One patient mentioned the following:

> *"I don't want to have anything else besides therapy. Otherwise, it's too much. I'd like to be able to stop thinking about my illness." (Pat_KG_FC4).* (extracted as free text comments).

3.4.5. IPOS Subscale for Communication and Practical Issues

In the subscale pertaining to communication and practical issues, the control patients exhibited slightly higher average scores at baseline in comparison to the intervention patients (M = 5.781 vs. M = 4.160), suggesting more prevalent issues in the control group within this domain. The observed difference at baseline was statistically significant (U = 259.000, Z = −2.303, $p = 0.010$).

At three months (T1), the intervention patients showed an increase in their scores (M = 4.889), indicating a greater need in this area, while control patients exhibited a decrease (M = 5.133). However, the observed difference at T1 was not statistically significant (U = 134.500, Z = −0.018, $p = 0.497$).

By six months (T2), the intervention patients demonstrated a notable decrease in reported communication and practical issues (M = 3.857), whereas the control patients' scores remained relatively stable (M = 5.143). The difference at T2 was statistically significant, with lower scores indicating fewer issues in the intervention group compared to the control group (U = 24.500, Z = −1.870, $p = 0.029$) (see Figure 8).

To further examine these differences while accounting for potential confounders, we conducted a linear mixed-effects model. The LMM did not reveal a significant group × time interaction ($F(2, 57.67) = 2.44$, $p = 0.096$). There were also no significant main effects of group ($F(1, 42.60) = 2.08$, $p = 0.157$) or time ($F(2, 56.31) = 0.47$, $p = 0.626$). None of the covariates were significant (all $p > 0.05$). Variance component estimates showed a residual variance of 4.20 and a random intercept variance of 0.75 (ICC ≈ 0.15). The AR(1) autocorrelation was non-significant (ρ = 0.06, $p = 0.872$; see Table A3).

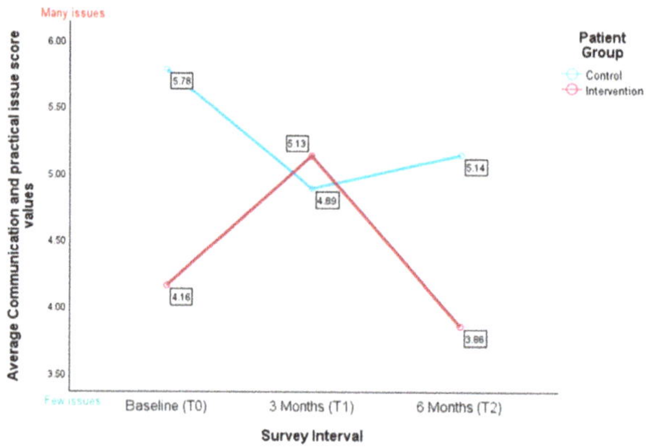

Figure 8. Average scores for the IPOS subscale for communication and practical issues ($n = 58$); the higher the score, the more perceived communication and practical issues.

The qualitative data revealed the communication challenges experienced by patients, aligning with the quantitative findings. In particular, some patients expressed difficulties in discussing their end-of-life care preferences and concerns with their families. For example, one patient shared the following:

> *"Can I do that to my wife, having her care for me at home until the end? I would rather die at home than in a nursing home or something like that, but I don't even dare to think about it or talk to her about it just yet"* (PAT_KG_CP15). (extracted as free text comments).

Another key concern raised by the patients was the need for continuous care from a fixed contact person to discuss problems and receive necessary information. A patient described their experience as follows:

> *"Although I've tried to discuss my worries and fears, it hasn't worked because I always see someone else. The main contact person is good, but you hardly see them as a patient because they have so little time. The constant change of doctors makes you feel like a number, so you can't really talk about your fears." [...] (PAT_IG_KR4).* (extracted as free text comments).

3.5. Cooperative Oncology Group (ECOG) Performance Status

The data indicate that, on average, patients in the control group had poorer performance scores and were potentially more reliant on assistance from others. While the mean ECOG scores of the intervention patients showed a slight decline, those of the control patients remained relatively stable between T1 and T2. A significant difference was observed between the control and intervention mean scores at three months (U = 77.000, Z = −2.234, $p = 0.011$) and six months (U = 21.000, Z = −2.054, $p = 0.044$). See Figure 9.

In addition, a linear mixed model revealed no significant group × time interaction (F(2, 44.48) = 1.32, $p = 0.278$; see Table 6B) or time effect (F(2, 44.00) = 0.95, $p = 0.394$). There was a trend towards a main effect of group (F(1, 56.03) = 3.04, $p = 0.087$). The specific group contrasts were significant (β = 0.78, $p = 0.040$; see Table 6A), with control patients scoring 0.78 points higher (i.e., worse PS) than intervention patients. Among the covariates, only ward was significant (β = 1.05, $p = 0.004$), indicating poorer PS in the internal medicine ward. Variance components revealed substantial between-patient variability (residual variance = 0.32, random intercept variance = 0.54, ICC ≈ 0.63) and a non-significant AR(1) autocorrelation (ρ = 0.19, $p = 0.561$; Table 6C).

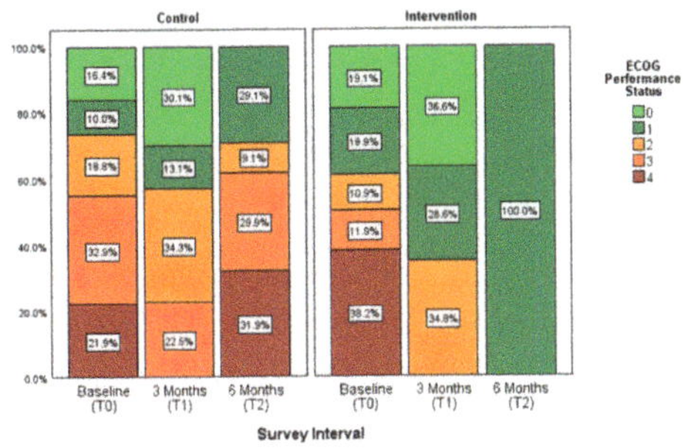

Figure 9. Average functional status of control and intervention group (n = 58); the higher the performance status (0–4), the lower the functional status.

Table 6. Mixed-effects model results for ECOG performance score.

Pannel A. Fixed-Effect Estimates						
Parameter	**β**	**Std. Error**	**df**	**t-Value**	***p*-Value**	**95% CI**
Intercept	1.19	0.50	69.92	2.39	0.020 *	[0.20, 2.18]
Group (control)	0.78	0.37	85.60	2.09	0.040 *	[0.04, 1.51]
Time (T0 vs. T2)	0.45	0.28	36.51	1.61	0.115	[−0.12, 1.02]
Time (T1 vs. T2)	0.24	0.27	51.66	0.87	0.386	[−0.31, 0.79]
Group × Time (control × T0)	−0.55	0.34	34.35	−1.62	0.115	[−1.25, 0.14]
Group × Time (control × T1)	-0.43	0.33	50.51	-1.30	0.200	[−1.10, 0.24]
Gender (female)	−0.02	0.39	51.18	−0.04	0.970	[−0.80, 0.77]
Ward (internal medicine)	1.05	0.35	51.01	3.00	0.004 *	[0.35, 1.74]
Age	0.00	0.01	45.79	0.37	0.712	[−0.02, 0.03]
Panel B. Type III Tests of Fixed Effects						
Parameters	**Num df**	**Den df**	**F**	***p*-value**		
Group	1	56.03	3.04	0.087		
Time	2	44.00	0.95	0.394		
Group × Time	2	44.48	1.32	0.278		
Gender	1	51.18	0.00	0.970		
Ward	1	51.01	9.02	0.004 *		
Age	1	54.79	0.14	0.712		
C. Variance Components and AR (1) Parameter						
Component	**Estimate**	**Std. Error**	**95% CI**			
Random-intercept variance	0.54	0.19	[0.27, 1.09]			
Residual variance	0.32	0.13	[0.15, 0.71]			
AR(1)	0.19	0.34	[−0.45, 0.71]			

Note CI = confidence interval; df = degrees of freedom; β = unstandardized coefficient; * $p < 0.05$. Reference categories: Group = intervention; Time = T2 6 months; Gender = male; Ward = gynecology.

4. Discussion

Our study evaluated the feasibility of implementing the MINI in two general university hospital wards with the primary objective of facilitating an earlier identification of terminally ill patients. This aimed to improve patient outcomes and foster sensitive, early communication regarding disease. We hypothesized that the intervention would enhance patient-reported outcomes, and our findings suggest a discernible positive trend supporting this. The intervention group demonstrated a greater improvement in their mental quality of life and generally exhibited a superior ECOG performance status. Conversely, the control group exhibited higher total IPOS scores, indicating a greater symptom burden, particularly in the physical and emotional domains. Although the intervention group initially reported more communication and practical issues, a marked improvement was observed by the six-month mark, suggesting potential long-term benefits even if short-term gains were less pronounced.

4.1. Allocation and General Sample Characteristics

In the control group, only senior physicians were asked the Surprise Question (SQ), whereas in the intervention group, all medical and nursing staff were instructed to do so. Additionally, the intervention phase introduced SPICT-DE^{TM} and an information hour, aiming to involve more staff and increase their awareness of palliative needs. These changes likely contributed to baseline differences between the two groups.

Identifying limited life expectancy appeared to be more straightforward for cancer patients, reflected in the intervention group's higher identification rate among this population. However, inviting more severely burdened patients also led to more individuals being too ill or dying before giving consent, especially in the non-cancer setting. Contrary to initial assumptions, broadening responsibility sometimes reduced ownership: recruitment declined once senior physicians were less involved. This "diffusion of responsibility" [36] highlights the importance of a designated lead, such as a senior physician, to effectively distribute responsibility. A higher proportion of female patients participated in both phases, largely due to recruitment from a gynecological ward. We deliberately included both a non-cancer ward and a cancer ward to address known gaps in early palliative identification, which is often pronounced in oncology [37,38] and among patients with chronic diseases. By covering both wards, we aimed to strengthen healthcare outputs for both cancer and non-cancer patients and expose systemic barriers to timely referral.

Finally, a greater proportion of patients in the intervention group reported having earlier knowledge of their condition's incurability. The MINI's systematic screening and proactive communication likely encouraged staff to speak directly with patients about their health status, aligning with studies indicating that training and a supportive environment facilitate earlier prognostic disclosure [39,40]. Moreover, the hospital context may have normalized these conversations, as staff were urged to identify terminally ill patients and address their diagnosis [41], and admission itself can serve as an opportunity to identify patients approaching the end of their life [5]. However, factors beyond the MINI, such as ward culture, physician communication styles, and individual patient circumstances, also affect when patients learn of their condition's incurability.

4.2. Outcome Measures

4.2.1. SF-12

In both groups, PCSs were consistently below the German standard mean (48.22 $\pm$ 8.77), reflecting their advanced disease status and the progressive nature of their disease. Neither the intervention nor the control group showed a distinct advantage in PCS at any time point, suggesting that, within this sample, the intervention did not confer a measurable benefit in terms of physical functioning over and above usual care. However, the initial improvement from T0 to T1 may highlight a short-term positive effect—whether from increased attention, symptom management, or other supportive measures. Disease progression likely overshadowed any gains in physical functioning over time, highlighting the need for robust symptom management and rehabilitation strategies alongside psychosocial interventions [42–44]. In contrast to the PCS, the MCS results showed more promising trends. In independent samples t-tests, the intervention group's MCS increased significantly from baseline to three months and remained higher at six months, though this latter difference did not reach statistical significance. However, in the mixed-model analysis, no significant treatment effect emerged, likely due to the small sample size and limited statistical power. Nevertheless, the MINI's emphasis on earlier identification and communication about palliative needs may have bolstered patients' sense of control, reduced anxiety, and improved coping, even if these benefits were not fully captured. Contrary to common concerns, talking about problems and illnesses and planning care can improve QoL [11]. Engaging both medical and nursing staff likely offered emotional and informational support, dispelling misconceptions and improving the overall mental well-being of patients and their caregivers. Overall, these findings are in line with other studies and suggest that while physical quality of life may remain relatively stable or even decline in the face of advancing illness, mental quality of life can be positively influenced by interventions that focus on issues beyond the patient's physical status and emphasize communication, emotional support, and early palliative care planning [43,45].

4.2.2. IPOS

The IPOS provides a comprehensive view of patients' palliative care needs including physical, emotional, and communication issues. Both groups reported multiple problems at baseline, reflecting the high burden of terminal illnesses. The results indicate that control patients consistently exhibited higher palliative care needs, as reflected in significantly higher IPOS scores at all time points. This aligns with previous findings that terminally ill individuals often experience a high symptom burden and unmet palliative care needs, not only due to physical symptoms but also because of the emotional distress associated with illness and its management [2,13]. Our findings reinforce the importance of structured palliative care approaches to address the complex needs of terminally ill patients. A modest effect on physical symptoms was observed. While the overall symptom burden tended to increase in both groups, the intervention group showed a less pronounced rise, consistent with the Mann–Whitney U test results at three months. In the mixed-model analysis, the group × time interaction trended towards significance, and the specific contrast indicated controls scoring higher on average. Although the small sample size limits definitive conclusions, these results indicate that the MINI may help mitigate the progression of physical symptoms in terminally ill patients.

We found that patients in the intervention group consistently reported fewer emotional symptoms than controls, with significant differences at baseline and six months, suggesting the MINI may alleviate emotional distress. The baseline advantage likely reflects the benefit of the staff training delivered to intervention personnel as part of the MINI. The mixed-model analysis confirmed a significant omnibus group effect, although the specific control vs. intervention contrast trended toward significance. Qualitative data further underscores patients' struggle with emotional burdens and their wish to avoid constant rumination about their illness. Together, these findings suggest that interventions such as the MINI may help meet these needs and highlights the value of structured psychosocial support [46], potentially enabled by earlier and more frequent conversations facilitated by the MINI. However, further research is required to confirm its long-term impact.

Although the data showed a modest increase in communication scores for the intervention at three months, by six months, they had decreased significantly below the control group's levels. This pattern suggests that while patients might initially feel overwhelmed by receiving a life-threatening diagnosis or discussions about care planning, over time, sustained engagement and communication pathways can help reduce barriers in communication and practical support and thus potentially increase QoL [47]. However, the linear mixed model did not reveal significant effects, suggesting that other factors may have influenced these results. Taken together, the IPOS findings suggest that targeted, proactive care planning may help mitigate certain palliative care needs [11].

4.2.3. ECOG

Performance status (PS) is crucial for terminally ill patients, particularly those with cancer, as patients with a greater PS are less likely to experience adverse events and have a greater likelihood of responding well to treatment [48]. Although PS often declines over time, patients in the intervention group exhibited a slight improvement or stabilization in ECOG scores compared to the control group at both three and six months. This pattern may suggest that the intervention has helped maintain PS. This could be attributed to structured support, including symptom monitoring, improved coping, and heightened disease awareness [49]. However, the linear mixed model only trended toward a significant main effect of group, despite the specific contrast showing an advantage for the intervention arm. Moreover, the significant ward effect suggest that site-specific factors may have also influenced PS. Taken together, these results suggest a potential positive impact of the intervention on preserving functional status, which is important because a greater PS could also enable patients to tolerate treatments more effectively, underscoring the importance of early palliative support that addresses both physical and psychosocial factors [50].

4.3. *Strengths, Limitations, and Lessons Learned*

Our study's prospective, mixed-method design provided direct, unbiased insights from terminally ill patients during the last year of their life, thereby overcoming the recall bias typical of retrospective studies. A further strength of this study is the diverse sample recruited, which included both cancer and non-cancer patients, alongside the active involvement of medical and nursing staff across multiple general hospital wards. This approach substantially enhances the real-world applicability of our findings.

Despite these strengths, our challenges included the limited sample size, data completeness, and the full implementation of the MINI. These challenges existed at individual (e.g., patient, family, and HCP), trial (e.g., recruitment barriers and workflow disruptions), and systemic (e.g., societal knowledge) levels.

A major limitation was gatekeeping by HCPs, a well-documented phenomenon in palliative care [51] often driven by concerns about patient distress and burden [52,53]. Staff sometimes explicitly discouraged referrals even when patients met the inclusion criteria. This reluctance aligns with findings that practitioners can experience intense emotional distress when breaking bad news, acting as a barrier to recruitment. Such concerns were exacerbated by limited time, resources, and training, with some HCPs worried that such conversations elicit physical and emotional responses, requiring more time and attention than they could realistically provide [39].

Furthermore, reluctance to use the SQ was observed. In the control phase, medical staff, particularly residents, often hesitated to answer 'no' for younger cancer patients or communicate the diagnosis' implications. For instance, a resident's decision to overrule a nurse's suggestion, despite the patient's metastases ("she was still so young...") and the nurse's reaction ("Are you saying this with your heart or with your mind?"), highlights this reluctance. Similarly, nurses, particularly in non-cancer wards, showed reluctance to use the SQ. This aligns with the literature noting prognostic issues as a substantial challenge for nurses, in which prognostication power is often still attributed solely to doctors [54,55]. This underscores the critical need for enhanced training to equip staff with confidence in identifying patients and discussing palliative care. Misconceptions that palliative care means immediate death, diminishing hope [3,56], or that offering non-curative treatment options signifies personal failure [57] further hindered SQ use and diagnosis discussions.

Data protection constraints also impacted recruitment. We could only recruit patients confirmed by their medical team as aware of their terminal illness. This is problematic, as HCPs' perception of prognosis discussions may differ from patients' and carers' perceptions [58]. Consequently, some patients declined to participate due to unawareness of their terminal illness, believing the study was inappropriate (e.g., one patient stated she had surgery recently and thus did not meet the criteria for being terminal ill).

Patient health status [59] significantly impacted consent and retention. Non-cancer inpatients, often with more advanced conditions [60], exhibited high dropout rates before the baseline assessment or within the first three months, frequently due to death or rapid health deterioration. This instability was observed in both non-cancer and cancer inpatients compared to cancer outpatients. Even relatively stable outpatient cancer patients frequently declined to participate, consistent with Walshe et al. [53]. Terminally ill patients experience significant emotional and organizational burden from their treatment, fostering "double awareness" [61]—a simultaneous need for hope and intermittent reprieves from the reality of their illness. This made many reluctant to commit to our four quarterly interviews, leading to withdrawals driven by study duration, workload, negative associations with palliative care, and uncertainty about future health status. External disruptions—including the COVID-19 pandemic, a prolonged nurses' strike (1 May 2022–20 July 2022), and the end of the funding phase (31 April 2023/31 October 2023)—prematurely curtailed the follow-up and impeded longitudinal data collection.

From the insights gained through this study's implementation, several actionable recommendations emerge for optimizing the implementation of future palliative care interventions. Specifically, fostering a clear sense of ownership among all healthcare professionals is paramount. This can be achieved through the precise delineation of roles and a continuous emphasis on the value of early palliative identification in routine clinical practice. Furthermore, comprehensive and ongoing training is essential. This training should systematically address emotional challenges, correct misconceptions about palliative care, and build confidence in using screening tools effectively and facilitating sensitive end-of-life conversations. To mitigate patient burden, particularly in data collection, strategies such as flexible follow-up schedules or the adoption of alternative, less intrusive methods (e.g., shorter interviews or remote surveys) are recommended. Optimizing recruitment procedures necessitates ensuring patients have a profound understanding of the study's aims, which can be achieved through its introduction by a familiar face they trust, and attention to appropriate researcher attire [62]. Finally, the establishment of robust contingency plans is critical to safeguard study continuity and resilience against unforeseen external disruptive events, such as pandemics or strikes. Adherence to these targeted strategies will facilitate a more effective integration of the MINI into existing hospital workflows, thereby fostering improved end-of-life care outcomes.

5. Conclusions

This pilot study indicates that system-wide change requires time and perseverance, but that the MINI can be a first step to meaningful change in healthcare. However, our findings must be interpreted with caution due to the inherently small sample size of this pilot study, even when the results appear significant. Notably, the intervention's full impact may take longer to manifest, underscoring the importance of extended intervention periods, staff training on comprehensive communication, and adaptive recruitment strategies in future trials. Future studies with larger cohorts should build on these preliminary findings, refining the MINI approach and avoiding the pitfalls identified here. Considering the specific context of our study within a single university hospital and with particular patient characteristics, the broader applicability of these findings needs careful consideration. By doing so, we can increase our understanding on how disease trajectory, patient preferences, and staff training collectively influence outcomes, paving the way for future research that can continue moving from "mini" interventions to create truly meaningful changes in palliative care.

Supplementary Materials: The following supporting information can be downloaded at: https://www.mdpi.com/article/10.3390/healthcare13162024/s1. STROBE Statement—checklist of items that should be included in reports of observational studies.

Author Contributions: Conceptualization, J.S., A.K. and R.V.; methodology, J.S. and J.S.G.; investigation, J.S.G. and A.K.; resources, J.S. and R.V.; data curation, J.S.G.; formal analysis, J.S.G.; writing—original draft preparation, J.S.G.; writing—review and editing, J.S.G., J.S., R.V. and A.K.; project administration, J.S.G., A.K., and J.S.; supervision, J.S. and R.V.; funding acquisition, J.S. and R.V. All authors have read and agreed to the published version of the manuscript.

Funding: This research was funded by the German Federal Ministry of Education and Research (BMBF); #01GY1916.

Institutional Review Board Statement: The study was conducted in accordance with the Declaration of Helsinki and approved by the Ethics Commission of the Medical Faculty of Medicine of Cologne University (20-1431; 12 November 2020). The trial was also registered in the German Clinical Trials Register (DRKS00022378, registration date: 10 February 2021).

Informed Consent Statement: Informed consent was obtained from all subjects involved in the study.

Data Availability Statement: The datasets used and/or analyzed during the current study are available from the corresponding author on reasonable request.

Acknowledgments: We would like to express our gratitude to Gloria Dust for her valuable contributions to the conceptualization and acquisition of funding. We would also like to thank Leonie Weyres and Belinda Werner for their excellent support during the data collection period. Our gratitude extends to the dedicated medical and nursing staff on the participating wards for their invaluable cooperation, and to the study nurse Sandra Scher for her outstanding support during the intervention phase. A special thanks to all the patients and their families for their valuable time and insights. We thank CoRe-Net for overseeing the overall project management tasks, including data safety, and to all the experts within the consortium for their valuable contributions to the study design. The authors acknowledge funding from the German Federal Ministry of Education and Research (BMBF).

Conflicts of Interest: The authors declare no conflicts of interest. The funders had no role in the design of the study; in the collection, analyses, or interpretation of data; in the writing of the manuscript; or in the decision to publish the results.

Abbreviations

The following abbreviations are used in this manuscript:

AaR	Attrition at random
ADD	Attrition due to death
ADI	Attrition due to illness
CG	Control group
ECOG	Eastern Cooperative Oncology Group Performance Status
HCPs	Healthcare professionals
IG	Intervention group
ICC	Intraclass Correlation Coefficient
IPOS	Integrated Palliative Care Outcome Scale
LYOL-C-II	Last Year of Life Study Cologne—Part 2
M	Mean
MCS-12	Mental Component Score
MINI	Minimally Invasive Intervention

PCS-12	Physical Component Score
PROMS	Patient-reported outcome measures
QoL	Quality of life
QPS	Question prompt sheets
SF12	Short-Form Health Service
SD	Standard deviation
SPICT-DETM	Supportive and Palliative Care Indicators Tool
SQ	Surprise Question
T (0-4)	Timepoints

Appendix A

Table A1. Average values for the physical and mental quality of life of control and intervention group, measured using the Short-Form Health Service Questionnaire (SF12).

	PCS		MCS	
	Control M (SD)	Intervention M (SD)	Control M (SD)	Intervention M (SD)
T0	31.34 (5.53)	33.40 (5.50)	38.63 (7.53)	38.09 (7.25)
T1	32.54 (6.51)	35.14 (7.20)	38.10 (7.06)	42.03 (4.82)
T2	29.24 (5.55)	29.74 (4.93)	39.68 (7.27)	44.67 (6.24)

Table A2. Mixed-effects model results of fixed parameters for the IPOS total score.

A. Fixed-Effect Estimates						
Parameter	β	Std. Error	df	t-Value	*p*-Value	95% CI
Intercept	20.30	5.01	71.41	4.05	<0.001	[10.31, 30.29]
Group (control)	8.77	3.99	95.46	2.20	0.030 *	[0.854, 16.69]
Time (T0 vs. T2)	4.53	3.23	42.63	1.40	0.168	[−1.98, 11.04]
Time (T1 vs. T2)	2.22	2.89	56.43	0.77	0.445	[−3.56, 8.00]
Group × Time (control × T0)	−2.97	4.05	39.41	−0.74	0.476	[−11.15, 5.21]
Group × Time (control × T1)	−3.39	3.56	54.27	−0.95	0.346	[−10.53, 3.75]
Gender (female)	1.59	3.92	51.78	0.41	0.687	[−6.29, 9.46]
Ward (internal medicine)	−0.31	3.59	51.63	−0.09	0.932	[−7.51, 6.89]
Age	0.21	0.11	44.75	1.87	0.068	[−0.016, 0.43]

B. Type III Tests of Fixed Effects				
Parameters	Num df	Den df	F	*p*-value
Group	1	56.79	6.44	0.014 *
Time	2	46.74	1.91	0.159
Group × Time	2	47.68	0.45	0.638
Gender	1	51.78	0.16	0.687
Ward	1	51.63	0.01	0.932
Age	1	44.75	3.50	0.068

C. Variance Components and AR (1) Parameter			
Component	Estimate	Std. Error	95% CI
Random-intercept variance	8.87	90.02	[0, 3.87×10^9] **
Residual variance	85.90	89.54	[11.14, 666.55]
AR(1)	0.62	0.39	[−0.48, 0.96]

Note CI = confidence interval; df = degrees of freedom; β = unstandardized coefficient; * $p < 0.05$. Reference categories: Group = intervention; Time = T2 6 months; Gender = male; Ward = gynecology. ** Variance CIs are Wald-type (estimate ± 1.96 × SE), truncated at zero, with large upper bounds shown in scientific notation.

Table A3. Mixed-effects model results for the IPOS subscale communication and practical issues.

A. Fixed-Effect Estimates						
Parameter	**β**	**Std. Error**	**df**	**t-Value**	***p*-Value**	**95% CI**
Intercept	4.05	1.14	77.12	3.55	0.001	[1.78, 6.31]
Group (control)	1.09	1.02	95.46	1.07	0.288	[−0.94, 3.12]
Time (T0 vs. T2)	0.22	0.91	40.63	0.24	0.812	[−1.62, 2.06]
Time (T1 vs. T2)	1.29	0.94	60.59	1.36	0.177	[−0.59, 3.17]
Group × Time (control × T0)	0.51	1.13	37.23	0.45	0.657	[−1.78, 2.80]
Group × Time (control × T1)	−1.46	1.18	55.73	−1.24	0.222	[−3.83, 0.91]
Gender (female)	0.07	0.81	46.96	0.08	0.936	[−1.57, 1.70]
Ward (internal medicine)	−0.33	0.74	48.15	−0.45	0.656	[−1.82, 1.16]
Age	0.03	0.02	35.29	1.54	0.133	[−0.01, 0.08]
B. Type III Tests of Fixed Effects						
Parameters	**Num df**	**Den df**	**F**	***p*-value**		
Group	1	42.60	2.08	0.157		
Time	2	56.31	0.47	0.626		
Group × Time	2	57.67	2.44	0.096		
Gender	1	46.96	0.01	0.936		
Ward	1	48.15	0.20	0.656		
Age	1	35.29	2.36	0.133		
C. Variance Components and AR (1) Parameter						
Component	**Estimate**	**Std. Error**	**95% CI**			
Random-intercept variance	0.75	1.61	[0.01, 50.49]			
Residual variance	4.20	1.61	[1.98, 8.92]			
AR(1)	0.06	0.37	[−0.58, 0.65]			

Note CI = confidence interval; df = degrees of freedom; β = unstandardized coefficient; Reference categories: Group = intervention; Time = T2 6 months; Gender = male; Ward = gynecology.

References

1. Voltz, R. *Palliativ … und Jetzt? 10 Erkenntnisse zum Umgang mit schwerer Krankheit und für die letzte Lebensphase*, 1st ed.; W. Kohlhammer: Stuttgart, Germany, 2022; ISBN 978-3-17-041178-4.
2. Kremeike, K.; Bausewein, C.; Freytag, A.; Junghanss, C.; Marx, G.; Schnakenberg, R.; Schneider, N.; Schulz, H.; Wedding, U.; Voltz, R. DNVF-Memorandum Versorgungsforschung im letzten Lebensjahr. *Gesundheitswesen* **2022**. [CrossRef] [PubMed]
3. Fliedner, M.C.; Zambrano, S.C.; Eychmueller, S. Public perception of palliative care: A survey of the general population. *Palliat. Care Soc. Pract.* **2021**, *15*, 26323524211017546. [CrossRef]
4. Knaul, F.M.; Arreola-Ornelas, H.; Kwete, X.J.; Bhadelia, A.; Rosa, W.E.; Touchton, M.; Méndez-Carniado, O.; Vargas Enciso, V.; Pastrana, T.; Friedman, J.R.; et al. The evolution of serious health-related suffering from 1990 to 2021: An update to The Lancet Commission on global access to palliative care and pain relief. *Lancet Glob. Health* **2025**, *13*, e422–e436. [CrossRef] [PubMed]
5. Voltz, R.; Dust, G.; Schippel, N.; Hamacher, S.; Payne, S.; Scholten, N.; Pfaff, H.; Rietz, C.; Strupp, J. Improving regional care in the last year of life by setting up a pragmatic evidence-based Plan-Do-Study-Act cycle: Results from a cross-sectional survey. *BMJ Open* **2020**, *10*, e035988. [CrossRef] [PubMed]
6. Strupp, J.; Kasdorf, A.; Dust, G.; Hower, K.I.; Seibert, M.; Werner, B.; Kuntz, L.; Schulz-Nieswandt, F.; Meyer, I.; Pfaff, H.; et al. Last Year of Life Study-Cologne (LYOL-C) (Part II): Study protocol of a prospective interventional mixed-methods study in acute hospitals to analyse the implementation of a trigger question and patient question prompt sheets to optimise patient-centred care. *BMJ Open* **2021**, *11*, e048681. [CrossRef]
7. Strupp, J.; Hanke, G.; Schippel, N.; Pfaff, H.; Karbach, U.; Rietz, C.; Voltz, R. Last Year of Life Study Cologne (LYOL-C): Protocol for a cross-sectional mixed methods study to examine care trajectories and transitions in the last year of life until death. *BMJ Open* **2018**, *8*, e021211. [CrossRef]
8. Kasdorf, A.; Dust, G.; Hamacher, S.; Schippel, N.; Rietz, C.; Voltz, R.; Strupp, J. The last year of life for patients dying from cancer vs. non-cancer causes: A retrospective cross-sectional survey of bereaved relatives. *Support. Care Cancer* **2022**, *30*, 4971–4979. [CrossRef]

9. Schippel, N.; Dust, G.; von Reeken, C.; Voltz, R.; Strupp, J.; Rietz, C. Can we determine burdensome transitions in the last year of life based on time of occurrence and frequency? An explanatory mixed-methods study. *Palliat. Support. Care* **2022**, *20*, 637–645. [CrossRef]
10. Scholten, N.; Günther, A.L.; Pfaff, H.; Karbach, U. The size of the population potentially in need of palliative care in Germany--an estimation based on death registration data. *BMC Palliat. Care* **2016**, *15*, 29. [CrossRef]
11. Goswami, P. Advance Care Planning and End-Of-Life Communications: Practical Tips for Oncology Advanced Practitioners. *J. Adv. Pract. Oncol.* **2021**, *12*, 89–95. [CrossRef]
12. Epstein, R.M.; Duberstein, P.R.; Fenton, J.J.; Fiscella, K.; Hoerger, M.; Tancredi, D.J.; Xing, G.; Gramling, R.; Mohile, S.; Franks, P.; et al. Effect of a Patient-Centered Communication Intervention on Oncologist-Patient Communication, Quality of Life, and Health Care Utilization in Advanced Cancer: The VOICE Randomized Clinical Trial. *JAMA Oncol.* **2017**, *3*, 92–100. [CrossRef]
13. Kasdorf, A.; Dust, G.; Vennedey, V.; Rietz, C.; Polidori, M.C.; Voltz, R.; Strupp, J. What are the risk factors for avoidable transitions in the last year of life? A qualitative exploration of professionals' perspectives for improving care in Germany. *BMC Health Serv. Res.* **2021**, *21*, 147. [CrossRef]
14. Debenedetti, S.; Cosmai, S.; Cattani, D.; Mancin, S.; Cangelosi, G.; Petrelli, F.; Mazzoleni, B. Language Validation and Cultural Adaptation of the Italian Version of the Family Caregiver Quality of Life Scale. *Nurs. Rep.* **2024**, *14*, 2302–2312. [CrossRef] [PubMed]
15. Braun, M.; Scholz, U.; Hornung, R.; Martin, M. Die subjektive Belastung pflegender Ehepartner von Demenzkranken. Hinweise zur Validität der deutschen Version des Zarit Burden Interviews. *Z. Gerontol. Geriatr.* **2010**, *43*, 111–119. [CrossRef]
16. Wagle, K.C.; Skopelja, E.N.; Campbell, N.L. Caregiver-Based Interventions to Optimize Medication Safety in Vulnerable Elderly Adults: A Systematic Evidence-Based Review. *J. Am. Geriatr. Soc.* **2018**, *66*, 2128–2135. [CrossRef]
17. Locatelli, G.; Zeffiro, V.; Occhino, G.; Rebora, P.; Caggianelli, G.; Ausili, D.; Alvaro, R.; Riegel, B.; Vellone, E. Effectiveness of Motivational Interviewing on contribution to self-care, self-efficacy, and preparedness in caregivers of patients with heart failure: A secondary outcome analysis of the MOTIVATE-HF randomized controlled trial. *Eur. J. Cardiovasc. Nurs.* **2022**, *21*, 801–811. [CrossRef]
18. Haroen, H.; Maulana, S.; Harlasgunawan, A.R.; Rahmawati, S.; Riansyah, A.; Musthofa, F.; Pardosi, J.F. Barriers and Facilitators of Early Palliative Care in the Trajectory of People Living with Chronic Condition: A Mini Review Using Socio-ecological Framework to Inform Public Health Strategy. *J. Multidiscip. Healthc.* **2024**, *17*, 4189–4197. [CrossRef] [PubMed]
19. Harnischfeger, N.; Rath, H.M.; Oechsle, K.; Bergelt, C. Addressing palliative care and end-of-life issues in patients with advanced cancer: A systematic review of communication interventions for physicians not specialised in palliative care. *BMJ Open* **2022**, *12*, e059652. [CrossRef] [PubMed]
20. Kasdorf, A.; Werner, B.; Grimm, J.S.; Dust, G.; Voltz, R.; Strupp, J.; on behalf of the Cologne Research and Development Network (CoRe-Net). Promising Concept, Challenging Implementation: Evaluating the Implementation of a Minimally Invasive Intervention (MINI) to Identify Patients in Their Last Year of Life: A Multi-Methods Feasibility Study with University Hospital Staff in Germany. Correspondence: Department of Palliative Medicine, University Hospital Cologne, Cologne, North Rhine-Westphalia, Germany. 2025; (manuscript in preparation).
21. Grimm, J.S.; Kasdorf, A.; Voltz, R.; Strupp, J.; on behalf of the Cologne Research and Development Network (CoRe-Net). "Alone it would be simply impossible to cope with the disease and the burdensome organization around it" Perceived care partner burden in end-of-life care.; Correspondence Department of Palliative Medicine, University Hospital Cologne, Cologne, North Rhine-Westphalia, Germany. 2025; (manuscript in preparation).
22. Ware, J.; Kosinski, M.; Keller, S.D. A 12-Item Short-Form Health Survey: Construction of scales and preliminary tests of reliability and validity. *Med. Care* **1996**, *34*, 220–233. [CrossRef]
23. Murtagh, F.E.; Ramsenthaler, C.; Firth, A.; Groeneveld, E.I.; Lovell, N.; Simon, S.T.; Denzel, J.; Guo, P.; Bernhardt, F.; Schildmann, E.; et al. A brief, patient- and proxy-reported outcome measure in advanced illness: Validity, reliability and responsiveness of the Integrated Palliative care Outcome Scale (IPOS). *Palliat. Med.* **2019**, *33*, 1045–1057. [CrossRef]
24. Oken, M.M.; Creech, R.H.; Tormey, D.C.; Horton, J.; Davis, T.E.; McFadden, E.T.; Carbone, P.P. Toxicity and response criteria of the Eastern Cooperative Oncology Group. *Am. J. Clin. Oncol.* **1982**, *5*, 649–655. [CrossRef]
25. van der Zee, E.N.; Noordhuis, L.M.; Epker, J.L.; van Leeuwen, N.; Wijnhoven, B.P.L.; Benoit, D.D.; Bakker, J.; Kompanje, E.J.O. Assessment of mortality and performance status in critically ill cancer patients: A retrospective cohort study. *PLoS ONE* **2021**, *16*, e0252771. [CrossRef]
26. von Elm, E.; Altman, D.G.; Egger, M.; Pocock, S.J.; Gøtzsche, P.C.; Vandenbroucke, J.P. The Strengthening the Reporting of Observational Studies in Epidemiology (STROBE) statement: Guidelines for reporting observational studies. *J. Clin. Epidemiol.* **2008**, *61*, 344–349. [CrossRef]
27. Aaronson, E.L.; George, N.; Ouchi, K.; Zheng, H.; Bowman, J.; Monette, D.; Jacobsen, J.; Jackson, V. The Surprise Question Can Be Used to Identify Heart Failure Patients in the Emergency Department Who Would Benefit from Palliative Care. *J. Pain Symptom Manag.* **2019**, *57*, 944–951. [CrossRef]

28. Afshar, K.; Feichtner, A.; Boyd, K.; Murray, S.; Jünger, S.; Wiese, B.; Schneider, N.; Müller-Mundt, G. Systematic development and asjustment of the German version of the Supportive and Palliative Care Indicators Tool (SPICT-DE). *BMC Palliat. Care* **2018**, *17*, 27. [CrossRef] [PubMed]
29. Afshar, K.; van Baal, K.; Schleef, T.; Frerichs, H.; Schneider, N. *Handlungsempfehlungen für die Versorgung von Menschen am Lebensende und ihren Angehörigen: Ergebnisse aus dem Projekt OPAL Optimale Versorgung am Lebensende*, 2nd ed.; Medizinische Hoschule Hannover, Intitute für Allgemeinmedizin und Palliativmedizin: Hanover, Germany, 2023. Available online: https://www.mhh.de/fileadmin/mhh/allgemeinmedizin/downloads/weitere_Downloadelemente/AllPallMed_Broschuere_OPAL.pdf (accessed on 5 March 2025).
30. Gandek, B.; Ware, J.E.; Aaronson, N.K.; Apolone, G.; Bjorner, J.B.; Brazier, J.E.; Bullinger, M.; Kaasa, S.; Leplege, A.; Prieto, L.; et al. Cross-validation of item selection and scoring for the SF-12 Health Survey in nine countries: Results from the IQOLA Project. International Quality of Life Assessment. *J. Clin. Epidemiol.* **1998**, *51*, 1171–1178. [CrossRef] [PubMed]
31. Drixler, K.; Morfeld, M.; Glaesmer, H.; Brähler, E.; Wirtz, M.A. Validierung der Messung gesundheitsbezogener Lebensqualität mittels des Short-Form-Health-Survey-12 (SF-12 Version 2.0) in einer deutschen Normstichprobe. *Z. Psychosom. Med. Psychother.* **2020**, *66*, 272–286. [CrossRef] [PubMed]
32. Wirtz, M.A.; Morfeld, M.; Glaesmer, H.; Brähler, E. Normierung des SF-12 Version 2.0 zur Messung der gesundheitsbezogenen Lebensqualität in einer deutschen bevölkerungsrepräsentativen Stichprobe. *Diagnostica* **2018**, *64*, 215–226. [CrossRef]
33. Miles, M.B.; Huberman, A.M.; Saldaña, J. *Qualitative Data Analysis: A Methods Sourcebook*, 3rd ed.; SAGE: Thousand Oaks, CA, USA, 2014; ISBN 978-1-4522-5787-7.
34. Higginson, I.J.; Evans, C.J.; Grande, G.; Preston, N.; Morgan, M.; McCrone, P.; Lewis, P.; Fayers, P.; Harding, R.; Hotopf, M.; et al. Evaluating complex interventions in end of life care: The MORECare statement on good practice generated by a synthesis of transparent expert consultations and systematic reviews. *BMC Med.* **2013**, *11*, 111. [CrossRef]
35. Oriani, A.; Dunleavy, L.; Sharples, P.; Perez Algorta, G.; Preston, N.J. Are the MORECare guidelines on reporting of attrition in palliative care research populations appropriate? A systematic review and meta-analysis of randomised controlled trials. *BMC Palliat. Care* **2020**, *19*, 6. [CrossRef]
36. Bandura, A. Social cognitive theory of self-regulation. *Organ. Behav. Hum. Decis. Process.* **1991**, *50*, 248–287. [CrossRef]
37. Adolfsson, K.; Kreicbergs, U.; Bratthäll, C.; Holmberg, E.; Björk-Eriksson, T.; Stenmarker, M. Referral of patients with cancer to palliative care: Attitudes, practices and work-related experiences among Swedish physicians. *Eur. J. Cancer Care (Engl.)* **2022**, *31*, e13680. [CrossRef]
38. Salins, N.; Ghoshal, A.; Hughes, S.; Preston, N. How views of oncologists and haematologists impacts palliative care referral: A systematic review. *BMC Palliat. Care* **2020**, *19*, 175. [CrossRef] [PubMed]
39. Francis, L.; Robertson, N. Healthcare practitioners' experiences of breaking bad news: A critical interpretative meta synthesis. *Patient Educ. Couns.* **2023**, *107*, 107574. [CrossRef] [PubMed]
40. Ratna, H. The Importance of Effective Communication in Healthcare Practice. *Harv. Public Health Rev.* **2019**, *23*, 1–6. [CrossRef]
41. Dale MacLaine, T.; Lowe, N.; Dale, J. The use of simulation in medical student education on the topic of breaking bad news: A systematic review. *Patient Educ. Couns.* **2021**, *104*, 2670–2681. [CrossRef]
42. Wang, X.; Liu, M.; Li, J.; Wang, Z.; Liang, Q.; Yan, Z.; Wang, J.; Luan, X. Relationship between quality of life, fear of disease progression, and coping styles in patients with pulmonary hypertension: A network analysis. *Res. Nurs. Health* **2023**, *46*, 546–557. [CrossRef]
43. Wang, C.; Bi, S.; Lu, Y.; Li, Y.; Han, B.; Xu, M.; Meng, G.; Zhou, Q. Availability and stability of palliative care for family members of terminally ill patients in an integrated model of health and social care. *BMC Palliat. Care* **2024**, *23*, 140. [CrossRef]
44. Marschner, N.; Zacharias, S.; Lordick, F.; Hegewisch-Becker, S.; Martens, U.; Welt, A.; Hagen, V.; Gleiber, W.; Bohnet, S.; Kruggel, L.; et al. Association of Disease Progression with Health-Related Quality of Life Among Adults with Breast, Lung, Pancreatic, and Colorectal Cancer. *JAMA Netw. Open* **2020**, *3*, e200643. [CrossRef]
45. Salamanca-Balen, N.; Merluzzi, T.V.; Chen, M. The effectiveness of hope-fostering interventions in palliative care: A systematic review and meta-analysis. *Palliat. Med.* **2021**, *35*, 710–728. [CrossRef]
46. Merluzzi, T.V.; Salamanca-Balen, N.; Philip, E.J.; Salsman, J.M.; Chirico, A. Integration of Psychosocial Theory into Palliative Care: Implications for Care Planning and Early Palliative Care. *Cancers* **2024**, *16*, 342. [CrossRef]
47. Tolstrup, L.K.; Ditzel, H.M.; Giger, A.-K.W.; Jørgensen, T.L.; Ryg, J.; Dieperink, K.B. Determinants of poor quality of life in older patients with cancer: A longitudinal mixed methods study (PROGNOSIS-Q). *J. Geriatr. Oncol.* **2023**, *14*, 101500. [CrossRef]
48. Käsmann, L.; Taugner, J.; Eze, C.; Roengvoraphoj, O.; Dantes, M.; Gennen, K.; Karin, M.; Petrukhnov, O.; Tufman, A.; Belka, C.; et al. Performance Status and Its Changes Predict Outcome for Patients with Inoperable Stage III NSCLC Undergoing Multimodal Treatment. *Anticancer Res.* **2019**, *39*, 5077–5081. [CrossRef] [PubMed]
49. Azam, F.; Latif, M.F.; Farooq, A.; Tirmazy, S.H.; AlShahrani, S.; Bashir, S.; Bukhari, N. Performance Status Assessment by Using ECOG (Eastern Cooperative Oncology Group) Score for Cancer Patients by Oncology Healthcare Professionals. *Case Rep. Oncol.* **2019**, *12*, 728–736. [CrossRef] [PubMed]

50. Kumar, D.; Neeman, E.; Zhu, S.; Sun, H.; Kotak, D.; Liu, R. Revisiting the Association of ECOG Performance Status with Clinical Outcomes in Diverse Patients with Cancer. *J. Natl. Compr. Canc. Netw.* **2024**, *22*, e237111. [CrossRef]
51. Dunleavy, L.; Preston, N.; Walshe, C. Health care professional recruitment of patients and family carers to palliative care randomised controlled trials: A qualitative multiple case study. *Palliat. Med.* **2023**, *37*, 1540–1553. [CrossRef]
52. LeBlanc, T.W.; Lodato, J.E.; Currow, D.C.; Abernethy, A.P. Overcoming recruitment challenges in palliative care clinical trials. *J. Oncol. Pract.* **2013**, *9*, 277–282. [CrossRef] [PubMed]
53. Walshe, C.; Dunleavy, L.; Preston, N.; Payne, S.; Ellershaw, J.; Taylor, V.; Mason, S.; Nwosu, A.C.; Gadoud, A.; Board, R.; et al. Understanding barriers and facilitators to palliative and end-of-life care research: A mixed method study of generalist and specialist health, social care, and research professionals. *BMC Palliat. Care* **2024**, *23*, 159. [CrossRef] [PubMed]
54. Kerr, D.; Milnes, S.; Ammentorp, J.; McKie, C.; Dunning, T.; Ostaszkiewicz, J.; Wolderslund, M.; Martin, P. Challenges for nurses when communicating with people who have life-limiting illness and their families: A focus group study. *J. Clin. Nurs.* **2020**, *29*, 416–428. [CrossRef]
55. Bruun, A.; Oostendorp, L.; Bloch, S.; White, N.; Mitchinson, L.; Sisk, A.-R.; Stone, P. Prognostic decision-making about imminent death within multidisciplinary teams: A scoping review. *BMJ Open* **2022**, *12*, e057194. [CrossRef]
56. Ramos, K.; Kaufman, B.G.; Winger, J.G.; Boggins, A.; van Houtven, C.H.; Porter, L.S.; Hastings, S.N. Knowledge, goals, and misperceptions about palliative care in adults with chronic disease or cancer. *Palliat. Support. Care* **2023**, *22*, 1707–1713. [CrossRef]
57. Kitta, A.; Hagin, A.; Unseld, M.; Adamidis, F.; Diendorfer, T.; Masel, E.K.; Kirchheiner, K. The silent transition from curative to palliative treatment: A qualitative study about cancer patients' perceptions of end-of-life discussions with oncologists. *Support. Care Cancer* **2021**, *29*, 2405–2413. [CrossRef] [PubMed]
58. Lelorain, S. Discussing Prognosis with Empathy to Cancer Patients. *Curr. Oncol. Rep.* **2021**, *23*, 42. [CrossRef]
59. Amroud, M.S.; Raeissi, P.; Hashemi, S.-M.; Reisi, N.; Ahmadi, S.-A. Investigating the challenges and barriers of palliative care delivery in Iran and the World: A systematic review study. *J. Educ. Health Promot.* **2021**, *10*, 246. [CrossRef]
60. Nipp, R.D.; El-Jawahri, A.; Moran, S.M.; D'Arpino, S.M.; Johnson, P.C.; Lage, D.E.; Wong, R.L.; Pirl, W.F.; Traeger, L.; Lennes, I.T.; et al. The relationship between physical and psychological symptoms and health care utilization in hospitalized patients with advanced cancer. *Cancer* **2017**, *123*, 4720–4727. [CrossRef]
61. Colosimo, K.; Nissim, R.; Pos, A.E.; Hales, S.; Zimmermann, C.; Rodin, G. "Double awareness" in psychotherapy for patients living with advanced cancer. *J. Psychother. Integr.* **2018**, *28*, 125–140. [CrossRef]
62. Petrilli, C.M.; Saint, S.; Jennings, J.J.; Caruso, A.; Kuhn, L.; Snyder, A.; Chopra, V. Understanding patient preference for physician attire: A cross-sectional observational study of 10 academic medical centres in the USA. *BMJ Open* **2018**, *8*, e021239. [CrossRef] [PubMed]

healthcare

MDPI

Article

Promising Concept, Challenging Implementation of a Minimally Invasive Intervention (MINI) to Identify Patients in Their Last Year of Life—A Multi-Methods Feasibility Study at a German University Hospital

Alina Kasdorf [1,*], Belinda Werner [2], Jana Sophie Grimm [1], Gloria Dust [1], Steffen T. Simon [1,3,4], Raymond Voltz [1,3,4] and Julia Strupp [1] on behalf of the Cologne Research and Development Network (CoRe-Net) Study Group

1 Department of Palliative Medicine, Faculty of Medicine and University Hospital, University of Cologne, 50937 Cologne, Germany; steffen.simon@uk-koeln.de (S.T.S.); raymond.voltz@uk-koeln.de (R.V.); julia.strupp@uk-koeln.de (J.S.)
2 Economics and Social Sciences, Institute of Sociology and Social Psychology (ISS), Faculty of Management, University of Cologne, 50937 Cologne, Germany
3 Center for Integrated Oncology Aachen Bonn Cologne Duesseldorf (CIO ABCD), Faculty of Medicine and University Hospital, University of Cologne, 50937 Cologne, Germany
4 Center for Health Services Research, Faculty of Medicine and University Hospital, University of Cologne, 50937 Cologne, Germany
* Correspondence: alina.kasdorf@uk-koeln.de; Tel.: +49-221-478-86910

Abstract: Background/Objectives: Identifying patients with palliative care needs can be challenging in clinical practice. This study reports on the tailoring and evaluation of a minimally invasive intervention (MINI) to support early planning of palliative care in acute hospitals. The MINI includes the Surprise Question (SQ) and the Supportive and Palliative Care Indicators Tool (SPICT™) for health and social care professionals, as well as a patient Question Prompt Sheet. **Methods**: A multi-method intervention study was conducted, including interviews and a pre–post survey of professionals on the development, implementation, and experiences with MINI. Interview data were analyzed inductively and survey data descriptively. **Results**: Data from 44 participants were included. MINI was generally considered acceptable and relevant, particularly the SQ, which prompted reflection among staff. Following the intervention, a significant improvement was observed in the presentation of regional specialist palliative care services for patients, as well as in the identification of psychosocial problems and their discussion with patients and relatives. While physicians reported increased confidence in initiating end-of-life conversations, other hospital staff showed mixed responses. Reported barriers for implementing MINI included limited time, the COVID-19 pandemic, staff strikes, emotional burden, and unclear responsibilities, indicating a low level of commitment. SPICT use was inconsistent, suggesting low integration into workflows. Interprofessional collaboration improved, particularly with external palliative care providers. Sustainability was hindered by a lack of institutional support, ongoing training, and formal routines. **Conclusions**: MINI may have the potential to shift the focus away from purely curative approaches. However, to guarantee success, future studies should ensure better alignment between intervention design, implementation and framework conditions.

Keywords: prognosis; surprise question; palliative care; end-of-life care; terminally ill; decision making; feasibility studies; patient-centered care; hospitals

1. Introduction

The timely identification of patients with palliative care needs remains a major challenge for hospital staff, often leading to late or missed opportunities for palliative care integration [1]. Early palliative care has been shown to improve quality of life, patient satisfaction, and even survival outcomes in various populations [2]. In recent years, Germany has expanded its specialized palliative care services, enabling the provision of such complex and comprehensive care and ensuring the highest possible quality of life for dying patients [3,4]. Although few people in Germany identify the hospital as their preferred place of death, most still die there [5,6]. The hospital plays a significant role as a healthcare setting in the last year of life, with around 9 out of 10 patients having been hospitalized at least once [5]. It is estimated that one in three patients die within a year of hospital admission, with nearly one in two elderly patients dying within this period [7]. Although the hospital plays a crucial role in transitions and care in the last year of life, relatives were the least satisfied with the care received in hospitals [5]. Other studies also showed that there are still discrepancies between palliative care recommendations and the care actually provided in hospitals [8,9].

In fact, recommendations for the care of patients with life-limiting illnesses emphasize the importance of integrating palliative care early on, rather than waiting until the dying phase. Patients themselves also want to be informed about the possibilities of palliative care, but there is a gap in communication with HCPs [10,11]. Palliative care is often only integrated into treatment at a late stage by hospital staff, if at all [9]. Previous studies suggest that a substantial proportion, estimated at around one quarter, of hospitalized patients may have palliative care needs [12–14]. In the acute inpatient setting, high workloads, an emphasis on curative treatments and life-sustaining treatments, and the challenge of making accurate prognoses can delay early identification of patients' palliative care needs by hospital staff [15,16].

Recent evidence evaluating minimally invasive prognostic tools for the identification of palliative needs in hospital settings shows that combining the 12-month Surprise Question (SQ) and the Supportive and Palliative Care Indicators Tool (SPICT™) is a promising method for identifying patients in their last year of life [17–20]. However, studies have shown that systematic approaches for identifying patients who might benefit from early palliative interventions are still inconsistently applied in hospital settings [21,22]. Building on existing screening tools such as the Surprise Question and SPICT™, this study addresses this gap by developing and evaluating a minimally invasive intervention (MINI) tailored to the acute hospital context.

2. Materials and Methods

This study is the second part of the Last Year of Life Study in Cologne (LYOL-C I), hereafter referred to as LYOL-C II. Both parts of the study were conducted in Cologne, Germany. Further information can be found in the published study protocols and related publications [23,24].

2.1. Ethical Approval

The study was approved by the Ethics Committee of the Medical Faculty of the University of Cologne (#20-1431), the Staff Council of the University of Cologne, the Equal Opportunities Officers, and the representatives of the severely disabled. This trial is registered in the German Clinical Trials Register (DRKS00022378).

2.2. Participants

A distinction is made between two groups of participants (see Figure 1). The first group consists of those who were interviewed to tailor the intervention to the specific inpatient settings (I). The second group consists of university hospital staff who received the intervention, including a training session and subsequent application, and were later evaluated (Phase II). The participants in part I were health and social care practitioners (HSCPs) providing care for patients in their last year of life. These practitioners were sampled from January to April 2021 and were recruited using a purposive sampling strategy. The participants in part II were hospital staff from two hospital wards at the University Hospital Cologne. These included the gynecology ward, including its outpatient clinic, and an internal medicine ward. Most of the patients were treated for illnesses related to oncology and nephrology. The hospital staff had agreed to attend a Minimally Invasive Intervention (MINI) training. These participants were sampled from April 2022 to January 2023. Information regarding the training was disseminated through the hospital's newsletter and through announcements by the research team and senior physicians.

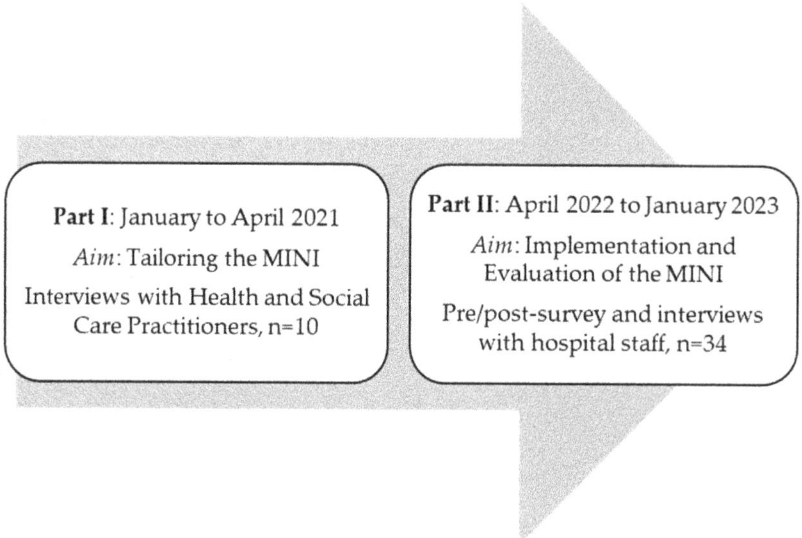

Figure 1. Study program.

All study participants were informed about the study and provided written informed consent.

2.3. Intervention

Part I: Tailoring MINI

To tailor the MINI to the planned study at a German acute University Hospital, a total of ten HSCP: seven experts (care providers from a predominantly inpatient medical setting) and three patient representatives from Cologne were interviewed. Due to the COVID-19 pandemic, the data collection was shifted to virtual, one-on-one interviews rather than the originally planned group sessions. This format contained in-depth insights into the care situation of patients in their last year of life and highlighted opportunities to improve both the identification of palliative care needs and the provision of care. In addition, determinants relevant to MINI and its implementation were identified to adapt the intervention to the hospital context and to derive targeted implementation strategies.

The interviews were also used to tailor the content and design of the newly developed Question Prompt Sheet (QPS) to the needs of patients in the last year of life.

Part II: Implementing MINI

Following the validation and adaptation of the intervention to the individual circumstances of the ward and the deliberately selected HSCP, the implementation of the intervention was planned. The conception and design of MINI aimed to facilitate the early identification of patients in their last year of life.

MINI involved the administration of two instruments: the 12-month Surprise Question (SQ: "Would I be surprised if this patient died within the next 12 months?") and the Supportive Palliative Care Indicator Tool (SPICT-DE^{TM}) for HSCP [25]. SPICT-DE^{TM} provides a structured set of general and disease-specific indicators to identify patients with deteriorating health who may need palliative care. A QPS titled "Conversation Guide for Your Healthcare" was also provided, intended for both patients and their care partners [23]. Both SQ and SPICT-DE^{TM} were available and validated in German [25,26]. The intervention study comprised two main components: HSCP-related and patient-related. HSCP-related components were aimed to enhance HSCPs' awareness of palliative needs by conducting MINI-training designed to equip them with the necessary skills to utilize the intervention. Patient-related components were to emphasize improving patient outcomes in comparison to the control group. As this study focuses on the HSCP-side intervention, the use of QPS is not explicitly evaluated herein (for further details regarding patient outcomes of MINI, see Grimm et al., 2025 [24]).

The intervention comprised providing diverse resources, such as updated posters, flyers, and an (online) MINI-training course for members of the ward staff, including physicians, nurses, and case managers. Key stages of implementation involve distributing materials at strategic points during care (e.g., after initial treatment or before physician consultations) and ensuring proper handovers of responsibility between staff, including healthcare providers and the study teams. The MINI training emphasized fundamental principles of palliative care, the importance of early integration, and effective communication strategies for discussing terminal diagnoses with patients and their families, utilizing the SPIKES communication model (Setting, Perception, Invitation, Knowledge, Emotions with Empathy and Strategy) [27], delivered by an experienced palliative care physician, among others. Following the training program, staff were guided to apply the SQ alongside the SPICT-DE^{TM} to identify patients in their last year of life. Each training, including the educational lecture, presentation of MINI, and case discussions, lasted approximately 60–90 min. A survey questionnaire was administered prior to and following the MINI training (pre–post survey).

2.4. Instruments

2.4.1. Interview Guide

Qualitative data were assessed for both groups of participants.

All interviews were audio recorded and transcribed verbatim. The STROBE checklist was used to guarantee thorough and transparent reporting of all critical elements of the quantitative investigation [28], while the COREQ Checklist (Consolidated criteria for Reporting Qualitative research) was used to report the qualitative data [29].

Tailoring interviews with HSCP n = 10: Interviews included the following questions: Presentation/discussion of MINI: In order to facilitate effective realization and implementation of the MINI, what is required? What design suggestions do you have? Does MINI meet the needs? How would you assess the feasibility of implementation? How do you rate the content of MINI? What additional information would you add? Is more disease-specific information/criteria considered important? In what form and how would you present this tool on the ward? Who should use the tool? How? And when? What do you think should be considered in the day-to-day use of the intervention? How can the long-term use of the tool be maintained? With regard to the implementation of the intervention, which barriers do you consider to be of significance, in order to be able to tailor our intervention as closely as possible to the requirements?

Evaluation interviews with hospital staff members n = 10: Interviews included the following questions: What does 'palliative care' mean to you? Have you used the intervention? Did applying the intervention change your perspective on palliative care needs? What could we have done better? Which patient groups do you use MINI for? How would you rate the intervention overall, i.e., the benefits of the intervention?

Purposive sampling was utilized to select participants for interviews, with the criteria including attendance at the training and a sufficient level of motivation to discuss their experience with MINI. The interview guide was presented and discussed in a qualitative research workshop with the research group in September 2022. A positive vote from the staff council was obtained in December 2022. The number of interviews conducted depended on reaching thematic saturation regarding the research question. A total of five interviews per hospital unit were planned, involving staff from different professional groups engaged in the intervention's implementation. Individual interviews were conducted due to scheduling constraints across professional groups with survey participants. The interviews were planned to take place at the University Hospital. The data collection took place from December 2022 to August 2023. The evaluation interviews were conducted by two female research associates of the Cologne Research and Development Network (CoRe-Net) study group members with experience in conducting qualitative research. It is noteworthy that the interviewer was not the presenter of the MINI training.

2.4.2. Questionnaire

To evaluate the MINI, hospital staff members underwent a pre–post survey by using a self-developed questionnaire consisting of 30 (pre-) and 36 (post-) items. The questionnaire was available both online and on paper, with the online survey conducted via the LimeSurvey platform at the University of Cologne. The data was collected between April 2022 and August 2023, as shown in Figure 1, via an online survey. The questionnaire was based on the German National S3 guideline for palliative care (providing recommendations for structured hospital conversations addressing patients' physical, emotional, social, and spiritual needs, life goals, and end-of-life care) and findings from the previous study [30,31]. It collected demographic data and assessed self-reported competencies in areas such as identifying patients in their last year of life and addressing patients' wishes and needs through communication with patients and involved caregivers. The response format for the self-developed items consisted of a 4-point Likert scale with the options: 'agree', 'somewhat agree', 'somewhat disagree', and 'disagree', as well as a 'no response' option. The questionnaire also included open-ended questions allowing participants to elaborate on their answers and provide further comments.

To assess palliative self-efficacy, the Palliative Competence Test for Physicians (Palliative Kompetenztest (PKT), a validated 52-item tool, was used [32]. The self-efficacy scale of PKT was adapted for use in an acute care setting and across different professional groups by removing 8 of the 10 original items. As the PKT is designed for formative rather than diagnostic purposes, no cut-off values were defined. Permission to use the adapted version was obtained from the author. Some questions about communication on death and dying were based on a doctoral thesis by Hauck (2007), with content adapted to the study's aims and the response format standardized to align with the rest of the questionnaire [33].

To ensure comprehensibility and practicality, the entire questionnaire was initially presented and discussed in a research workshop with staff from the Department of Palliative Medicine at the University Hospital of Cologne. A revised version was pre-tested using the think-aloud technique, resulting in changes to wording and response format.

Data collection was pseudonymized. Participants created a personal code that could only be traced back to them, to allow them to exclude their data if they wished, as well as to analyze individual differences in the pre–post survey.

2.5. Analyses

The qualitative data were analyzed by following the principles of qualitative content analysis [34]. The analysis followed Mayring's structured approach to qualitative content analysis, consisting of summarizing, explicating, and structuring the material to derive inductive categories that reflect the essential content in a systematic and transparent manner. A common deductive framework was applied, reflecting the research questions of the evaluation. The Consolidated Framework for Implementation Research (CFIR) was used to analyze contextual determinants during the tailoring phase [35]. Proctor's and colleagues' implementation outcomes framework guided the evaluation of the implementation phase [36]. The subcategories of acceptability, appropriateness, feasibility, fidelity, and sustainability were derived deductively from Proctor's and colleagues' framework and categorized using the available interview material. Although the overall dataset also included inductively coded material, only the deductive categories were used for this publication to ensure theoretical consistency with the implementation focus. A detailed codebook was developed and applied consistently across all interviews to ensure transparency and reliability. Two researchers (AK and JS) had regular coder meetings to ensure the precise classification of categories. The sample size was considered sufficient based on the concept of information power [37], as the interviews provided rich, relevant, and specific information to address the research questions.

Quantitative data was analyzed descriptively using IBM SPSS Statistics 28. Responses "Don't know" were treated as a missing value; for other responses, the answers have been summarized in a dichotomous format ("Agree" including the responses "agree" and "somewhat agree", "disagree" including the responses "somewhat disagree" and "disagree"). Pre–post comparisons were conducted using the Wilcoxon signed-rank test. Statistical significance was assessed using unadjusted p-values, with an alpha level of 0.05. No correction for multiple comparisons (e.g., Bonferroni) was applied, as the analyses were exploratory in nature.

Due to the limited sample size, inferential testing (Wilcoxon signed-rank test) was conducted in an exploratory manner, and results are interpreted descriptively without claims of generalizability.

The results are presented according to Proctor et al.'s implementation outcome categories (acceptability, adoption, appropriateness, feasibility, fidelity, implementation cost, penetration and sustainability), reflecting the deductive coding of the qualitative data [30]. To provide a structured overview of the implementation experience, all data were translated into numeric scores (0 = not achieved, 1 = partially achieved, 2 = fully achieved; n/a = not applicable). The scoring was developed inductively based on the qualitative interview data and the corresponding quantitative survey trends, following researcher consensus. Each score represents the extent to which an implementation outcome, as defined by Proctor and colleagues' framework, was evident across data sources. For example, partially achieved indicates that the respective implementation criterion (e.g., feasibility or acceptability) was supported by some, but not all, qualitative statements or quantitative indicators.

3. Results

Part I: Tailoring MINI

The interviews were conducted to explore possible barriers to the implementation and necessary tailoring of the intervention and implementation strategies with regard to the hospital setting and resources. We assumed that a successful implementation of the SQ and SPICT intervention requires a well-planned combination of clear training, regular reminders, intensive interdisciplinary collaboration, and a clearly structured process. Employee motivation and open, transparent communication within the team were identified as key factors in this process.

The tailoring of MINI focused on addressing multiple categories to enhance accessibility and relevance for hospital staff. Tailored strategies included the continuous availability and presence of study staff, as well as regular updates of materials. The implementation strategy was designed to be flexible and patient-centered, ensuring that the intervention could be adapted to the needs of hospital staff and seamlessly integrated into their workflows.

Key barriers for a successful intervention were identified in the areas of content, language, format, and implementation strategies. The content of MINI was tailored to include diverse examples, clear language, and updated contact information. The layout was designed for readability, with appropriate font sizes and high contrast to improve accessibility. Long-term accessibility was ensured through regular updates and the dissemination of MINI through various channels, including digital formats and printed copies in staff areas.

Part II: Implementing MINI

3.1. Study Population

In total, there were 66 HSCPs, including 20 doctors, 40 nurses, and six other professionals (study nurse, case manager), as shown in Figure 2. The pre-survey was completed by 34 people, representing 51.5% of those invited. At baseline (t0), the sample size was already smaller (n = 34) than expected (n = 66), and by the follow-up (t1), a substantial number of participants had dropped out (n = 14). Thus, only 41.2% of participants from the pre-survey completed the post-survey.

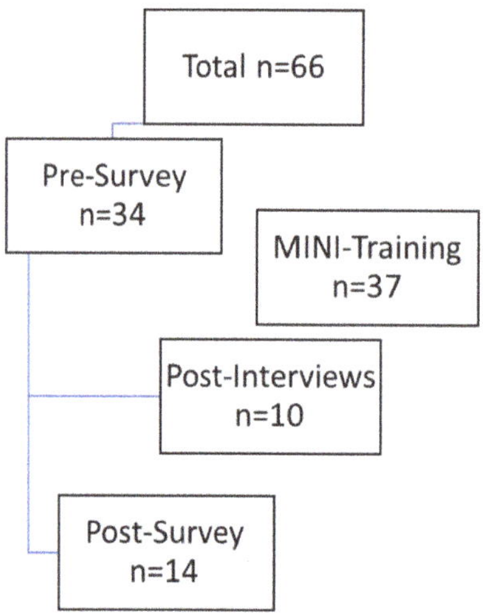

Figure 2. Data generation process.

The lower number of participants was due to some employees switching to other wards, leaving the organization, or being unavailable by email or telephone. Employees received an incentive of €25 in the form of a voucher for participating in both surveys. Five (35.7%) of the 14 participants who completed the post-survey indicated that they had moved to a different ward, which made it difficult to assess how the intervention had worked. In conclusion, a total of ten interviews were conducted with participants following their participation in the MINI training program. Six HSCPs worked on the non-oncology ward and four on the oncology ward. Table 1 presents the sociodemographic profile of the study participants.

Table 1. Sociodemographic data of the participants.

Characteristic	Total Pre N = 34 (%)	Total Post N = 14(%)
Age		
Under 20 years	1 (2.9)	0 (0)
21–30 years	13 (38.2)	8 (57.1)
31–40 years	10 (29.4)	2 (14.3)
41–50 years	5 (14.7)	3 (21.4)
51–60 years	5 (14.7)	1 (7.1)
Gender		
Female	20 (58.8)	9 (64.3)
Male	14 (41.2)	5 (35.7)
Hospital ward		
Nephrology	18 (52.9)	9 (64.3)
Gynecology	16 (47.1)	5 (35.7)
Profession		
Physician	13 (38.2)	6 (42.9)
Nurse	17 (50.0)	6 (42.9)
Other [1]	4 (11.8)	2 (14.2)
Work experience		
Under 1 year	5 (14.7)	3 (21.4)
1 to 5 years	9 (26.5)	5 (35.7)
6 to 10 years	4 (11.8)	1 (7.1)
11 to 20 years	11 (32.4)	4 (28.6)
More than 20 years	5 (14.7)	1 (7.1)
Experience in the treatment of seriously ill patients in the last year of life		
Under 1 year	6 (17.6)	4 (28.6)
1 to 5 years	9 (26.5)	6 (42.9)
6 to 10 years	9 (26.5)	0 (0)
11 to 20 years	6 (17.6)	3 (21.4)
More than 20 years	4 (11.8)	1 (7.1)
Additional qualification in palliative care		
Yes	4 (11.8)	0 (0)
No	30 (88.2)	14 (100)

[1] Case management and psychologists.

3.2. *Evaluating MINI*

The evaluation of the MINI reveals substantial variation across implementation dimensions, highlighting both conceptual potential and operational limitations.

3.2.1. Acceptability

Definition. *How well is MINI accepted by the involved HSCP?*

Overall, the MINI was well accepted, although experiences varied across professional groups and intervention components (Table 2). In the quantitative survey, a total of 90.0% of respondents found the SQ helpful, with the satisfaction rate among physicians at 100.0%. In qualitative interviews, however, views were more ambivalent. While some participants valued the SQ as a stimulus for reflection and collegial exchange, others described it as emotionally demanding, particularly when confronted with the tension between clinical responsibility and the acknowledgment of dying:

> *"And then you have to deal with your inner level, so to speak, and say: 'Well, no, so if I really look at it very closely and soberly, then it's actually like that, yes."* (Interview 10)

Table 2. Acceptability: critical appraisal of implementation outcomes *, Proctor et al. 2011 [36].

Category	Critical Appraisal of Implementation Outcomes	SQ	SPICT	QPS
Acceptability	The MINI was well accepted, especially the SQ, which is seen as stimulating interprofessional exchange and reflection, while SPICT and QPS were predominantly rejected by physicians due to their complexity and lack of suitability for everyday use; the intervention promoted external cooperation, but showed ambivalent outcomes on internal communication within the team.	2 ***	0 **	0 **

* This scoring is inductively derived from the mixed-methods findings of this study. This scoring provides a rapid overview of the extent to which MINI was successfully implemented. ** 0: Not achieved; *** 2: Fully achieved.

Among physicians, the supplementary tools (SPICT, QPS) were not seen as helpful at all (0% positive feedback). Overall, only 14.3% of participants found them useful. Barriers included limited applicability in routine workflows and perceived complexity, as reported by the respondents:

> *"It's good to read up on, I think, but in parts it's a bit much* [. . .]*"* (Interview 05)

Despite such reservations, overall satisfaction with the intervention was high (91.7%). A majority (71.4%) considered the time investment worthwhile, particularly physicians (83.4%). The intervention also had an influence on interprofessional communication. One interviewee emphasized the SQ's potential to initiate conversations across professional hierarchies.

> *"But the fact is that deliberately posing the question definitely draws attention to the topic, which is a good thing, it enables people to engage with seriously ill people or with the illness situation and that you can then also discuss it with younger colleagues, for example, and that you can then pass it on as CULTURE. So in that respect, the intervention was good. It woke things up. And now it would be good if we could stabilize it, so to speak. I would say that. So the question is definitely important, and the issue is right. We just need to be able to anchor it more firmly, yes."* (Interview 10)

Quantitative findings on interprofessional exchange showed mixed trends. Communication about patient needs within the ward team declined overall (from 58.8% to 50.0%), mainly due to a marked drop in physician-reported rates (from 61.5% to 33.3%). In contrast, non-medical staff reported stable or improved communication (from 57.1% to 66.7%). Notably, collaboration with external providers increased across nearly all domains: communication with specialists rose from 58.8% to 81.8%, with general practitioners from 22.6% to 36.4%, and with specialized outpatient palliative care from 53.3% to 66.7%. Contact with palliative care services and relatives remained consistently high (82.4% to 91.7% and 91.2% to 92.3%, respectively).

In terms of patient-centered care, physicians reported increased, though not statistically significant, engagement in key end-of-life conversations: regarding advance directives, power of attorney, upcoming decisions (84.6% to 100%, respectively), and preferred place of death (from 53.8% to 83.3%). Among non-medical staff, these changes were less pronounced.

3.2.2. Adoption

Definition. *To what extent is MINI implemented in practice?*

The adoption of the MINI into routine clinical practice was heterogeneous (Table 3).

Table 3. Adoption: critical appraisal of implementation outcomes *, Proctor et al. 2011 [36].

Category	Critical Appraisal of Implementation Outcomes	SQ	SPICT	QPS
Adoption	The adoption of the MINI was inconsistent and remained limited in routine practice. The SQ was used regularly and widely, leading to measurable increases in competence, particularly in the psychosocial area. SPICT and QPS, on the other hand, were rarely used due to unclear procedures and a lack of instructions and therefore had little outcome.	2 ***	0 **	0 **

* This scoring is inductively derived from the mixed-methods findings of this study. This scoring provides a rapid overview of the extent to which the MINI was successfully implemented. ** 0: Not achieved; *** 2: Fully achieved.

Although general willingness to engage was high particularly among physicians, its consistent implementation remained limited. Competing clinical priorities often leads to de-prioritization, especially among nursing staff and assistant physicians. While the intervention tools were available and known, they were frequently viewed as ancillary to core clinical tasks. A lack of defined follow-up structures and unclear responsibilities further impeded implementation:

> *"That's not easy to do more often. We have a meeting with the physicians here in the morning, we'll discuss it then. But it's only being touched on lightly. So it's not satisfactory. [...] They're there, everyone knows them [...] But anything additional is massively cut back right now. That really has to come from the top."* (Interview 02)

Self-assessments of palliative care competencies showed improvement, particularly in psychosocial domains (Table 4). Confidence in recognizing and addressing psychosocial concerns increased significantly (from 73.5% to 84.6%, $p = 0.026$), with the largest gains observed among non-medical staff (from 57.1% to 87.5%). Familiarity with regional specialized palliative care services improved (from 38.2% to 50.0%, $p = 0.020$), as did the ability to initiate referrals (from 57.6% to 69.2%). All participants reported post-intervention confidence in identifying complex needs at the end of life (100%). Other indicators demonstrated less consistent patterns. Among physicians, confidence in presenting local palliative care options declined slightly (from 38.5% to 33.3%), as did confidence in advising on advance directives (from 61.5% to 50.0%). In contrast, other staff reported gains, for instance, confidence in discussing living wills rose from 33.3% to 66.7%.

Participants also reported improvements in the identification and management of patients in the last year of life. Knowledge of relevant criteria for patients being in their last year of life increased from 82.4% to 92.9%, and confidence in recognizing such patients rose from 73.5% to 84.6%. While perceived ability to provide care improved modestly (from 72.7% to 78.6%), more pronounced gains were observed in participants' confidence in communicating life-limiting diagnoses (from 58.8% to 75.0%). These improvements were most pronounced among physicians, although other professional groups also reported positive changes.

Table 4. Self-assessment scale with focus on responses of participants who agreed or partly agreed to the statement. Palliative Competence Test for Physicians (Palliative Kompetenztest (PKT)) [26].

I Think That I Am Capable	Pre n (%)			Post n (%)		
	Physicians Only	Other Medical Staff Only	Overall	Physicians Only	Other Medical Staff Only	Overall
to collect data that describe a patient's pain in a differentiated way, n = 34/14.	11 (84.6)	19 (90.5)	30 (88.2)	5 (83.3)	6 (75.0)	11 (78.6)
to present the regional offers of specialized palliative care, n = 34/14. $p = 0.020$	5 (38.5)	8 (38.1)	13 (38.2)	2 (33.3)	5 (62.5)	7 (50.0)
to convince a colleague of the need for palliative support, n = 34/14.	12 (92.3)	19 (90.5)	31 (91.2)	6 (100)	7 (87.5)	13 (92.9)
recognize psychosocial problems and discuss them with patients and relatives, n = 34/14. $p = 0.026$	13 (100)	12 (57.1)	25 (73.5)	6 (100)	7 (87.5)	13 (92.9)
to organize a referral to hospice and palliative care services, n = 34/13.	7 (58.3)	12 (57.1)	19 (57.6)	5 (83.3)	4 (57.1)	9 (69.2)
to recognize the complex needs of a dying person and to react appropriately to them, n = 34/13.	9 (69.2)	16 (76.2)	25 (73.5)	6 (100)	7 (100)	13 (100)
to remain in conversation when the wish for euthanasia is expressed. n = 34/12.	9 (75.0)	12 (57.1)	21 (63.6)	5 (83.3)	5 (83.3)	10 (83.3)
to integrate cultural and spiritual aspects of dying and death into the treatment of seriously ill people, n = 34/12.	7 (53.8)	14 (66.7)	21 (61.8)	4 (66.7)	5 (83.3)	9 (75.0)
to recognize whether a person is suffering, even if the possibilities of communication are limited, n = 34/14.	12 (92.3)	19 (90.5)	31 (91.2)	5 (83.3)	8 (100)	13 (92.9)
to advise a patient on the framework of the living will and to draw one up with him/her, n = 34/12.	8 (61.5)	7 (33.3)	15 (44.1)	3 (50.0)	4 (66.7)	7 (58.3)

3.2.3. Appropriateness

Definition. *How suitable is MINI for the target group and the context?*

The appropriateness of the MINI appears to be highly context dependent (Table 5).

Interview data highlighted that successful implementation relied strongly on who initiated the intervention, when, and in which clinical setting. A sensitive, individualized approach was considered crucial, particularly by nursing staff, who often maintain closer emotional proximity to patients. At the same time, physicians were perceived to hold the greatest authority, especially regarding prognostic or conclusive statements, thereby reinforcing existing role hierarchies:

> "*[. . .] There are emotional hierarchies: When a doctor says something, it's different from when a nursing staff or case manager does.*" (Interview 02)

Application of the SQ varied across departments and was seen as less useful in certain contexts. For example, in nephrology or chronic care settings, the SQ was often perceived as insufficiently specific, given the high proportion of patients with poor but fluctuating prognoses. Even when criteria were met, the subsequent steps toward care planning were often lacking, indicating a disconnect between assessment and actionable change.

Interviewees emphasized that the relevance of the MINI was closely tied to the disease stage and the patient's willingness or ability to engage in prognostic conversations. Some patients avoided such discussions, while others were too emotionally or physically compromised to participate. Although MINI occasionally prompted earlier reflection, its introduction frequently occurred too late. The hospital environment, described as reactive and crisis-driven, was perceived as suboptimal for adopting such interventions by the respondents, especially when compared to primary care, where longer-term, continuous relationships could enable earlier engagement.

Table 5. Appropriateness: critical appraisal of implementation outcomes *, Proctor et al. 2011 [36].

Category	Critical Appraisal of Implementation Outcomes	SQ	SPICT	QPS
Appropriateness	While the conceptual relevance of MINI was broadly acknowledged, its practical appropriateness proved highly context-dependent. Successful application hinged on the constellation of who introduced the intervention, when, and in which setting. Physicians were generally attributed greater authority, particularly regarding prognostic communication, whereas nursing staff were seen as emotionally closer to patients. These role dynamics created ambiguity in responsibility and communication pathways. Moreover, variability in patient trajectories, especially outside oncology, posed challenges to the selective and meaningful application of MINI. The intervention's perceived relevance was largely restricted to cancer care, limiting its broader applicability.	1 ***	0 **	0 **

* This scoring is inductively derived from the mixed-methods findings of this study. This scoring provides a rapid overview of the extent to which the MINI was successfully implemented. ** 0: Not achieved; *** 1: Partially achieved.

Relational dynamics were also identified as key to acceptance. Nursing staff were viewed as more emotionally attuned facilitators, while physicians were seen as more credible in delivering prognostic information. This dual perception created a structural tension: the effectiveness of communication was shaped not only by what was said, but also by who delivered the message.

Despite these challenges, the intervention may have contributed to more favorable perceptions. Over half of the respondents (57.1%) reported that MINI had changed their view of palliative care needs, mainly through improved interdisciplinary communication and earlier recognition of relevant issues. In parallel, the proportion of staff who considered the hospital an appropriate setting for end-of-life discussions increased (from 78.8% to 92.9%). Furthermore, the belief that patients struggle to express fears about dying to hospital physicians declined (from 91.2% to 71.4%), indicating a potential shift in communication culture.

3.2.4. Feasibility

Definition. *How feasible is the implementation of MINI?*

The feasibility of the MINI varied considerably across its individual components (Table 6).

The SQ was still rated most positively: most respondents considered it comprehensible (90.0%), applicable (90.0%), and manageable in terms of time (90.0%). In contrast, the SPICT and, particularly, the QPS received substantially lower ratings. Only one-third of respondents were satisfied with the time investment required for SPICT (33.3%) and 40.0% for QPS. These instruments were also rated lower in terms of being comprehensible (57.1% and 66.7%) and applicable (42.9% and 50.0%).

Table 6. Feasibility: critical appraisal of implementation outcomes *, Proctor et al. 2011 [36].

Category	Critical Appraisal of Implementation Outcomes	SQ	SPICT	QPS
Feasibility	The SQ was widely accepted as a low-threshold, time-efficient tool. In contrast, SPICT and the QPS were considered impractical due to time constraints, low applicability, and limited uptake, particularly in fast-paced inpatient settings. Structural challenges, including shift work, limited staff resources, and a lack of dedicated coordination mechanisms, further impeded interdisciplinary collaboration. Implementation often remained improvised and lacked systematic integration into clinical routines.	2 ***	0 **	0 **

* This scoring is inductively derived from the mixed-methods findings of this study. This scoring provides a rapid overview of the extent to which the MINI was successfully implemented. ** 0: Not achieved; *** 2: Fully achieved.

A major barrier to implementation lies in the structural and organizational context, as reported by respondents. Shift work, staff shortages, and limited time windows hinder continuous and interprofessional coordinated application. Coordinating between nursing staff, physicians, and case management was frequently described as demanding. Although there was repeated interest in regular, structured meetings, the current implementation remains largely ad hoc and dependent on individual commitment, arguing against sustainable routine integration.

A particularly critical issue is the discrepancy between the perceived theoretical value of the intervention and its practical applicability. While the MINI is considered conceptually suitable, its application often fails due to the realities of everyday clinical practice. Without structural adjustments, such as defined time slots, clear responsibilities, and simplified materials, the intervention remains difficult to scale, as reported by the participants.

3.2.5. Fidelity

Definition. *To what extent is MINI being implemented in accordance with the original specifications?*

Several components, in particular SPICT, were modified in the application by being used selectively or omitted entirely (Table 7).

Table 7. Fidelity: critical appraisal of implementation outcomes *, Proctor et al. 2011 [36].

Category	Critical Appraisal of Implementation Outcomes	SQ	SPICT	QPS
Fidelity	Implementation fidelity was low. The MINI was rarely applied as designed but rather reduced to its most feasible components or adapted informally. SPICT, in particular, was frequently omitted. The COVID-19 pandemic and a months-long nursing strike severely disrupted implementation and training processes, contributing to fragmentation and inconsistencies. Without dedicated structures and prioritization within the clinical workflow, adherence to the original protocol remained limited.	1 ***	0 **	0 **

* This scoring is inductively derived from the mixed-methods findings of this study. This scoring provides a rapid overview of the extent to which the MINI was successfully implemented. ** 0: Not achieved; *** 1: Partially achieved.

These adjustments were often made to navigate profession-specific barriers or to enhance practical applicability in day-to-day routines. Qualitative data suggests that the intervention was primarily used as a cognitive prompt rather than as a standardized protocol. Especially among experienced nursing staff, the content was reportedly internalized to such a degree that formal application became less relevant in practice. One physician stated:

"So we can't avoid asking ourselves the question: palliative care or not? And I'm happy to take this note with me again. [...] As I said, I don't think I'll go into the patients' [...] ask myself point by point: Does this apply or not?" (Interview 03)

These findings are supported by quantitative data: while the SQ was used regularly by 75.0% of respondents, the use of SPICT remained maximally inconsistent, with 0.0% agreement in this item. This variation in adherence underscores a central challenge: the intervention was not applied as an integrated package, but rather in a fragmented and context-dependent manner.

External factors further contributed to limited fidelity. The COVID-19 pandemic significantly disrupted study procedures: hygiene restrictions, visitation bans, staff shortages, and the loss of key personnel led to gaps in implementation, evaluation, and training. In addition, the multi-month nursing strike (April–July 2022) had substantial consequences. Wards participating in the study were temporarily closed, untrained staff had to take over, and systematic application of the MINI became virtually impossible. As a result, implementation was highly fragmented and largely dependent on the initiative of individual staff members and the research team.

3.2.6. Implementation Costs

Definition. *What financial resources are required for implementation?*

Financial resources were hardly discussed (Table 8).

Table 8. Implementation Costs: critical appraisal of implementation outcomes *, Proctor et al. 2011 [36].

Category	Critical Appraisal of Implementation Outcomes	SQ	SPICT	QPS
Implementation Costs	While financial costs were not a dominant issue, the intervention was highly sensitive to staff and time constraints. Without sustained investment in training, coordination, and protected time for patient engagement, MINI remained a marginal and non-prioritized addition to existing duties. Notably, time spent with patients either remained unchanged or increased, raising questions about added workload in the absence of systemic support.	n/a **	n/a **	n/a **

* This scoring is inductively derived from the mixed-methods findings of this study. This scoring provides a rapid overview to what extent the MINI was successfully implemented. ** n/a: not applicable.

However, it became clear that the introduction and maintenance of the intervention require human resources, in particular time and coordination. Establishment as a standard process was only considered realistic if continuous personnel resources, e.g., through trained specialists or regular further training measures, could be provided. With regard to indirect cost efficiency, the survey data shows that the average time required for patients who are presumably in the last year of life has changed from 7.36 min (SD 8.5) to 13.07 min (SD 14.9) for respondents as a result of the intervention. Accordingly, for 23.1% of respondents, the time required has increased, and for 7.7% it has been considerably extended. 71.4% considered the intervention to have been worth the time invested, while 28.6% rated it as neutral.

3.2.7. Penetration

Definition. *How widespread is the MINI within the target population?*

The visibility and reach of the MINI within the target population were heterogeneous and partially low (Table 9).

Table 9. Penetration: critical appraisal of implementation outcomes *, Proctor et al. 2011 [36].

Category	Critical Appraisal of Implementation Outcomes	SQ	SPICT	QPS
Penetration	MINI was adopted selectively, mainly in oncology-related units and by senior medical staff. Broader dissemination was hampered by professional hierarchies, high workload, and low engagement from non-physician staff. The intervention failed to gain traction across diverse departments and patient groups, limiting its reach and systemic impact.	1 ***	0 **	0 **

* This scoring is inductively derived from the mixed-methods findings of this study. This scoring provides a rapid overview of the extent to which the MINI was successfully implemented. ** 0: Not achieved; *** 1: Partially achieved.

The intervention's penetration within the clinical setting appears to be limited to specific departments and patient groups (e.g., predominantly tumor patients). Despite some integration in routine practice, broader dissemination is hampered by logistical issues and varying levels of staff engagement. One interviewee criticized the non-uniform application of the intervention, which was developed on the basis of HSCP input. This selective penetration limits the impact on a broad level. It was found that the intervention was primarily implemented by senior physicians, potentially excluding other professional groups from active use. Change in responsibilities, the general workload and hierarchical structures in everyday hospital life also made it difficult to implement the intervention. Many HSCPs who were introduced to the intervention and were supposed to suggest patients for the study team by use of the MINI were difficult to reach, left the participating wards after some time or stated that they did not have time to implement MINI in addition to patient care.

3.2.8. Sustainability

Definition. *To what extent can the MINI be maintained in the long term?*

A number of prerequisites were identified as being necessary for the long-term implementation of the intervention (Table 10).

Table 10. Sustainability: critical appraisal of implementation outcomes *, Proctor et al. 2011 [36].

Category	Critical Appraisal of Implementation Outcomes	SQ	SPICT	QPS
Sustainability	While MINI generated reflective impulses, it failed to establish sustainable practice change. Its continued use was largely dependent on motivated individuals and external project support. In the absence of binding structures, ongoing training, and clearly defined responsibilities, long-term integration appeared unlikely. Prospects for cultural change remained aspirational rather than observable.	0 **	0 **	0 **

* This scoring is inductively derived from the mixed-methods findings of this study. This scoring provides a rapid overview of the extent to which the MINI was successfully implemented. ** 0: Not achieved.

The implementation of recurrent training sessions, designated meeting times within the team, and the utilization of visible reminder formats, including posters and displays, were identified as conducive to effective team functioning. Materials such as posters and SPICT displays were present on the ward; their perception was strongly influenced by individual attention focus and context (e.g., proximity to the workstation). The personal presence of the research team was described as crucial for recall and use.

At the same time, it became clear that the hospital requires structural routines to ensure widespread adoption of new instruments. Respondents generally indicated a high level of willingness to retain elements of the intervention but emphasized the difference between individual motivation and systematic implementation.

Continued interest in using the MINI was high, reported by 75.0% of all respondents (83.3% among physicians; 66.7% among other staff).

MINI appeared to initiate reflective processes within some teams, which occasionally extended beyond the study period. In selected settings, elements of the intervention were embedded into routine ward rounds and interdisciplinary case discussions, facilitating more differentiated and collaborative care planning.

4. Discussion

This study describes the evaluation of a low-threshold intervention aimed at supporting the early initiation of palliative care planning in acute hospital settings. The findings of the present study suggest that MINI may provide a minimally invasive stimulus for reflection on the ethos of curative care. However, while the SQ is regarded as a pragmatic and accessible catalyst for introspection, it has been demonstrated that SPICT and QPS are employed only sporadically as a preliminary guideline for the initial implementation. An analysis of the intervention's outcomes at the patient level, as reported by Grimm et al. (2025), suggests that MINI may influence aspects of the curative mindset [24], though results from the current study remain preliminary.

The intervention was generally well-received. MINI may foster interdisciplinary discourse and could support engagement with the subject of serious illness, dying, and death. Physicians showed indications of increased knowledge and self-awareness regarding the identification and management of patients in their last year of life compared to other medical staff. Some improvements were observed in recognizing relevant criteria and caring for these patients. The involvement of trained personnel may support patient communication and inter-team collaboration.

Satisfaction with the intervention is also reflected in its future prospects, with 80% of physicians expressing a desire to continue with the intervention. Physicians reported some increases in confidence in utilizing the intervention and in addressing palliative care aspects, including psychosocial concerns.

As indicated in previous studies on the SQ [38,39], its function as a low-threshold trigger for prognostic considerations has been emphasized. The results of our study lend further support to this finding. However, it is crucial to emphasize that the prognostic quality of MINI was not a subject of intervention, and no measurements were taken to ascertain the accuracy of the identification of a last year of life patient at any point in time. Internationally, the combination of the SQ with the Supportive and SPICT has received empirical support as a feasible and clinically valuable approach to identifying patients in their last year of life [20,40]. Research conducted in the domains of acute care and oncology has demonstrated the capacity for seamless integration of these instruments into established clinical workflows [41,42]. The extant results indicate that the service providers benefited exclusively from the use of the SQ. SPICT was utilized to a negligible extent, despite its adaptation and validation for the German healthcare system [25]. However, it can be hypothesized that the outcomes would have been even more favorable if SPICT had been digitally integrated into the hospital information system, as was the case in the study by Van Wijmen et al. [18].

MINI can trigger ambivalent reactions among medical staff, especially if it is understood as an implicit request to limit healing efforts. This is consistent with the findings that prognostic tools can trigger emotional discomfort and ethical uncertainty in clinicians, potentially leading to moral distress. These are recognized barriers to the adoption of prognostic tools as they can cause moral discomfort in healthcare professionals [43–45].

Our findings confirm this and highlight the emotional challenges faced by staff when engaging in end-of-life conversations.

International findings also show that the implementation of such interventions is associated with specific challenges. These barriers include lack of confidence in dealing with prognostic assessments, lack of time, cultural barriers, "rescue culture" in the hospital and concerns about the potential impact on the doctor-patient relationship [46–48]. At the same time, a dilemma arises: the structural conditions in inpatient care (lack of time, multi-bed rooms, crisis orientation) hinder early and individualized implementation, a problem described in another study on palliative care in hospitals [49]. In contrast to previous research, respondents had no mistrust in the prognostic qualities of the tool, which would rule out lack of trust as a cause of failed implementation [42]. Nevertheless, the positive changes in the communication climate indicate potential for development. MINI may have the potential to support a shift towards a more open approach to dying and death, provided that structural barriers are actively addressed.

As our data suggests, MINI uptake tends to be higher when interventions are linked to specific courses of action and can be meaningfully integrated into existing processes, such as ward rounds or interdisciplinary meetings. The low uptake of SPICT and QPS highlights that inadequate guidance and uncertainty in use are significant barriers, a challenge also identified in advance care planning interventions, where patients often experience decision uncertainty due to complex information and a lack of clarity [50,51].

Our results highlight that organizational and hierarchical structures have a significant influence on who feels responsible for implementation, a circumstance that tends to hinder the active participation of nurses and residents. The crucial role of cross-team implementation is well documented and underlines that interprofessional collaboration increases the effectiveness of palliative care interventions [52]. Our results are consistent with this observation and suggest that cohesive teamwork may facilitate better integration of tools such as MINI [53]. The deviations from the original implementation of MINI, in particular the selective application of the SPICT criteria and the flexible use of intervention as a reflection tool, are common in practice, especially in complex clinical situations [54]. In comparison, however, it is evident that in addition to its function as a cognitive stimulus, MINI may also contribute to interprofessional communication processes and role perceptions. The intervention has been demonstrated to elicit individual reflection, whilst, under certain conditions, also promoting coordination within teams and across sectors. This aspect has received little attention in the literature to date. Despite the modest scale of this preliminary study, future research could explore confirmatory testing to further investigate these trends.

At the same time, similar hurdles to implementation are evident as in other studies on advanced care planning or identification tools in the last year of life [51]. This supports earlier criticism that complex interventions are often difficult to put into practice in clinical settings. In contrast to studies that attribute low adherence to a lack of acceptance [55], our study shows that the MINI was not successful due to organizational bottlenecks and unclear responsibilities despite general acceptance. In retrospect, we suspect that recruiting a person employed on the ward to the research team would have been a solution to the problem of a lack of responsibility. This would have ensured the presence of a constant reminder to the participants of the study. With regard to sustainability, our observation of the strong dependence on key persons is consistent with the results of numerous implementation studies [49]. While selective integration is successful, systematic anchoring in routines, e.g., through training, reminder systems or standard processes, remains a key challenge. In particular, the selective application of SPICT criteria and QPS reflects the findings that the scope and complexity of instruments are critical success factors for their long-term use.

A particular added value of this study lies in the differentiated analysis of occupational group-specific differences. Instead of examining physicians or nurses in isolation, the chosen approach enables a comparative perspective on both professional groups. The only moderate or even declining outcomes among non-physician staff, particularly with regard to legal issues such as living wills or powers of attorney, raise questions about the profession-sensitive design of such measures. The literature increasingly emphasizes that interprofessional interventions need to be developed and trained from multiple perspectives in order to be effective in heterogeneous teams [56], an aspect that is also supported by our results.

Moreover, the partial decline in the perceived responsibility of non-medical professionals for conversations about dying and death indicates a potential unintentional reinforcement of conventional role patterns. While some studies point to an increasing openness for end-of-life content [57], our data rather show a re-traditionalization in which physicians are again clearly perceived as the primary actors. This indicates that without explicit role clarification and structural support, interventions such as MINI could potentially reinforce existing hierarchies. This should be given greater consideration in future studies.

In summary, MINI appears to be a context-sensitive intervention that may help initiate conversations about prognosis and end-of-life care after minor adaptations. In this feasibility study, some indications were observed that the intervention supports prognostic thinking and stimulates interprofessional communication. These findings highlight the importance of structured, professionally sensitive implementation strategies and appropriate institutional framework conditions. Given the small sample size, feasibility design, and implementation challenges, results should be interpreted cautiously, and further research is needed to confirm effectiveness and generalizability.

Limitations

This study is limited by external challenges. The implementation of the intervention exposed a multitude of challenges. The COVID-19 pandemic led to a significant reduction in recruitment, as happened to numerous other research projects during the same period [58]. This interruption was due to factors such as lockdowns and the reallocation of resources. Also, the application of the intervention was not always consistent, and there were challenges in integrating it into everyday clinical practice, particularly due to the lack of clear guidance and structural barriers. The extent to which the intervention is implemented within teams depends on the dedication of individual key personnel. This commitment is reflected in the variations in progress observed among different professional groups.

This study was designed as a feasibility study, which inherently limits the generalizability of the findings due to the small sample size across all evaluation components. Moreover, reported improvements are based on self-reported data, which may be subject to social desirability bias or influenced by the participants' subjective self-perceptions. All results must be viewed with caution due to the small sample size and the high loss of participants from the pre- to the post-survey. It is reasonable to assume that there is a bias in the post-survey, as it was particularly those HSCPs who were in favor of the intervention who took part. The actual values may therefore deviate from the values surveyed.

The findings are also subject to selection bias, as the interview results reflect the experiences and subjective assessments of ward staff who were directly involved in the implementation. Due to data protection regulations, we were not able to assess the accuracy of the MINI in identifying eligible patients, which limits the evaluation of implementation quality. However, it is important to emphasize that the aim of this study was not to assess the prognostic validity of the MINI, but rather to explore the feasibility of introducing a palliative care perspective on a curative ward. Furthermore, the study design did not include a validation of the healthcare professionals' assessments trained in the use of

MINI. As a result, staff had no feedback on the accuracy of their patient identification. A validation of these assessments by study personnel was not possible due to data protection constraints. Future studies should address these conditions in advance of implementation to allow for a more robust evaluation of both feasibility and prognostic validity.

However, variations in the effectiveness of the intervention across different professional groups suggest that further exploration is needed to understand why physicians benefited more than other medical staff. Additionally, the self-reported nature of these findings calls for further validation through objective assessments of participants' actual competencies.

Implications

The findings suggest that the MINI represents a promising tool for raising awareness and facilitating communication about limited life expectancy, particularly when embedded within structural processes and supported by interprofessional communication. For long-term integration, complementary measures such as regular training, reflective practice opportunities, and stronger institutional support are essential.

Sustainable implementation of the intervention requires its stable and routine integration into daily clinical practice. This includes regular training sessions, structured team meetings, and the use of reminder systems. Long-term anchoring in routine care can only be achieved if institutional structures and clearly defined responsibilities actively support the use of interventions.

Future research should explore the specific effectiveness of individual components of the intervention across various care settings to better understand their respective contributions and contextual adaptability.

5. Conclusions

MINI may have the potential to encourage a more palliative-aware approach when treating seriously ill and dying patients. However, to realize its full potential and ensure long-term success, it is important to adapt the approach to a specific context, adjust the interventions as necessary, and integrate it thoughtfully and participatory within each setting.

Author Contributions: Conceptualization, J.S., A.K. and R.V.; methodology, J.S., A.K., G.D. and J.S.G.; investigation, J.S.G., B.W., G.D., A.K., J.S. and R.V.; data curation, A.K.; formal analysis, A.K.; writing—original draft preparation, A.K.; writing—review and editing, J.S.G., J.S., R.V., S.T.S. and A.K.; project administration, J.S.G., A.K., G.D. and J.S.; supervision, J.S. and R.V.; funding acquisition, J.S. and R.V. Recruitment and data collection were conducted by B.W. All authors have read and agreed to the published version of the manuscript.

Funding: This research was funded by the German Federal Ministry of Education and Research (BMBF) #01GY1916.

Institutional Review Board Statement: This study was conducted in accordance with the Declaration of Helsinki and was approved by the Ethics Committee of the Medical Faculty of the University of Cologne (#20-1431), the Staff Council of the University of Cologne, the Equal Opportunities Officers, and the representatives of the severely disabled (approved date: 12 November 2020). This trial is registered in the German Clinical Trials Register (DRKS00022378).

Informed Consent Statement: Written informed consent was obtained from all subjects involved in the study.

Data Availability Statement: The authors will provide datasets generated and analyzed during the current study upon reasonably request.

Acknowledgments: The authors would like to acknowledge all the participants who took part in this study, in particular the hospital staff of the participating wards at University Hospital of Cologne.

We would also like to thank CoRe-Net study group members Christian Albus, Frank Jessen, Ludwig Kuntz, Ingo Meyer, Holger Pfaff, Nadine Scholten, Frank Schulz-Nieswandt, Stephanie Stock, and Ute Karbach. We would like to thank Melissa Ulmer, Lisa Bach, Christin Herrmann, Sophie Peter, Leonie Weyres and Kira Hower for their support during the data collection and analysis period.

Conflicts of Interest: The funders had no role in the design of the study; in the collection, analysis, or interpretation of data; in the writing of the manuscript; or in the decision to publish the results.

Abbreviations

The following abbreviations are used in this manuscript:

HSCP	Health and Social Care Practitioner
LYOL I/II	Last Year of Life (Part I and Part II)
MINI	Minimal Invasive Intervention
SQ	Surprise Question
SPICT^{TM}	Supportive & Palliative Care Indicators Tool

References

1. Adamidis, F.; Baumgartner, N.S.; Kitta, A.; Kum, L.; Ecker, F.; Bär, J.; Marosi, C.; Kreye, G.; Fischer, C.; Zeilinger, E.L.; et al. Timely integration of palliative care. the reality check. A retrospective analysis. *Support Care Cancer* **2024**, *32*, 518. [CrossRef] [PubMed]
2. Vanbutsele, G.; Pardon, K.; Van Belle, S.; Surmont, V.; De Laat, M.; Colman, R.; Eecloo, K.; Cocquyt, V.; Geboes, K.; Deliens, L. Effect of early and systematic integration of palliative care in patients with advanced cancer: A randomised controlled trial. *Lancet Oncol.* **2018**, *19*, 394–404. [CrossRef]
3. Arias-Casais, N.; López-Fidalgo, J.; Garralda, E.; Pons, J.J.; Rhee, J.Y.; Lukas, R.; de Lima, L.; Centeno, C. Trends analysis of specialized palliative care services in 51 countries of the WHO European region in the last 14 years. *Palliat. Med.* **2020**, *34*, 1044–1056. [CrossRef] [PubMed]
4. Gesell, D.; Hodiamont, F.; Bausewein, C.; Koller, D. Accessibility to specialist palliative care services in Germany: A geographical network analysis. *BMC Health Serv. Res.* **2023**, *23*, 786. [CrossRef] [PubMed]
5. Voltz, R.; Dust, G.; Schippel, N.; Hamacher, S.; Payne, S.; Scholten, N.; Pfaff, H.; Rietz, C.; Strupp, J. Improving regional care in the last year of life by setting up a pragmatic evidence-based Plan–Do–Study–Act cycle: Results from a cross-sectional survey. *BMJ Open* **2020**, *10*, e035988. [CrossRef]
6. Dasch, B.; Zahn, P.K. Place of death trends and utilization of outpatient palliative care at the end of life: Analysis of death certificates (2001, 2011, 2017) and pseudonymized data from selected palliative medicine consultation services (2017) in Westphalia, Germany. *Dtsch. Ärzteblatt Int.* **2021**, *118*, 331.
7. Clark, D.; Armstrong, M.; Allan, A.; Graham, F.; Carnon, A.; Isles, C. Imminence of death among hospital inpatients: Prevalent cohort study. *Palliat. Med.* **2014**, *28*, 474–479. [CrossRef]
8. Bakitas, M.A.; Tosteson, T.D.; Li, Z.; Lyons, K.D.; Hull, J.G.; Li, Z.; Dionne-Odom, J.N.; Frost, J.; Dragnev, K.H.; Hegel, M.T.; et al. Early Versus Delayed Initiation of Concurrent Palliative Oncology Care: Patient Outcomes in the ENABLE III Randomized Controlled Trial. *J. Clin. Oncol.* **2015**, *33*, 1438–1445. [CrossRef]
9. Dalgaard, K.M.; Bergenholtz, H.; Nielsen, M.E.; Timm, H. Early integration of palliative care in hospitals: A systematic review on methods, barriers, and outcome. *Palliat. Support Care* **2014**, *12*, 495–513. [CrossRef]
10. Volberg, C.; Schrade, S.; Heers, H.; Carrasco, A.J.P.; Morin, A.; Gschnell, M. End-of-life wishes and care planning for patients with advanced skin cancer. *JDDG J. Dtsch. Dermatol. Ges.* **2023**, *21*, 1148–1155. [CrossRef]
11. Heuser, N.; Heers, H.; Gschnell, M.; Urhahn, F.; Schrade, S.; Volberg, C. Do We Have a Knowledge Gap with Our Patients?—On the Problems of Knowledge Transfer and the Implications at the End of Life. *Int. J. Environ. Res. Public Health* **2025**, *22*, 247. [CrossRef]
12. Gott, M.C.; Ahmedzai, S.H.; Wood, C. How many inpatients at an acute hospital have palliative care needs? Comparing the perspectives of medical and nursing staff. *Palliat. Med.* **2001**, *15*, 451–460.
13. To, T.H.M.; Greene, A.G.; Agar, M.R.; Currow, D.C. A point prevalence survey of hospital inpatients to define the proportion with palliation as the primary goal of care and the need for specialist palliative care. *Intern. Med. J.* **2011**, *41*, 430–433. [CrossRef]
14. Scholten, N.; Günther, A.L.; Pfaff, H.; Karbach, U. The size of the population potentially in need of palliative care in Germany—An estimation based on death registration data. *BMC Palliat. Care* **2016**, *15*, 29. [CrossRef]
15. Rubbai, Y.S.; Chong, M.C.; Tang, L.Y.; Abdullah, K.L.; Mohammad, W.T.; Mohajer, S.; Namazinia, M. Barriers in providing quality end-of-life care as perceived by nurses working in critical care units: An integrative review. *BMC Palliat. Care* **2024**, *23*, 217. [CrossRef] [PubMed]

16. Sheward, K.; Clark, J.; Marshall, B.; Allan, S. Staff perceptions of end-of-life care in the acute care setting: A New Zealand perspective. *J. Palliat. Med.* **2011**, *14*, 623–630. [CrossRef] [PubMed]
17. Mudge, A.M.; Douglas, C.; Sansome, X.; Tresillian, M.; Murray, S.; Finnigan, S.; Blaber, C.R. Risk of 12-month mortality among hospital inpatients using the surprise question and SPICT criteria: A prospective study. *BMJ Support. Palliat. Care* **2018**, *8*, 213–220. [CrossRef] [PubMed]
18. van Wijmen, M.P.S.; Schweitzer, B.P.M.; Pasman, H.R.; Onwuteaka-Philipsen, B.D. Identifying patients who could benefit from palliative care by making use of the general practice information system: The Surprise Question versus the SPICT. *Fam. Pract.* **2020**, *37*, 641–647. [CrossRef]
19. Highet, G.; Crawford, D.; Murray, S.A.; Boyd, K. Development and evaluation of the Supportive and Palliative Care Indicators Tool (SPICT): A mixed-methods study. *BMJ Support Palliat. Care* **2014**, *4*, 285–290. [CrossRef]
20. Moss, A.H.; Lunney, J.R.; Culp, S.; Auber, M.; Kurian, S.; Rogers, J.; Dower, J.; Abraham, J. Prognostic significance of the 'surprise' question in cancer patients. *J. Palliat. Med.* **2010**, *13*, 837–840. [CrossRef]
21. Roch, C.; Heckel, M.; van Oorschot, B.; Alt-Epping, B.; Tewes, M. Screening for Palliative Care Needs: Pilot Data from German Comprehensive Cancer Centers. *JCO Oncol. Pract.* **2021**, *17*, e1584–e1591. [CrossRef]
22. Xie, Z.; Ding, J.; Jiao, J.; Tang, S.; Huang, C. Screening instruments for early identification of unmet palliative care needs: A systematic review and meta-analysis. *BMJ Support Palliat. Care* **2024**, *14*, 256–268. [CrossRef]
23. Strupp, J.; Kasdorf, A.; Dust, G.; Hower, K.I.; Seibert, M.; Werner, B.; Kuntz, L.; Schulz-Nieswandt, F.; Meyer, I.; Pfaff, H.; et al. Last Year of Life Study-Cologne (LYOL-C) (Part II): Study protocol of a prospective interventional mixed-methods study in acute hospitals to analyse the implementation of a trigger question and patient question prompt sheets to optimise patient-centred care. *BMJ Open* **2021**, *11*, e048681.
24. Grimm, J.S.; Kasdorf, A.; Voltz, R.; Strupp, J. From MINI to Meaningful Change—A German Pilot Study to Improve Patient Outcomes in End-of-life care. *Healthcare* **2025**, *13*, 2024. [CrossRef] [PubMed]
25. Afshar, K.; Feichtner, A.; Boyd, K.; Murray, S.; Jünger, S.; Wiese, B.; Schneider, N.; Müller-Mundt, G. Systematic development and adjustment of the German version of the Supportive and Palliative Care Indicators Tool (SPICT-DE). *BMC Palliat. Care* **2018**, *17*, 27. [CrossRef] [PubMed]
26. Gupta, A.; Burgess, R.; Drozd, M.; Gierula, J.; Witte, K.; Straw, S. The Surprise Question and clinician-predicted prognosis: Systematic review and meta-analysis. *BMJ Support. Palliat. Care* **2025**, *15*, 12–35. [CrossRef]
27. Baile, W.F.; Buckman, R.; Lenzi, R.; Glober, G.; Beale, E.A.; Kudelka, A.P. SPIKES—A Six-Step Protocol for Delivering Bad News: Application to the Patient with Cancer. *Oncologist* **2000**, *5*, 302–311. [CrossRef] [PubMed]
28. von Elm, E.; Altman, D.G.; Egger, M.; Pocock, S.J.; Gøtzsche, P.C.; Vandenbroucke, J.P. The Strengthening the Reporting of Observational Studies in Epidemiology (STROBE) statement: Guidelines for reporting observational studies. *J. Clin. Epidemiol.* **2008**, *61*, 344–349. [CrossRef]
29. Booth, A.; Hannes, K.; Harden, A.; Noyes, J.; Harris, J.; Tong, A. COREQ (Consolidated Criteria for Reporting Qualitative Studies). In *Guidelines for Reporting Health Research: A User's Manual*; John Wiley & Sons, Ltd.: Hoboken, NJ, USA, 2014; pp. 214–226.
30. Dust, G.; Schippel, N.; Stock, S.; Strupp, J.; Voltz, R.; Rietz, C.; CoRe-Net Co-Applicants. Quality of care in the last year of life: Adaptation and validation of the German "Views of Informal Carers' Evaluation of Services—Last Year of Life—Cologne". *BMC Health Serv. Res.* **2022**, *22*, 1433. [CrossRef]
31. Deutsche Krebshilfe, A.W.M.F. Leitlinienprogramm Onkologie. Palliativmedizin für Patienten mit Einer Nicht-Heilbaren Krebserkrankung. Available online: https://www.leitlinienprogramm-onkologie.de/leitlinien/palliativmedizin/ (accessed on 8 October 2025).
32. Mosich, V.; Sellner-Pogány, T.; Wallner, J. PKT–der Palliative Kompetenztest für Ärzte. *Der Schmerz.* **2017**, *31*, 375–382. [CrossRef]
33. Hauck, M. Eine Befragung von Patienten, Ärzten und Pflegekräften über die Bedingungen zu Einem Guten "Sterben". Doctoral Dissertation, (Albert-Ludwigs-Universität Freiburg) University of Freiburg, Breisgau, Germany, 2025. Available online: https://nbn-resolving.org/urn:nbn:de:bsz:25-opus-45880 (accessed on 8 October 2025).
34. Mayring, P. Qualitative Content Analysis. Forum Qualitative Sozialforschung. *Forum Qual. Soc. Res.* **2000**, *1*, 2.
35. Damschroder, L.J.; Reardon, C.M.; Opra Widerquist, M.A.; Lowery, J. Conceptualizing outcomes for use with the Consolidated Framework for Implementation Research (CFIR): The CFIR Outcomes Addendum. *Implement. Sci.* **2022**, *17*, 7. [CrossRef] [PubMed]
36. Proctor, E.; Silmere, H.; Raghavan, R.; Hovmand, P.; Aarons, G.; Bunger, A.; Griffey, R.; Hensley, M. Outcomes for Implementation Research: Conceptual Distinctions, Measurement Challenges, and Research Agenda. *Adm. Policy Ment. Health* **2011**, *38*, 65–76. [CrossRef]
37. Malterud, K.; Siersma, V.D.; Guassora, A.D. Sample Size in Qualitative Interview Studies: Guided by Information Power. *Qual. Health Res.* **2016**, *26*, 1753–1760. [CrossRef]
38. Downar, J.; Goldman, R.; Pinto, R.; Englesakis, M.; Adhikari, N.K.J. The "surprise question" for predicting death in seriously ill patients: A systematic review and meta-analysis. *CMAJ* **2017**, *189*, E484–E493. [CrossRef] [PubMed]

39. White, N.; Kupeli, N.; Vickerstaff, V.; Stone, P. How accurate is the 'Surprise Question' at identifying patients at the end of life? A systematic review and meta-analysis. *BMC Med.* **2017**, *15*, 139. [CrossRef] [PubMed]
40. Owusuaa, C.; van Beelen, I.; van der Heide, A.; van der Rijt, C.C.D. Physicians' views on the usefulness and feasibility of identifying and disclosing patients' last phase of life: A focus group study. *BMJ Support. Palliat. Care* **2024**, *14*, e1903–e1908. [CrossRef]
41. Le, K.; Lee, J.; Desai, S.; Ho, A.; van Heukelom, H. The Surprise Question and Serious Illness Conversations: A pilot study. *Nurs. Ethics* **2021**, *28*, 1010–1025. [CrossRef]
42. Haydar, S.A.; Almeder, L.; Michalakes, L.; Han, P.K.J.; Strout, T.D. Using the Surprise Question to Identify Those with Unmet Palliative Care Needs in Emergency and Inpatient Settings: What Do Clinicians Think? *J. Palliat. Med.* **2017**, *20*, 729–735. [CrossRef]
43. Bennardi, M.; Diviani, N.; Gamondi, C.; Stüssi, G.; Saletti, P.; Cinesi, I.; Rubinelli, S. Palliative care utilization in oncology and hemato-oncology: A systematic review of cognitive barriers and facilitators from the perspective of healthcare professionals, adult patients, and their families. *BMC Palliat. Care* **2020**, *19*, 47. [CrossRef]
44. Lund, S.; Richardson, A.; May, C. Barriers to Advance Care Planning at the End of Life: An Explanatory Systematic Review of Implementation Studies. *PLoS ONE* **2015**, *10*, e0116629. [CrossRef]
45. Periyakoil, V.S.; Neri, E.; Kraemer, H. No Easy Talk: A Mixed Methods Study of Doctor Reported Barriers to Conducting Effective End-of-Life Conversations with Diverse Patients. *PLoS ONE* **2015**, *10*, e0122321. [CrossRef]
46. Porter, I.; Gonçalves-Bradley, D.; Ricci-Cabello, I.; Gibbons, C.; Gangannagaripalli, J.; Fitzpatrick, R.; Black, N.; Greenhalgh, J.; Valderas, J.M. Framework and guidance for implementing patient-reported outcomes in clinical practice: Evidence, challenges and opportunities. *J. Comp. Eff. Res.* **2016**, *5*, 507–519. [CrossRef]
47. McDermott, E.; Selman, L.E. Cultural Factors Influencing Advance Care Planning in Progressive, Incurable Disease: A Systematic Review with Narrative Synthesis. *J. Pain Symptom Manag.* **2018**, *56*, 613–636. [CrossRef] [PubMed]
48. Gravel, K.; Légaré, F.; Graham, I.D. Barriers and facilitators to implementing shared decision-making in clinical practice: A systematic review of health professionals' perceptions. *Implement. Sci.* **2006**, *1*, 16. [CrossRef] [PubMed]
49. Damschroder, L.J.; Aron, D.C.; Keith, R.E.; Kirsh, S.R.; Alexander, J.A.; Lowery, J.C. Fostering implementation of health services research findings into practice: A consolidated framework for advancing implementation science. *Implement. Sci.* **2009**, *4*, 50. [CrossRef] [PubMed]
50. Sudore, R.L.; Schillinger, D.; Knight, S.J.; Fried, T.R. Uncertainty about advance care planning treatment preferences among diverse older adults. *J. Health Commun.* **2010**, *15* (Suppl. S2), 159–171. [CrossRef]
51. Brinkman-Stoppelenburg, A.; Rietjens, J.A.C.; van der Heide, A. The effects of advance care planning on end-of-life care: A systematic review. *Palliat. Med.* **2014**, *28*, 1000–1025. [CrossRef]
52. Kesonen, P.; Salminen, L.; Kero, J.; Aappola, J.; Haavisto, E. An Integrative Review of Interprofessional Teamwork and Required Competence in Specialized Palliative Care. *Omega* **2024**, *89*, 1047–1073. [CrossRef]
53. van Riet Paap, J.; Vernooij-Dassen, M.; Sommerbakk, R.; Moyle, W.; Hjermstad, M.J.; Leppert, W.; Vissers, K.; Engels, Y. Implementation of improvement strategies in palliative care: An integrative review. *Implement Sci.* **2015**, *10*, 103. [CrossRef]
54. Sun, L.; Booth, A.; Sworn, K. Adaptability, Scalability and Sustainability (ASaS) of complex health interventions: A systematic review of theories, models and frameworks. *Implement Sci.* **2024**, *19*, 52. [CrossRef]
55. Zwakman, M.; Milota, M.M.; van der Heide, A.; Jabbarian, L.J.; Korfage, I.J.; Rietjens, J.A.C.; van Delden, J.J.M.; Kars, M.C. Unraveling patients' readiness in advance care planning conversations: A qualitative study as part of the ACTION Study. *Support Care Cancer* **2021**, *29*, 2917–2929. [CrossRef] [PubMed]
56. Kirkpatrick, A.J.; Donesky, D.; Kitko, L.A. A Systematic Review of Interprofessional Palliative Care Education Programs. *J. Pain Symptom Manag.* **2023**, *65*, e439–e466. [CrossRef] [PubMed]
57. Wildfeuer, J.; Schnell, M.W.; Schulz, C. Talking about dying and death: On new discursive constructions of a formerly postulated taboo. *Discourse Soc.* **2015**, *26*, 366–390. [CrossRef]
58. Bratan, T.; Aichinger, H.; Brkic, N.; Rueter, J.; Apfelbacher, C.; Boyer, L.; Loss, J. Impact of the COVID-19 pandemic on ongoing health research: An ad hoc survey among investigators in Germany. *BMJ Open* **2021**, *11*, e049086. [CrossRef]

healthcare

MDPI

Article

The Practices of Portuguese Primary Health Care Professionals in Palliative Care Access and Referral: A Focus Group Study

Camila Barreto [1,2], Marcelle Miranda da Silva [3], Ana Fátima Carvalho Fernandes [4], Romel Jonathan Velasco Yanez [4] and Carlos Laranjeira [2,5,6,*]

1 USF Buarcos, Local Health Unit of Baixo Mondego, Av. Dr. Mário Soares 64, 3080-254 Figueira da Foz, Portugal; camilajbarreto17@gmail.com

2 School of Health Sciences, Polytechnic University of Leiria, Campus 2, Morro do Lena, Alto do Vieiro, Apartado 4137, 2411-901 Leiria, Portugal

3 Escola de Enfermagem Anna Nery (EEAN), Universidade Federal do Rio de Janeiro (UFRJ), Afonso Cavalcanti Street, Rio de Janeiro 21211-110, Brazil; marcellemsufrj@gmail.com

4 Department of Nursing, Federal University of Ceará, Fortaleza 60430-160, Brazil; afcana@ufc.br (A.F.C.F.); romebarce_95@hotmail.com (R.J.V.Y.)

5 Centre for Innovative Care and Health Technology (ciTechCare), Polytechnic University of Leiria, Campus 5, Rua das Olhalvas, 2414-016 Leiria, Portugal

6 Comprehensive Health Research Centre (CHRC), University of Évora, 7000-801 Évora, Portugal

* Correspondence: carlos.laranjeira@ipleiria.pt

Abstract: Background/Objectives: The prevalence of people with incurable and progressive diseases in primary health care is high. Family doctors and nurses must be active agents in the early identification of palliative needs and the implementation of palliative approaches in cases of low to intermediate complexity. While there is a need for early referral of more complex palliative care (PC) cases to specialized teams, primary health care (PHC) professionals lack the confidence or skill to describe their role. This study sought to explore and describe (a) the practices of PHC professionals regarding their PC provision; (b) the barriers regarding access and referral of patients to specialized PC services; and (c) the strategies used or recommended to mitigate difficulties in accessing and referring to specialized PC. **Methods**: A descriptive qualitative study was carried out, using five focus groups conducted with nursing and medical staff at three local health units in the central region of Portugal. Semi-structured interviews were conducted, and then recorded, transcribed, and analyzed through a thematic analysis approach. The reporting of this research follows the COREQ checklist. **Results**: In total, 34 PHC professionals participated in this study. The majority of participants were women ($n = 26$) and family doctors ($n = 24$). Their mean age was 43.8 ± 11.9 (range: 29 to 65 years). The findings were organized into three core themes: (1) the contours of palliative action developed by PHC teams; (2) barriers to access and safe transition between PHC and specialized PC; and (3) ways to mitigate difficulties in accessing and referring to specialized PC. **Conclusions**: Our findings highlight the fundamental role of PHC professionals in providing primary PC, and in identifying PC needs and referring patients to PC early on, while exposing the systemic and interpersonal challenges that hinder these processes. To overcome these challenges, it is essential to invest in the development of integrated care models that promote practical, low-bureaucratic referral processes and capture the human resources necessary for the adequate follow-up of users.

Keywords: palliative care; primary health care; professionals; access; referral; qualitative study; Portugal

1. Introduction

Over the last few decades, exponential population aging has been a trend observed worldwide, and the number of deaths occurring at older ages is expected to continue to increase [1,2]. This reality is especially notable in developed and developing countries, and also applies to the Portuguese population [3–6]. In parallel, today's societies exhibit a high prevalence and incidence of chronic, incurable, and progressive diseases [2,7]. The rising prevalence of multimorbidities exerts escalating pressure on health and social institutions, which encounter difficulties in accommodating the evolving requirements of shifting populations and necessitate unique health considerations, especially toward the end-of-life (EoL) [1,2,7]

This scenario requires a palliative care (PC) approach to enhance patients' quality of life, resulting in a heightened need and demand for such care [7–10]. Palliative interventions and early referral practices are known to reduce costs, improve the care experiences of people in PC and their caregivers, enable patients to make choices about their EoL care, and in some cases, increase life expectancy [9,11–13]. In particular, home-based PC has demonstrated significant benefits in meeting the needs of people with advanced diseases, in addition to reducing hospital admissions and emergency department visits, thus emphasizing person-centered care and reinforcing the sustainability of the health system [14,15].

The care model, composed of specialized community palliative care teams (CPCT), has been shown to improve the experience of EoL care, namely, by reducing the use of emergency services by around 50% [16]. In addition, it offers patients the possibility of dying at home: results found that 39% of patients with CPCT died in a hospital compared to 74.8% without CPCT [15,16]. In fact, the home is the preferred location for EoL care, both for patients and their families, with preferences varying between 11% and 89%. The home is also the preferred place of death, with preferences varying between 51% and 55% [17].

The World Health Organization estimated that, overall, only 14% of people who need PC currently receive it [18]. PC delivery differs significantly across countries, health systems, and communities. PC access is widely available in most high-income countries, where there has been a steady growth in the availability of specialized PC services, but it remains limited in low- and middle-income countries [19,20]. Even so, while the availability of specialized services has grown across Europe, the ratios per 100,000 people remain below the recommendations set by the European Association for Palliative Care (EAPC) [21]. In the Portuguese context, according to the 2023 Autumn Report of the Portuguese Palliative Care Observatory, universal coverage of PC resources in the country is far from being achieved. Data also reveal profound asymmetries among districts/regions and typologies. According to the EAPC recommendations and across the different types, Portugal requires an estimated total of 793 beds for PC at the national level (90 beds per million inhabitants). However, there are presently only 423 beds, which represents a national coverage rate of 53% (with 72% in acute care and 45% in non-acute care). Regarding CPCTs, the coverage rate at the population/structural level is 46% [22]. Clearly, in Portugal, access to PC still falls short of patient needs [22,23].

Given the increasing palliative needs and the deficient coverage of specialized PC, the teaching and training of skills for primary health care (PHC) professionals is necessary for earlier, more accessible, and global PC [7,11]. In this sense, family physicians and nurses must be active agents in the early identification of palliative needs and in the implementation of palliative approaches in cases of low to intermediate complexity [7,24], as they are often the first point of contact between patients and health care [19,25,26]. In more complex cases, they play an important role in early referral to specialized PC teams [24].

PHC covers most of an individual's health needs throughout their lifespan, including prevention, treatment, rehabilitation, and EoL care [25–27]. It provides comprehensive care in the community, allowing access to care and dealing with all health problems (regardless of age, sex, or any other characteristic of the person in question) [25,26,28], from the individual's conception until their death (and extending into the mourning period) [19,24,25]. Furthermore, the proximity of family doctors and nurses to users and families favors the therapeutic relationship, and the involvement of these teams in PC is associated with greater patient satisfaction [29]. The skills and characteristics of PHC teams are based on principles and objectives that are common to the PC paradigm. Both seek health care that is centered on the person (and not just the disease), with continuous care, with a global and holistic vision, and both highlight the importance of addressing physical, psychological, social, and spiritual issues of the ill person and their family unit [25–27,30].

Critically, PHC professionals need to understand how they can provide PC in their context, and when they should refer to specialized PC, within a collaborative and integrated network [10,24,28,31]. Although studies highlight the challenges in referring and providing PC by PHC professionals [19,30,32,33], there are no known studies that focus on the Portuguese reality, justifying the present study. Thus, we intend to explore the following: (a) the practices of PHC professionals regarding their PC provision; (b) barriers regarding access and referral of patients to specialized PCs; and (c) the strategies used or recommended to mitigate difficulties in accessing and referring to specialized PCs. In this way, we hope to contribute to a better understanding of the articulation of PHC and PC in the Portuguese reality to understand what difficulties professionals face and how clinical practice could be improved.

2. Materials and Methods

2.1. Study Design

This is a qualitative, exploratory, and descriptive study using focus groups (FGs), following the proposal of Krueger and Casey [34]. The study is anchored in a subjective view of the subject and linked to a constructivist perspective of reality, exploring perceptions in a categorized way and integrating their theoretical references [35]. Qualitative research is an evolutionary and adaptive approach that focuses on people's experiences, behaviors, and opinions. It seeks to answer "why" and "how" questions, providing detailed insight and understanding that quantitative methods cannot achieve [36,37].

Focus groups (FGs), in particular, are a form of interview designed to gather multiple perceptions on a particular topic/area of interest and are an increasingly used qualitative research method [38,39]. Unlike individual interviews, FGs provide the additional dimension of interactions between group members [40]. In the context of health care and medical research, FGs are particularly relevant, as they suggest explanations for behaviors that could have a sociocultural context [40].

The study followed the consolidated criteria for reporting qualitative research (COREQ) checklist [41] (Supplementary File S1).

2.2. Setting and Participants

Five FGs were organized with primary health care doctors and nurses from three local health units (LHUs) in the central region of Portugal. Each FG was composed of professionals assigned to the same LHU, with a number varying between six and eight participants (out of a total of 34). For the recruitment process, a purposive sampling strategy was used [42], and the following inclusion criteria were established: (1) doctors and nurses with at least one year of experience in PHC; (2) professionals who provide direct care to patients and their families, particularly to people who routinely required referral to PC. Exclusion criteria: professionals absent from work at the time of data collection (due to illness, training, or vacation). The application of eligibility criteria was assessed by the principal investigator. The data saturation criterion was used to determine the number of participants [43]. Recruitment ceased when data no longer provided meaningful information [44]. To obtain maximum sample variation, no restrictions were imposed on sex, age, and professional seniority.

2.3. Data Collection

Data were collected using semi-structured interviews, between October and November 2024, during working hours to facilitate attendance. FGs were moderated by an experienced female doctor (C.B.) and assisted by a faculty researcher (C.L.) and had an average duration of 75 min (range: 30 to 100 min). The participants were unfamiliar with the researchers before data collection. Data were collected in each clinical site, and the choice of location for the in-person interviews followed FG recommendations [34] in terms of accessibility, comfort for participants, as well as the confidentiality of the information shared.

Potential participants were contacted by the principal investigator via email, who provided details about the study and FG scheduling, including time and location. Consent was obtained from contacts who were willing to participate in the study. Each participant completed a sociodemographic and professional characterization with questions about their age, gender, professional category, qualifications, years of professional experience in primary health care, years of overall professional experience, training in PC, and self-assessment of the level of perceived competence for PC practice (on a scale of 0 = no level to 10 = high level).

A guiding script was followed for each FG session, consisting of four distinct parts: introduction, when the main researcher/moderator thanked the group for their availability and participation and presented the study's components; FG legitimacy, obtaining authorization to record the audio of the session, providing the informed consent form and ensuring the confidentiality of the information; development, presenting the purpose and objectives of the study, and posing questions to encourage discussion and group discussion; and finally the conclusion, when the researcher thanked everyone for their availability and collaboration, made themself available for future clarifications and guaranteed that the findings would be available for consultation [34].

A pilot FG discussion was performed to evaluate the interview guide questions and to facilitate effective collaboration between the moderator and the observer. The final study incorporated data from the pilot FG, as only minimal modifications were applied to the interview guide.

The main researcher/moderator encouraged participants to openly share their experiences and stressed the importance of confidentiality of observations made during discussions and tolerance of different perspectives. The discussion in each FG was initiated using the presentation of a clinical vignette, which consisted of a clinical case of a user with several palliative needs, requiring a reflective analysis by the participants. Participants are more willing to share their views when using the vignette approach as it allows some distance between their own experience and the given scenario [34]. This vignette served as an "icebreaker", followed by the question, "What palliative needs do you identify in this clinical case?" Thereafter, the moderator introduced open questions from the interview script, guided by the literature and primary study objectives, and refined by discussions among the authors. Questions covered the following topics: (1) intervention practices in PC; (2) access and referral to specialized PC; (3) facilitating factors and barriers; and (4) strategies used or to be implemented for referral [7,45–47]. Encouraging affirmations and direct inquiries were employed to facilitate interaction and stimulate additional debate on these subjects of interest. The moderator's assistant noted privileged information about facial expressions, gestures, tone of voice, and the context in which the discourse was delivered. These aspects are fundamental in the process of decoding, interpreting, and analyzing data. No repeat interviews were carried out. Participants were neither provided with the transcripts for feedback or changes nor solicited for commentary on the outcomes.

2.4. Data Analysis

Thematic analysis of the data was performed according to the proposal by Braun and Clarke [48,49] (Figure 1).

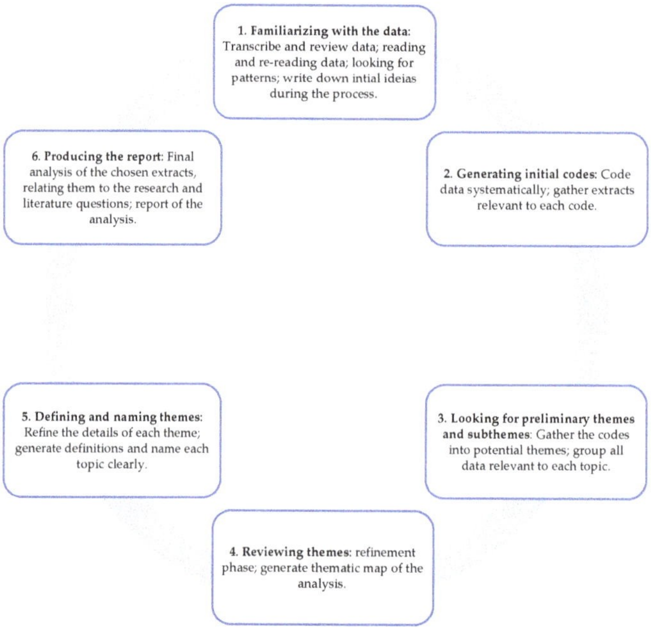

Figure 1. Six-step Braun and Clarke [48,49] thematic analysis.

The interviews were audio-recorded and manually transcribed to maintain the authenticity of the original meanings. The first and last authors thoroughly analyzed the transcripts and familiarized themselves with the data, including the context in which extracts were produced; thus, the interpretation was supported by a systematic analysis of the data. Preliminary codes were categorized into themes and refined following each interview. An endeavor was undertaken to transition from descriptive to interpretative codes to discern wider links among participant experiences. After each interview, the coding matrix was rigorously analyzed to identify the most pertinent elements of participant experiences, culminating in an agreement among researchers through discussion [44].

The interviews were loaded into the qualitative data analysis program WebQDA (Version 3.0, University of Aveiro, Aveiro, Portugal) for data storage and administration. After the analytical procedure, the textual excerpts, initially in European Portuguese, were translated and subsequently "back-translated" to ensure the retention of their original meaning.

2.5. Trustworthiness

The Guba and Lincoln criteria were used to maintain study rigor [50]. To ensure credibility, we used quotes from participants that faithfully expressed their narrative.

Qualitative data from other sources, such as transcripts and researcher notes, were also used. Triangulation of researchers was used to refine the findings and respective thematic analysis. To ensure transferability, the study design, participants, context, sampling methods, data collection, and analysis were described in detail. To ensure reliability, the work was subjected to an external audit by independent researchers. Finally, confirmability was achieved by maintaining reflective reporting throughout the data collection and analysis phases. Through peer debriefing and reflective journaling, biases and reflections were documented, increasing transparency and minimizing subjectivity.

The research team used a hybrid approach (i.e., including both deductive and inductive coding strategies) to form thematic categories [48,49]. Several research meetings were conducted to facilitate the sharing and comparison of findings, helping to identify recurring themes. When differing opinions arose, a consensus was reached through discussion. The main researcher is a resident physician in general and family medicine, with clinical experience with chronic and palliative patients, and is undergoing postgraduate training in PC. The fourth author (R.J.V.Y.) is a registered nurse with experience in PHC and PC. The remaining authors (M.M.S., A.F.C.F., and C.L.) hold PhD degrees and are faculty members with expertise in using qualitative research. Before collecting and analyzing the data, each author documented and acknowledged their preconceptions, thus allowing their conscious use, particularly in the development of the interview guide, and thereby fostering enhanced and/or novel insights into the subject of study.

2.6. Ethical Considerations

The present study was carried out in accordance with the principles of the Declaration of Helsinki and after the favorable opinion of the Local Ethics Committee (CE/IPLEIRIA/87/2024). Participation was voluntary and was accompanied by the completion of the informed consent form. The study's goal was clearly articulated to all participants, and confidentiality of their identity and reports was guaranteed. The interview recordings were stored in a password-protected file accessible solely to the researchers and will be deleted one year after the project's conclusion. The lead researcher informed participants that they could interrupt the interview at any time without any associated consequences. Participants received no benefit and incurred no risks of harm or costs for their participation in this study. Alphanumeric codes (FG1, FG2, ...) were used, thus ensuring transparency in the documentation of observations and expressing consensus among participants.

3. Results

3.1. Sample Description

In total, 34 primary health care professionals participated in this study. The majority of the participants were women (n = 26), and the mean age was 43.8 ± 11.9 (range: 29 to 65 years). Regarding the professional category, most participants were doctors (n = 24), and the rest were nurses (n = 10). Most participants had no training in PC (n = 23). Notably, the average level of self-perceived competence in PC was low (3.9 ± 1.7). A sample background is provided in Table 1.

3.2. Findings Overview

The findings were articulated through three themes and ten subthemes (Table 2) that bring together the key elements to respond to the study's objectives. Initially, the practices of primary health care professionals regarding their provision of PC were explored. Subsequently, how professionals ensure access and referral of patients and families to specialist PC was described. This exploration resulted in the identification of barriers that

Professionals who have completed postgraduate studies in PC recognize gains in their clinical activity in terms of managing more complex cases and the need for referral to specialized units. The rest of the team also ends up benefiting from the presence of trained professionals, fostering numerous debriefing moments that allow discussion of cases.

FG2: Training undoubtedly facilitates referencing itself. Those who have undergone training in the area are more sensitive to the problem and end up referring it much more, compared to colleagues who have not. . .
FG4: We have learned from those who are doing postgraduate studies within our unit. We ask a lot of questions and discuss the most problematic situations.

(b) Customization of services to the needs of people with palliative needs

Participants reported that it was necessary to dedicate more consultation time to meet the needs of palliative patients, since the time available in a "normal" consultation is not sufficient for monitoring the needs of patients and families.

FG4: The truth is that a consultation time of 15 to 20 min is clearly not enough to deal with the complexity of the needs of the palliative patient and their family. Which means rescheduling after rescheduling, and families are left dissatisfied.
FG1: We fall short in terms of psychological and emotional support, largely due to the time constraints we face. It is necessary to manage the schedule to allow more consultation time to be reserved for these users.

While some professionals can easily control the scheduling of appointments, others do not have this possibility. To solve this problem, participants mentioned the creation of a specific consultation in palliative care, as is already done for hypertensive, diabetic, pregnant patients, etc.

FG1: Sometimes we don't have control over appointment schedules. Therefore, only by creating a specific query in PC is it be possible to improve the quality of our current care provision.
FG3: The main problem is that we have to respond to the constant pressure we suffer from patients, family caregivers, coworkers and managers. We have to create priorities and there is not time for everything. The possibility of a PC consultation as part of the PHC service portfolio could be a solution similar to what we do in other areas. However, this implies the secure allocation of human resources.

The need for an integrative care model was highlighted as an ideal model of action in which early referral to palliative care is combined with primary health care. The possibility of PHC teams including professionals with training in PC would facilitate intervention with palliative patients, as well as serve as a bridge between PHC services and specialized teams in PC.

FG4: Basic palliative care units should be created in primary health care. Just as there are additional portfolios for alcoholism, smoking cessation, obesity, etc., there should be a basic palliative consultation by trained colleagues to help manage symptoms, provide psychological first aid, etc. It would be an easy and relatively cheap way for the Unified Health System to democratize access to palliative care for a large part of the population that is currently unable to benefit from it.
FG3: Create teams. . . for example, in each LHU a team should be created to carry out specific palliative consultations. This was envisaged a long time ago, but it never happened.
FG2: Having the possibility of shared monitoring makes perfect sense. (. . .). We don't have the time that community palliative care support teams offer, they have visits lasting two hours. . . We don't have that time, we can't provide that support. Therefore, we need an integrated approach and greater proximity between generalist care and specialized PC care.

participants face in this process, as well as the strategies they use or would recommend to mitigate the difficulties experienced.

Table 1. Participants' background (N = 34).

			FG1	FG2	FG3	FG4	FG5
Participants number			6	7	7	6	8
Age (Mean ± SD)			35.8 (7.0)	42.9 (13.4)	50.9 (10.6)	44.5 (8.9)	46.2 (5.3)
Sex	Female		5	6	6	5	4
	Male		1	1	1	1	4
Profession	Family Doctor	Specialist	3	5	4	2	5
		Resident	3	2	0	0	0
	Nurse	Specialized Family Nurse	0	0	0	2	3
		Without Specialty	0	0	3	2	0
Years of professional experience (Mean ± SD)	In health care, globally		9.5 (7.8)	17.1 (15.9)	26 (11.3)	21.3 (11.2)	19.6 (6.3)
	In Primary Care		8.2 (7.6)	15.7 (15.5)	20.4 (11.2)	13.2 (4.2)	13.8 (6.9)
Training in PC	No		2	6	5	4	6
	Yes		4	1	2	2	2
Perceived competence level for PC on a scale from 0 to 10 (Mean ± SD)			3.5 (1.2)	2.9 (1.5)	4.3 (1.1)	5.3 (1.9)	5.8 (2.4)

FG: focus group; PC: palliative care; SD: standard deviation.

Table 2. An overview of the themes and subthemes.

Themes	Subthemes
Theme 1—The contours of palliative action developed by PHC teams	(a) Identification of palliative needs (b) The primacy of the therapeutic relationship (c) Limitations in response capacity
Theme 2—Barriers to access and safe transition between PHC and specialized PC	(a) Myths and misconceptions regarding PC (b) Early referral conditioned by the heterogeneity of disease trajectories (c) Bureaucratization of processes and difficulties in the transition of care (d) Scarcity of resources.
Theme 3. Ways to mitigate difficulties in accessing and referring to specialized PC	(a) Investment in PC training for PHC professionals (b) Customization of services to the needs of people with palliative needs (c) Strengthening specialized community palliative care teams.

3.2.1. Theme 1—The Contours of Palliative Action Developed by PHC Teams

A consensus developed among FGs that PC targets individuals with incurable diseases, characterized by a limited life expectancy, where alleviation of suffering is paramount to the therapeutic approach. The participants indicated that palliative principles were beneficial, regardless of diagnosis, whether the patient had slowly progressing dementia or an advanced cancer. This theme includes three subthemes: (a) identification of palliative needs; (b) the primacy of the therapeutic relationship; and (c) limitations in response capacity.

(a) Identification of palliative needs

Participants described ease in identifying and assessing palliative needs through the use of decision-making support tools. However, most participants revealed ambivalence in the process of assessing non-oncological palliative needs, particularly in patients with dementia, heart failure, or chronic respiratory diseases.

FG1: When assessing palliative needs, sometimes the difficulty is not so much with cancer, but with non-oncological diseases, namely heart failure, COPD, dementia, which could benefit from some (palliative) monitoring. We have some difficulty understanding these needs.
FG2: The first step is to demystify the idea that palliative care is only for oncological diseases, which is what we hear about most. There is no doubt that for these conditions we are much more aware to identify palliative needs.
FG4: Oncological situations are easy to identify. Perhaps, if we think more about chronic diseases, for example heart failure with decompensation, then it might be more difficult. These are situations that people don't associate with palliative care.
FG5: The use of instruments such as the Edmonton Symptom Assessment, the Performance Palliative Scale, or the surprise question are important resources for assessing needs.

Furthermore, participants highlighted that, in cases of chronic non-oncological diseases, the response often underestimates the severity of the situation, due to the long course of the disease and the aging process.

FG4: That's definitely more difficult, because we end up devaluing it. As a rule, they are also older people. It is much easier to assess an oncological situation than a non-oncological chronic disease.

(b) The primacy of the therapeutic relationship

Another aspect that was consensual among the FGs is related to the proximity of primary health care professionals to patients and families. Being a PHC professional means having the opportunity to accompany different generations of the same family throughout their life cycle, allowing one to build lasting therapeutic relationships that impact the quality of care offered.

FG1: The fact that we follow people throughout their lives makes it easier for us to reach the person. Many times, patients accept it better when we tell them, even if we don't have to be the ones to do it, even if the diagnosis was provided elsewhere. Also, because we don't really know what has been said or not... Other times they come to clarify things that the hospital doctor didn't convey, or that they didn't hear or didn't understand.
FG4: It's giving support. It's knowing how to listen. It's giving that hug. The user may be trying to deal with the situation alone, but then their daughter, their wife comes to us to support them in the background.
FG2: Often, being family doctors and nurses can be an advantage, because we know the person better.

Communication is an important catalyzer in promoting a person's self-determination. Participants highlighted the need for active listening and information management about what the person wants to know about their illness or what they intend to share about the illness with their family support network.

FG5: There are many people who prefer not to know, and this is not always respected (...). We must always ask what the person knows and what they want to know. We have to give the patient space, they may not want the family to get involved, so the family doesn't suffer. We must demystify this with them, but at the same time respect their decision.

(c) Limitations in response capacity

The professionals mentioned several situations in which they provided general PC, with emphasis on symptomatic control in the initial phases, referral and mobilization of resources/support in the community, as well as involvement of families.

FG1: With our approach we achieve initial pain control, but in more advanced situations this no longer happens. Also for constipation and nausea, if applicable. We can answer simpler questions, even if they are not in situations of terminal illness, but in which the principles of palliative care apply.

FG2: We can manage pain and some symptoms in the earliest stages. In social terms, users often have doubts, particularly about the support and benefits they may be entitled to. As we are not social workers and do not know how to clarify all doubts, we refer the person to the Social Worker and make ourselves available for whatever is necessary.
FG3: We adjust medication, mobilize some social resources and provide support to the family.
FG4: We can and should provide palliative care! It is the only way to give access to the population (...). We monitor low complexity situations or pass this responsibility on to specialized care in moderate to high complexity situations given our limitations.

Despite existing efforts, there is a feeling that little is being done to help people die at home (the location preferred by most patients).

FG5: Despite everything, we do very little. Most of our users die in the hospital. If we don't issue death certificates, it's because they die in hospital... the truth is that we are doing little, especially in this matter of allowing people to do this journey at home, which we know will not be for everyone, but perhaps the vast majority would be able to do so (...).

3.2.2. Theme 2—Barriers to Access and Safe Transition Between PHC and Specialized PC

Primary health care professionals face several barriers when it comes to the transition of care and the referral process. Four subthemes were identified: (a) myths and misconceptions regarding PC; (b) early referral conditioned by the heterogeneity of disease trajectories; (c) bureaucratization of processes and difficulties in the transition of care; and (d) scarcity of resources.

(a) Myths and misconceptions regarding PC

Professionals acknowledged that there are several myths and misconceptions among patients, families, and the wider community regarding PC. The myth that PC hastens death, as well as the association of PC with terminality and abandonment, constitute barriers to timely referral. According to participants, it is necessary to invest in community awareness about PC, its benefits, and its person-centered approach.

FG1: People often associate palliative care with people who are dying, so we sometimes face reservations about speaking openly as we may not be well interpreted (...). The lack of literacy in palliative care is very significant. Talking about death is still taboo.
FG2: People really associate palliative care with terminality and the idea that there is nothing more to offer. But after receiving PC, patients feel very good and appreciate this support.
FG3: Talking about palliative care is scary for many and there are many prejudices. We had a user who only accepted treatment here with us in the treatment room, and did not accept care at home (...). Families themselves also experience uncertainty and fear of dealing with losses... and this greatly affects adherence.
FG4: It is important to demystify the word "palliative" for the community in general. We recently had a case of a user who was an informed person, but who got it into his head that when he was referred to palliative care it was the end for him... he internalized that we were, in a way, giving up on him. Later, the family team went home after he was integrated into palliative care and he is now grateful because he is in his natural environment, in his home.

(b) Early referral conditioned by the heterogeneity of disease trajectories

The teams described the different moments in which they felt the need to refer more complex cases to specialized teams. In all FGs, it was evident that the lack of symptomatic control, a worsening functional state, and an increase in psycho-emotional and spiritual needs make it difficult for family teams to monitor the situation.

FG1: Referral is necessary when we can no longer control the symptoms, when multiple decompensations or hospitalizations begin to occur. Certain types of therapeutic formulations are not available in PHC, for example, subcutaneous and transdermal or transmucosal medication.
FG2: When the pain is no longer controllable, or multiple side effects of the medication appear: constipation, dyspnea, lack of appetite and nausea.... We try to control it, but at a certain point we need help from specialized teams.

Although participants describe the transition of care related to patient complexity, specific tools are not used for their assessment. At the same time, the difficulty in interpreting the assessment scales used by specialized PC teams was also mentioned.

FG1: We know that there are tools that can be used to assess the complexity of patients, but they are also very extensive and not easy to apply (...). Sometimes we look at the palliative care team's records and we see that they use a lot of scales, but then having to interpret or validate that assessment is sometimes difficult.

On the other hand, the responsibility of professionals in the late transition to specialized PC was highlighted.

FG5: We referred too late, we thought about it too late. Perhaps we don't have the sensitivity to understand that it makes sense to refer right at that initial stage. And perhaps an initial assessment is more advantageous than an assessment "just to die", so to speak.

(c) Bureaucratization of processes and difficulties in the transition of care

The bureaucracy associated with referral processes, the slow response times, and the limited response from the National Network of Integrated Continuing Care (RNCCI) constitute significant barriers for participants.

FG3: On the computer platform, the social worker has to fill out one part, the nurse fills out another part, the family doctor fills out another part... All of this is a time-consuming process and the user is waiting, with the possibility of the request being denied.... The delay is a problem!
FG5: The referral form is terrible to fill out and our response capacity should be faster. There shouldn't be so much bureaucracy, because patients and families are suffering...

Professionals also criticize the lack of a user-friendly platform for referral to the RNCCI, which requires filling out a series of questions that, in most cases, are poorly adapted to reality.

FG4: Very difficult and there are questions that don't fit very well, details that are unnecessary, without relevance. Mandatory questions arise of a sexual nature that seem unnecessary to us, at least at the time of referral. It might make sense at a later stage, but not at that moment.

These participants also expressed the lack of a proximity of care in a collaborative and integrated network where they could obtain advice and support in decision-making regarding patients with palliative needs.

FG3: There are not enough community teams in PC to help us with the most complex cases. There is no proximity and this also makes it difficult to access answers.
FG4: We have the RNCCI, but we do not have a Community Palliative Care Support Team. We can only count on the in-hospital team, but we do not have access to them, only the hospital services can refer patients there.

Another barrier to the safe transition of care results from the lack of coordination between primary and hospital health care, hindering the user's integrated monitoring.

FG1: Just think that when a person is hospitalized, they often lose contact with their family doctor, and communication between the two levels of care does not always exist.

(d) Scarcity of resources

The shortage of human resources in essential primary care to support palliative patients, such as psychologists and social workers, is a difficulty faced by participants.

FG2: We lack resources, we realize the importance of psychosocial support and then, in practice, we lack the support of psychologists.

FG3: Social prescription here is still a myth, it is still a goal to be achieved. Obviously, it is through the social worker that the family often mobilizes home hygiene support, support for meals, transport and other benefits to which the user may be entitled. But the social worker is "general", not just involved in the referral process or the palliative care team. It's the only one that exists here, (...) and it ends up being overloaded.

FG4: We have very few resources. We have had a psychologist here at the Health Center for a short time now, but she is clearly not, in any way, sufficient for what we need. Therefore, either families have the possibility to appeal on their own, or unfortunately they are left without answers.

The need to adequately understand the disease trajectories for early referral was also recognized. However, participants state that response capacity is largely determined by available resources.

FG5: According to the person's diagnosis, it is possible to anticipate their needs and we try to prevent the situation from evolving into symptomatic loss of control. We try to ensure that the person has the greatest comfort and the best care possible. However, we have a limited response capacity due to a lack of resources.

FG4: This is very unpredictable. It is obvious that there are situations, especially in cancer, when we can predict better, but others... it is very difficult to perceive when the person will start to decline. And so ideally we would have a faster response capacity. In other words, we risk referring people who didn't exactly need it at that moment.

3.2.3. Theme 3–Ways to Mitigate Difficulties in Accessing and Referring to Specialized PC

The professionals suggested several strategies that could be used (and some that are already used) to mitigate difficulties in accessing and referring to specialized PC. In this context, the following subthemes emerged: (a) investment in PC training for PHC professionals; (b) customization of services to the needs of people with palliative needs; and (c) strengthening specialized community palliative care teams (CPCT).

(a) Investment in PC training for PHC professionals

The disinvestment in PC in undergraduate training was recognized by all groups. Consequently, investing in training was considered a priority with an impact on both the quality of care offered and the referral process.

FG2: It is very likely that things would be better if we had basic training in PC. Mandatory palliative care training should even be part of the General and Family Medicine internship. (...) It may even be necessary to decide whether it is time to make a referral or even to be more alert to the activities that we can or cannot do.

FG3: It is the general feeling that we do not have adequate training. In the case of younger professionals, only those who seek training at the master's level are more up-to-date. Furthermore, mandatory training is insufficient or even non-existent (...) It is one of the areas in which we need ongoing training and updating.

FG4: The big issue here is that most of us don't have PC training and we are on the front line! Until patients reach specialized teams, we are the ones who deal with them and their families. What we learn is based on acquired experience, and also on our sensitivity. Therefore, it would have been important to have some investment in the continued training of professionals.

(c) **Strengthening specialized community palliative care teams (CPCT)**

In all FGs, participants reported added value in strengthening CPCTs, as they support decision-making and provide consultancy when necessary.

FG1: I have already had conversations with colleagues at CPCTs about pain control therapy, using co-analgesics that we do not usually use. With these teams, we don't feel helpless.
FG2: They have the team's cell phone, to provide support, both for patients and for us, colleagues. Fortunately, we have the community team and a good relationship with them. We are a privileged unit and I think this has a lot of influence on our performance.

Another positive aspect described by participants is the speed of the CPCT response. Although CPCTs have limitations in offering home care to all palliative patients, they offer other services such as consultancy, telephone support, and teleconsultation.

FG5: They are quick to respond, often responding within the same week. Sometimes they suggest a first joint visit with the family doctor, who in this case is the person who already knows the patient and who proposes the referral. Even if they are not able to make a home visit, there are other forms of support such as telephone assistance and teleconsultation.

4. Discussion

Family doctors and nurses play a central role in accessing and referring patients to PC, since the response provided by specialized palliative care does not meet the needs of the population [12]. The skills of these professionals include approaching the patient's suffering, basic symptom management, and developing a treatment plan aligned with the person's preferences, thus respecting their autonomy [51,52]. Although participants described relative ease in identifying and assessing palliative needs, the majority revealed ambivalence in the process of assessing non-oncological palliative needs, with difficulty in identifying the needs of these patients and the apparent devaluation of situations associated with aging and long disease trajectories. In fact, according to the available evidence, frail older people, people with non-malignant diseases, and people from ethnic minorities have unequal access to PC. Given that they tend to access these services later and with less functional reserve, many are never identified as having palliative needs [33,53,54]. PHC professionals developed a person-centered approach, which has demonstrated positive effects on health outcomes, including better patient–professional relationships and higher patient satisfaction rates [55]. According to the literature, family doctors and nurses are essential for providing EoL care, due to the strong, close relationship built over time, which allows for detailed knowledge of the patient and family's history [8]. Although participants consider themselves to be in a privileged position of proximity to users (which facilitates communication), they admit to difficulties in communicating bad news and the need for training in this area [56].

The findings highlighted several difficulties in accessing and referring to specialized PC. Emphasis was placed on myths and misconceptions regarding PC, so it is essential to invest in PC literacy among patients, caregivers, and the wider community [57–60]. Although professionals acknowledge the increased complexity of patients and lack of symptom control as the main reasons for referral to specialized PC, they recognize that these are often late. According to previous studies, this fact may be related to difficulties in estimating prognosis, disease trajectory, and timely recognition of the end of life [19,30,32,33,59]. Other barriers include the scarcity of resources, bureaucratization of referral processes, and difficulties in communication between health professionals, conditioning the fluidity in the articulation of care [7,61].

Investment in training was identified by participants as an improvement strategy with an impact on the care they offered and also on referral processes. The education and training of health professionals in PC have been reported as inadequate in several studies carried out in different populations, particularly with regard to the complexity of care and the diagnosis of palliative needs [30,61]. To improve professionals' skills, it is necessary to provide learning opportunities and educational resources [8]. Customizing services for people with palliative needs was also a strategy proposed by participants, as a way of overcoming the lack of consultation time at PHCs to meet the needs of these patients in the best and most complete way possible [57,62]. These strategies involve adapting the medical or nursing schedule to increase the consultation time allocated to these patients or implementing a specific consultation model for this type of patient [63]. It was also suggested that a consultation be implemented by primary health care teams with specialized training in palliative care. This could serve as a bridge between family doctors and nurses and specialized hospital care. The possibility of consultancy, the use of effective communication channels, collaborative work, and the existence of an integrated care network are tools that increase the responses of health professionals [64,65]. In the present study, participants recognized the importance of CPCT as teams that meet these criteria, given their collaborative work model and proximity to the community [66]. Furthermore, participants highlighted the need to increase the number of these teams, which provide more rapid responses, as an improvement strategy to be implemented.

4.1. Strengths and Limitations

The present study presents a set of strengths and limitations. Given the lack of research in Portugal on this topic, this study contributes to the expansion of available knowledge regarding the experiences of PHC professionals. This study highlights the role of family doctors and nurses as key elements in ensuring global access to PC, both due to their fundamental role in providing PC and their importance in referrals to specialized teams. Furthermore, the integration of the subjective perspectives of professionals provides a comprehensive view of the reality of PC in Portugal. In methodological terms, the researchers rigorously followed the different phases of the research. To ensure the credibility of the study, the researchers maintained reflexivity throughout the research process, and each research phase was discussed and documented in detail. In parallel, the sample provided variations in the experiments and attained data saturation.

Regarding the limitations of the study, the fact that the participants within each FG knew each other could have influenced their interactions. FGs can exhibit subject bias, given that dominant participants or the moderator can influence individual and group opinions, which may result in the non-expression of some individual perceptions and experiences. To mitigate the risk of social desirability bias, data collectors used techniques to establish rapport with participants, such as using probing questions, requesting stories and examples, and providing assurances. While focus groups can be valuable for exploring specific topics and understanding group dynamics, relying solely on them without methodological triangulation can lead to a less comprehensive and potentially biased understanding of the research question. Further mixed methods may identify convergent or divergent patterns of phenomena. Although using a qualitative vignette is an effective projecting strategy, this can elicit answers from participants that they prefer to withhold. To address this claim, participants were assured they were not required to connect the scenario to their personal experiences unless they chose to do so. Although the present study involved three different local health units in the central region of the country, we admit that the practices of PHC and PC professionals, as well as the organization of these services, vary with geographic context, limiting the transferability of the findings.

4.2. Implications for Practice

This study offers a deeper understanding of the Portuguese reality in terms of the articulation between primary health care and PC. It identified the main challenges faced by PHC health professionals when providing PC and in the transition of care, highlighting strategies that they apply or recommend for improving clinical practice. In Portugal, PC education in undergraduate programs, particularly within the nursing and medical fields, is being developed but still faces challenges in terms of curriculum integration and practical experience. While there is growing awareness of the need for PC education due to an increased prevalence of chronic diseases, there is a gap between theoretical knowledge and practical application that reinforces the need for better curricula integration of PC. This study also highlighted the importance of training and continuous professional development in PC for PHC providers. Improving education and support for PHC teams may enable them to be more proactively involved in identifying patients with palliative needs and initiating early referral. The stereotypes that exist in the community regarding PC make it urgent to invest in health literacy, in order to highlight the work carried out by PC services [67,68]. Furthermore, research highlights the need to strengthen communication and collaboration among healthcare professionals. Fragmentation and lack of integration are often expressed as barriers, suggesting the need for more structured interprofessional collaboration and shared care models [69,70]. The scarcity of resources and the bureaucratization of processes are important issues on the political agenda, and it is necessary to invest in financing PHC and simplifying referral processes.

5. Conclusions

To the best of our knowledge, so far, no other studies have analyzed the practices, access, and referral to PC from the perspective of PHC professionals. The findings were organized into three core themes: (1) the contours of palliative action developed by PHC teams; (2) barriers to access and safe transition between PHC and specialized PC; and (3) ways to mitigate difficulties in accessing and referring to specialized PC. This study highlights the fundamental role of PHC professionals in providing primary PC, identifying PC needs, and referring patients to PC early, while exposing the systemic and interpersonal challenges that hinder these processes. To overcome these challenges, it is essential to invest in the development of integrated care models that promote practical, low-bureaucratic referral processes and capture the human resources necessary for adequate follow-up of users. Measures should strengthen collaboration between PHC and PC services, as well as promote the improvement of professional training, particularly in communication skills. Health education must be promoted to demystify PC among the population. The findings also highlight the importance of CPCTs in PC as fundamental agents to improve access and support PHC professionals in care decisions and practices. By recognizing and acting on these implications, health systems can move toward a more equitable, timely, and person-centered PC, anchored in strong primary health care and supported by informed and empowered communities.

Supplementary Materials: The following supporting information can be downloaded at: https://www.mdpi.com/article/10.3390/healthcare13131576/s1. Supplementary Table S1: Consolidated criteria for reporting qualitative studies (COREQ): 32-item checklist. The reference (Tong et al., 2007 [41]) is cited within the Supplementary Materials.

Author Contributions: Conceptualization, C.B. and C.L.; methodology, C.B. and C.L.; software, C.B. and C.L.; validation, C.B. and C.L.; formal analysis, C.B. and C.L.; investigation, C.B. and C.L.; resources, C.B. and C.L.; data curation, C.B. and C.L.; writing—original draft preparation, C.B. and C.L.; writing—review and editing, C.B., M.M.d.S., A.F.C.F., R.J.V.Y. and C.L.; visualization, C.B.,

M.M.d.S. and C.L.; supervision, C.L.; project administration, C.L.; funding acquisition, C.L. All authors have read and agreed to the published version of the manuscript.

Funding: This work is supported by national funds through FCT—Fundação para a Ciência e a Tecnologia, I.P. (UID/05704/2023)—and under the Scientific Employment Stimulus-Institutional Call (https://doi.org/10.54499/CEECINST/00051/2018/CP1566/CT0012, accessed on 20 June 2025).

Institutional Review Board Statement: This study was conducted in accordance with the Declaration of Helsinki and approved by the Research Ethics Committee of Polytechnic University of Leiria (CE/IPLEIRIA/87/2024; approval date: 20 September 2024).

Informed Consent Statement: Informed consent was obtained from all subjects involved in the study.

Data Availability Statement: All data generated or analyzed during this study are included in this article. This article is based on the first author's Master's dissertation in palliative care at the School of Health Sciences—Polytechnic University of Leiria (supervised by Carlos Laranjeira).

Acknowledgments: The authors express their profound gratitude to the professionals who generously contributed to this study.

Conflicts of Interest: The authors declare no conflicts of interest. The funders had no role in the design of the study; in the collection, analyses, or interpretation of data; in the writing of the manuscript; or in the decision to publish the results.

Abbreviations

COPD	Chronic Obstructive Pulmonary Disease
FG	Focus Group
LHU	Local Health Unit
PHC	Primary Health Care
PC	Palliative Care
CPCT	Community PC Teams
RNCCI	National Network of Integrated Continuing Care (Rede Nacional de Cuidados Continuados Integrados *in Portuguese*)

References

1. Proietti, M.; Cesari, M. Frailty: What Is It? In *Frailty and Cardiovascular Diseases: Research into an Elderly Population*, 1st ed.; Veronese, N., Ed.; Springer: Cham, Switzerland, 2020.
2. Aker, N.; Griffiths, S.; Kupeli, N.; Frost, R.; Nair, P.; Walters, K.; Melo, L.J.; Davies, N. Experiences and access of palliative and end of life care for older people from minority ethnic groups: A scoping review. *BMC Palliat. Care* **2024**, *23*, 228. [CrossRef] [PubMed]
3. Xi, J.Y.; Liang, B.H.; Zhang, W.J.; Yan, B.; Dong, H.; Chen, Y.Y.; Lin, X.; Gu, J.; Hao, Y.T. Effects of population aging on quality of life and disease burden: A population-based study. *Glob. Health Res. Policy* **2025**, *10*, 2. [CrossRef] [PubMed]
4. INE. Estatísticas Territoriais: Estimativas de População Residente. Available online: https://www.ine.pt/xportal/xmain?xpid=INE&xpgid=ine_destaques&DESTAQUESdest_boui=645507713&DESTAQUESmodo=2&xlang=pt (accessed on 17 April 2025).
5. INE. Estatísticas Territoriais: População residente (N.º) por Local de Residência (NUTS—2013), Sexo e Grupo Etário; Anual. Available online: https://www.ine.pt/xportal/xmain?xpid=INE&xpgid=ine_indicadores&indOcorrCod=0008273 (accessed on 17 April 2025).
6. Marques, P.; Rêgo, F.; Nunes, R. Palliative Care in Portugal—From Intention to Reality, What Is Yet to Be Accomplished. *Nurs. Rep.* **2023**, *13*, 1477–1485. [CrossRef] [PubMed]
7. Carey, M.L.; Zucca, A.C.; Freund, M.A.; Bryant, J.; Herrmann, A.; Roberts, B.J. Systematic review of barriers and enablers to the delivery of palliative care by primary care practitioners. *Palliat. Med.* **2019**, *33*, 1131–1145. [CrossRef]
8. Hui, D.; Heung, Y.; Bruera, E. Timely Palliative Care: Personalizing the Process of Referral. *Cancers* **2022**, *14*, 1047. [CrossRef]
9. Hughes, M.C.; Vernon, E.; Hainstock, A. The effectiveness of community-based palliative care programme components: A systematic review. *Age Ageing* **2023**, *52*, afad175. [CrossRef]
10. Devik, S.A.; Lersveen, G.L. Specialist and Primary Physicians' Experiences and Perspectives of Collaboration While Caring for Palliative Patients-A Qualitative Study. *Healthcare* **2023**, *11*, 2188. [CrossRef]

11. World Health Organization. Integrating Palliative Care and Symptom Relief into Primary Health Care: A WHO Guide for Planners, Implementers and Managers. Available online: https://iris.who.int/bitstream/handle/10665/274559/9789241514477%20eng.pdf?sequence=1&isAllowed=y (accessed on 17 April 2025).
12. Godrie, F.; Van Zuilekom, I.; Onwuteaka-Philipsen, B.; Van Os-Medendorp, H.; Schoonmade, L.; Metselaar, S. Specialized expertise among healthcare professionals in palliative care—A scoping review. *BMC Palliat. Care* **2024**, *23*, 170. [CrossRef]
13. Pini, S.; Hackett, J.; Taylor, S.; Bekker, H.L.; Kite, S.; Bennett, M.I.; Ziegler, L. Patient and professional experiences of palliative care referral discussions from cancer services: A qualitative interview study. *Eur. J. Cancer Care* **2021**, *30*, e13340. [CrossRef]
14. Feliciano, D.R.; Reis-Pina, P. Enhancing End-of-Life Care with Home-Based Palliative Interventions: A Systematic Review. *J. Pain. Symptom Manag.* **2024**, *68*, e356–e372. [CrossRef]
15. Bergqvist, J.; Ljunggren, G. The Impact of Integrated Home Palliative Care Services on Resource Use and Place of Death. *J. Palliat. Med.* **2020**, *23*, 67–73. [CrossRef] [PubMed]
16. McCarroll, S.; Avsar, P.; Moore, Z.; O'Connor, T.; Nugent, L.; Patton, D. The Impact of Specialist Community Palliative Care Teams on Acute Hospital Admission Rates in Adult Patients Requiring End of Life Care: A Systematic Review. *Eur. J. Oncol. Nurs.* **2022**, *59*, 102168. [CrossRef] [PubMed]
17. Pinto, S.; Lopes, S.; de Sousa, A.B.; Delalibera, M.; Gomes, B. Patient and Family Preferences About Place of End-of-Life Care and Death: An Umbrella Review. *J. Pain Symptom Manag.* **2024**, *67*, e439–e452. [CrossRef] [PubMed]
18. World Health Organization. Palliative Care. Available online: https://www.who.int/health-topics/palliative-care (accessed on 18 April 2025).
19. Peeler, A.; Afolabi, O.; Adcock, M.; Evans, C.; Nkhoma, K.; Van Breevoort, D.; Farrant, L.; Harding, R. Primary palliative care in low- and middle-income countries: A systematic review and thematic synthesis of the evidence for models and outcomes. *Palliat. Med.* **2024**, *38*, 776–789. [CrossRef]
20. World Health Organization. Assessing the Development of Palliative Care Worldwide: A Set of Actionable Indicators. Available online: https://www.who.int/publications/i/item/9789240033351 (accessed on 18 April 2025).
21. Arias-Casais, N.; López-Fidalgo, J.; Garralda, E.; Pons, J.J.; Rhee, J.Y.; Lukas, R.; De Lima, L.; Centeno, C. Trends analysis of specialized palliative care services in 51 countries of the WHO European region in the last 14 years. *Palliat. Med.* **2020**, *34*, 1044–1056. [CrossRef]
22. Observatório Português dos Cuidados Paliativos. Relatório de Outono 2023: Cobertura e Caracterização das Equipas e Profissionais das Equipas de Cuidados Paliativos. Available online: https://fcse.lisboa.ucp.pt/asset/12366/file (accessed on 18 April 2025).
23. Comissão Nacional de Cuidados Paliativos (CNCP). Relatório de Implementação do Plano Estratégico para o Desenvolvimento dos Cuidados Paliativos: Biénio 2019–2020. Available online: http://www.aenfermagemeasleis.pt/2019/04/03/plano-estrategico-para-o-desenvolvimento-dos-cuidados-paliativos-para-o-bienio-2019-2020/ (accessed on 18 April 2025).
24. Gouveia, M.; Reis-Pina, P. A atuação do médico de família e os cuidados paliativos: O método ACERTAR. *Rev. Med. Geral Fam.* **2023**, *39*, 84–90. [CrossRef]
25. World Family Doctors Cring for People (WONCA). The European Definition of General Practice/Family Medicine. Available online: https://www.woncaeurope.org/file/41f61fb9-47d5-4721-884e-603f4afa6588/WONCA_European_Definitions_2_v7.pdf (accessed on 18 April 2025).
26. Justino, E.T.; Kasper, M.; Santos, K.D.S.; Quaglio, R.C.; Fortuna, C.M. Palliative care in primary health care: Scoping review. *Rev. Lat. Am. Enfermagem.* **2020**, *28*, e3324. [CrossRef]
27. World Health Organization. Cuidados de Saúde Primários. Available online: https://www.who.int/world-health-day/world-health-day-2019/fact-sheets/details/primary-health-care (accessed on 19 April 2025).
28. McCormick, E.; Chai, E.; Meier, D.E. Integrating palliative care into primary care. *Mt. Sinai J. Med.* **2012**, *79*, 579–585. [CrossRef]
29. Aguiar, H. Os cuidados paliativos nos cuidados de saúde primários—O desafio para o século XXI. *Rev. Port. Med. Geral Fam.* **2012**, *28*, 442–447. [CrossRef]
30. Silva, T.C.D.; Nietsche, E.A.; Cogo, S.B. Palliative care in Primary Health Care: An integrative literature review. *Rev. Bras. Enferm.* **2021**, *75*, e20201335. [CrossRef]
31. Vitorino, J.V.; Duarte, B.V.; Laranjeira, C. When to initiate early palliative care? Challenges faced by healthcare providers. *Front. Med.* **2023**, *10*, 1220370. [CrossRef] [PubMed]
32. Kawashima, A.; Evans, C.J. Needs-based triggers for timely referral to palliative care for older adults severely affected by noncancer conditions: A systematic review and narrative synthesis. *BMC Palliat. Care* **2023**, *22*, 20. [CrossRef] [PubMed]
33. Stow, D.; Matthews, F.E.; Hanratty, B. Timing of GP end-of-life recognition in people aged ≥75 years: Retrospective cohort study using data from primary healthcare records in England. *Br. J. Gen. Pract.* **2020**, *70*, e874–e879. [CrossRef] [PubMed]
34. Krueger, R.A.; Casey, M.A. *Focus Groups: A Practical Guide for Applied Research*, 5th ed.; SAGE Publications: Thousand Oaks, CA, USA, 2015; p. 252.
35. Lee, C.G. Reconsidering Constructivism in Qualitative Research. *Educ. Philos. Theory* **2012**, *44*, 403–412. [CrossRef]

36. Gill, P.; Baillie, J. Interviews and focus groups in qualitative research: An update for the digital age. *Br. Dent. J.* **2018**, *225*, 668–672. [CrossRef]
37. Bender, D.E.; Ewbank, D. The Focus Group as a Tool for Health Research: Issues in Design and Analysis. *Health Transit. Rev.* **1994**, *4*, 63–80.
38. Pyo, J.; Lee, W.; Choi, E.Y.; Jang, S.G.; Ock, M. Qualitative Research in Healthcare: Necessity and Characteristics. *J. Prev. Med. Public Health* **2023**, *56*, 12–20. [CrossRef]
39. Hudson, P. Focus Group Interviews: A Guide for Palliative Care Researchers and Clinicians. *Int. J. Palliat. Nurs.* **2003**, *9*, 202–207. [CrossRef]
40. Wong, L.P. Focus Group Discussion: A Tool for Health and Medical Research. *Singap. Med. J.* **2008**, *49*, 256–260.
41. Tong, A.; Sainsbury, P.; Craig, J. Consolidated Criteria for Reporting Qualitative Research (COREQ): A 32-Item Checklist for Interviews and Focus Groups. *Int. J. Qual. Health Care* **2007**, *19*, 349–357. [CrossRef]
42. Patton, M.Q. *Qualitative Research and Evaluation Methods. Integrating Theory and Practice*, 4th ed.; Sage Publications Inc.: Thousand Oaks, CA, USA, 2015.
43. Rego, A.; Pina e Cunha, M.; Meyer, V. Quantos participantes são necessários para um estudo qualitativo? Linhas práticas de orientação. *Rev. Gestão Países Língua Port.* **2019**, *17*, 43–57. [CrossRef]
44. Moser, A.; Korstjens, I. Series: Practical Guidance to Qualitative Research. Part 3: Sampling, Data Collection and Analysis. *Eur. J. Gen. Pract.* **2018**, *24*, 9–18. [CrossRef] [PubMed]
45. Rhee, J.J.; Grant, M.; Senior, H.; Monterosso, L.; McVey, P.; Johnson, C.; Aubin, M.; Nwachukwu, H.; Bailey, C.; Fallon-Fergunson, J.; et al. Facilitators and Barriers to General Practitioner and General Practice Nurse Participation in End-of-Life Care: Systematic Review. *BMJ Support. Palliat. Care*, 2020; *online ahead of print*. [CrossRef]
46. Balasundram, S.; Holm, A.; Benthien, K.S.; Waldorff, F.B.; Reventlow, S.; Overbeck, G. Increasing the Chance of Dying at Home: Roles, Tasks and Approaches of General Practitioners Enabling Palliative Care—A Systematic Review of Qualitative Literature. *BMC Prim. Care* **2023**, *24*, 77. [CrossRef] [PubMed]
47. Suntai, Z.; Won, C.R.; Noh, H. Access Barrier in Rural Older Adults' Use of Pain Management and Palliative Care Services: A Systematic Review. *Am. J. Hosp. Palliat. Care* **2021**, *38*, 494–502. [CrossRef]
48. Braun, V.; Clarke, V. Using Thematic Analysis in Psychology. *Qual. Res. Psychol.* **2006**, *3*, 77–101. [CrossRef]
49. Braun, V.; Clarke, V. *Successful Qualitative Research: A Practical Guide for Beginners*, 1st ed.; Sage: London, UK, 2013.
50. Korstjens, I.; Moser, A. Series: Practical Guidance to Qualitative Research. Part 4: Trustworthiness and Publishing. *Eur. J. Gen. Pract.* **2018**, *24*, 120–124. [CrossRef]
51. Buss, M.K.; Rock, L.K.; McCarthy, E.P. Understanding Palliative Care and Hospice: A Review for Primary Care Providers. *Mayo Clin. Proc.* **2017**, *92*, 280–286. [CrossRef]
52. Ghosh, A.; Dzeng, E.; Cheng, M.J. Interaction of Palliative Care and Primary Care. *Clin. Geriatr. Med.* **2015**, *31*, 207–218. [CrossRef]
53. Lau, C.; Meaney, C.; Morgan, M.; Cook, R.; Zimmermann, C.; Wentlandt, K. Disparities in Access to Palliative Care Facilities for Patients with and without Cancer: A Retrospective Review. *Palliat. Med.* **2021**, *35*, 1191–1201. [CrossRef]
54. Leach, I.; Mayland, C.R.; Turner, N.; Mitchell, S. Understanding Patient Views and Experiences of the IDENTIfication of PALLiative Care Needs (IDENTI-PALL): A Qualitative Interview Study. *Br. J. Gen. Pract.* **2024**, *74*, e88–e95. [CrossRef]
55. Ahmed, A.; van den Muijsenbergh, M.E.T.C.; Vrijhoef, H.J.M. Person-Centred Care in Primary Care: What Works for Whom, How and in What Circumstances? *Health Soc. Care Community* **2022**, *30*, e3328–e3341. [CrossRef] [PubMed]
56. Ruiz Sancho, E.; Pérez Nieto, M.Á.; Román, F.J.; León Mateos, L.; Sánchez Escamilla, F.; Enrech Francés, S.; Pérez Escutia, M.A.; Juez Martel, I.; Pérez-Segura, P.; Aguirre Herrero, A.; et al. Differences in the Communication of Cancer Diagnoses by Different Health Professionals and the Impact of Oncologist Communication on Patients' Emotions. *Cancers* **2024**, *16*, 2444. [CrossRef] [PubMed]
57. Kim, H. Barriers to Effective Communication About Advance Care Planning and Palliative Care: A Qualitative Study. Available online: https://www.e-jhpc.org/journal/view.html?uid=516&vmd=Full (accessed on 19 April 2025).
58. Enguidanos, S.; Rahman, A. *Identifying Challenges to Using Home-Based Palliative Care for Patients with Serious Illness*; Patient-Centered Outcomes Research Institute (PCORI): Washington, DC, USA, 2021.
59. Cardenas, V.; Rahman, A.; Zhu, Y.; Enguidanos, S. Reluctance to Accept Palliative Care and Recommendations for Improvement: Findings from Semi-Structured Interviews with Patients and Caregivers. *Am. J. Hosp. Palliat. Care* **2022**, *39*, 189–195. [CrossRef] [PubMed]
60. Patra, L.; Ghoshal, A.; Damani, A.; Salins, N. Cancer Palliative Care Referral: Patients' and Family Caregivers' Perspectives—A Systematic Review. *BMJ Support. Palliat. Care*, 2022; *online ahead of print*. [CrossRef]
61. Pitzer, S.; Kutschar, P.; Paal, P.; Mülleder, P.; Lorenzl, S.; Wosko, P.; Osterbrink, J.; Bükki, J. Barriers for Adult Patients to Access Palliative Care in Hospitals: A Mixed Methods Systematic Review. *J. Pain Symptom Manag.* **2023**, *67*, e16–e33. [CrossRef]
62. Kuckel, D.P.; Jones, A.L.; Smith, D.K. The Spiritual Assessment. *Am. Fam. Physician* **2022**, *106*, 415–419.

63. Cardoso, C.S.; Prazeres, F.; Oliveiros, B.; Nunes, C.; Simões, P.; Aires, C.; Rita, P.; Penetra, J.; Lopes, P.; Alcobia, S.; et al. Feasibility and Effectiveness of a Two-Tiered Intervention Involving Training and a New Consultation Model for Patients with Palliative Care Needs in Primary Care: A Before-After Study. *Palliat. Med.* **2024**, *38*, 842–852. [CrossRef]
64. Atreya, S.; Datta, S.S.; Salins, N. Views of General Practitioners on End-of-Life Care Learning Preferences: A Systematic Review. *BMC Palliat. Care* **2022**, *21*, 162. [CrossRef]
65. Zhang, S.; Li, Z.; Yue, P. Healthcare Providers' Attitudes and Associated Factors on Palliative Care Referral: A Qualitative Systematic Review and Meta-Aggregation. *J. Clin. Nurs.* **2024**, *33*, 3355–3380. [CrossRef]
66. Caetano, P.; Querido, A.; Laranjeira, C. Preparedness for Caregiving Role and Telehealth Use to Provide Informal Palliative Home Care in Portugal: A Qualitative Study. *Healthcare* **2024**, *12*, 1915. [CrossRef]
67. Marrazes, V.; Gonçalves, L.; Querido, A.; Laranjeira, C. Informal Palliative Care at Home: A Focus Group Study Among Professionals Working in Palliative Care in Portugal. *Healthcare* **2025**, *13*, 978. [CrossRef]
68. Monteiro, A.; Ali, A.M.; Laranjeira, C. Lived Experiences of Physiotherapists in Caring for People with Advanced Amyotrophic Lateral Sclerosis in Portugal: A Phenomenological Study. *Behav. Sci.* **2025**, *15*, 510. [CrossRef] [PubMed]
69. Vitorino, J.V.; Duarte, B.V.; Ali, A.M.; Laranjeira, C. Compassionate engagement of communities in support of palliative and end-of-life care: Challenges in post-pandemic era. *Front. Med.* **2024**, *11*, 1489299. [CrossRef] [PubMed]
70. Laranjeira, C.; Dixe, M.A.; Coelho, A.; Reigada, C.; Carneiro, R.; Querido, A. The needs of family caregivers providing palliative home care in Portugal: A multi-stage mixed methods study protocol. *Front Public Health* **2025**, *13*, 1596657. [CrossRef] [PubMed]

healthcare

MDPI

Article

Volunteer Services in Palliative Care by Third Age University Students

Gönül Düzgün [1,*], Yasemin Kılıç Öztürk [2], Gökşen Polat [1] and Sevnaz Şahin [3]

1 Vocational School First Aid and Emergency Program, Izmir Tınaztepe University, Buca, 35400 Izmir, Türkiye; goksen.polat@tinaztepe.edu.tr
2 Izmir Medical Faculty, University of Health Sciences, Tepecik Training and Research Hospital, 35020 Izmir, Türkiye; yasemin.ozturk2@saglik.gov.tr
3 Department of Internal Medicine, Division of Geriatrics, Ege University Hospital, 35100 Izmir, Türkiye; drsevnaz@gmail.com
* Correspondence: gonul.duzgun@tinaztepe.edu.tr; Tel.: +90-0544-779-35-97

Abstract: Background: Volunteering is a type of support that provides high motivation and supports social participation during the active aging process without any financial reward. Volunteering services provided by an active older person not only provide free services to the community where needed but also help individuals feel valued by creating a social environment, thereby increasing their resilience. The aim of this study was to determine the views on volunteering in palliative care services among older individuals over the age of sixty who attend the Ege University of the Third Age [U3A] and outline the volunteer profile of older students after receiving palliative care training. Methods: This study was conducted using a qualitative research method. The study population consisted of seventy students from the Ege U3A in İzmir who met the inclusion criteria. Before the training, the U3A students were given a brief pre-test about palliative care and volunteering, followed by 2-day, 16 h basic palliative care training. After the training, the students were asked to respond to written questions about volunteering in palliative care, and their responses were collected in their own handwriting. For the data analysis, a thematic content analysis was conducted using MAXQDA 20, a qualitative data analysis program. Results: In this study, the average age of the 70 University of the Third Age students were 67.47 (60–89) years. The participants were 75% women; 85% were married, 40% lived with their spouse, and 37.14% had been students at the University of the Third Age for 3 years. After the thematic analysis, six main themes emerged: physical and social support, educational support, medical/clinical support, financial support, spiritual support, and caregiving for pediatric patients. Conclusions: In our study, it was clearly observed that older students enrolled in the Ege U3A, who had a high potential for volunteering, were willing to work voluntarily in palliative care within the limits of their physical abilities and resources. This research, which aimed to create a volunteer profile in palliative care, allowed older students to find suitable roles for themselves and increased their motivation to provide this unpaid service. Based on this, it aimed to establish an effective start and an encouraging practice for the development of a pilot study, which is needed for Türkiye.

Keywords: palliative care; active aging; volunteer training; qualitative research

1. Introduction

"Before meeting the patient, I learn about their preferences and needs to make appropriate preparations. If permitted, I can dress them in clothes that suit their taste and set aside some for them to wear once they have recovered, hoping to make them happy and give them hope by telling them they will be able to wear these clothes later. I find out their favorite music in advance and record it on my phone; if they wish, I can listen to the recorded music with them and sing along. I learn about books they like and, if they want, I can read them, then leave the books for their own reading later. I listen to their stories and try to engage in conversation. If there is a family photo album, I would obtain it from their relatives, look through it with them, and listen to their memories if they wish to share. At the end of the day, I review the time we spent together and make sure to convey my intention to return. The hope of spending another day together in a better and healthier way will be beneficial for both them and me."

The statements above are expressions from a volunteer who participated in our study, written exactly as they were originally provided. We believe that the time has come to transform this potential that older individuals have for healthy aging into a real dynamic, especially for a developing country such as Türkiye in the field of palliative care.

Volunteer work can best be defined as a free, non-profit activity that usually serves the common good. Working as a volunteer supports a person's positive attitude towards life. Helping someone else for free at any age provides a high level of motivation. Conducting volunteer work feels like therapy to a person and provides motivation to engage in it constantly [1]. The World Health Organization [WHO] classifies chronological ages as follows: older adults between the ages of 65 and 74 years as the youngest-old, those between the ages of 75 and 84 years as the middle-old, and those aged over 85 years as the oldest-old [2]. Being able to live actively during old age is an important criterion for successful aging [3]. Active aging is a multi-dimensional concept influenced by several factors, such as lifelong learning, physical health and functionality, lifestyle, environmental conditions, and social inclusion.

The most productive way of active aging for the elderly is to participate in volunteer work. The volunteer work of this population group can be understood as a valuable resource, as older people have freer time availability and can contribute a wealth of experience. Furthermore, volunteering is seen as an opportunity for older people, as it offers opportunities to participate in social life, experience social inclusion as well as recognition, and able to engage in meaningful activities. Therefore, it is not surprising that in Austria too, the highest volunteering participation rate of 57% occurred for the 60–69 age group and that 43% of 70–79-year-olds still volunteer [4]. Furthermore, the engagement of older people benefits not only volunteer organizations and society but also the individuals themselves. Many studies have shown that volunteering by older people is associated with better physical and mental health [5], a lower probability of illness, better mental well-being, greater life satisfaction, lower mortality, and better general well-being. This list includes aspects that people want for old age or need for successful aging [1].

Lifelong learning plays a key role in older individuals expressing themselves, participating in community life and employment, and developing skills and experience, and it also strengthens intergenerational communication and experience transfer. Studies indicate that there is a linear relationship between active aging and lifelong learning. U3A is one of the best examples of these studies [6]. U3A opened its doors to individuals over the age of 60 in 2016 as part of a lifelong learning initiative under a social responsibility project at Ege University. The Ege U3A, coordinated by the Department of Geriatrics at Ege University and involving volunteer academics from various faculties of the university, is a social responsibility project that includes both theoretical and practical courses. The theoretical courses cover a wide range of topics, from health preservation and vaccination to cosmology and history. Some of the practical courses include folk dance, psychodrama, choir, and knitting. The duration of the program is 3 years. U3A not only strengthens individuals physiologically, psychologically, and socially but it also contributes to the development of new roles [7]. These universities first emerged in France in 1973 [6,8]. Since the training programs are shaped according to regional needs, there is no standard curriculum. When examining examples in our country, no palliative care training specifically aimed at the older population has been found. It is important for older individuals to understand the concept, scope, and purpose of palliative care.

Particularly, in the aging global population, deaths caused by infections have been replaced by deaths due to chronic diseases. Consequently, aging individuals appear to be at a higher risk for chronic illnesses, and their need for symptomatic care related to these diseases has become more prominent. Understanding the content of this care forms a preliminary preparation phase for evaluating how well the provided services will meet expectations and for identifying the required areas of care. In particular, collaborating with healthcare professionals will provide an advantage in meaningfully maintaining social support for patients [9].

One of the best examples of creating a strong social support network through individuals who volunteer to join a team in palliative care in Germany. In Germany, individuals who volunteer to join a team in palliative care are representatives of normal life within the interdisciplinary team. They support the care team, establish connections between the institution and daily life, bring various skills and experiences to the team, and take on tasks such as conversing with patients or their families, reading books, going for walks, accompanying patients at night, and indirectly participating in bureaucratic tasks and other activities [10,11]. U3A students receive services from volunteer academics and observe what it means to serve in a voluntary job. Therefore, they are a very suitable group for volunteering, as they provide social and psychological motivation. The desire of U3A students to engage in active aging, their free time, and their high instinct to be useful to society after receiving education increase their volunteering potential.

In Türkiye, involving older individuals as volunteers in palliative care is highly valuable for promoting positive outcomes, such as continuing to produce based on healthy aging, strengthening social connections, and providing motivation through voluntary work. It allows older individuals to find and maintain a meaningful place in life to the extent that their competencies permit at every age. The aim of our research was to identify the views of U3A students who aim for active aging regarding volunteering in palliative care after receiving training on the subject and to outline the profile of older individuals in Türkiye who are interested in volunteering in palliative care.

2. Methods

This study used a qualitative research method. The study population consisted of Ege U3A students. A total of 70 students from Ege U3A, who were enrolled and had received 16 h of theoretical training in palliative care, were included in the study. The theoretical training program included the following topics: "Definition of palliative care (what is palliative care and what is it not?), palliative care practices in Türkiye, palliative care practices in the world, symptom management in palliative care, making a medical will, end-of-life care and communication with the dying patient, the health of caregivers in palliative care, and volunteer work in palliative care".

The following inclusion criteria were used for this study:

- Being a U3A student;
- Being 60 years of age or older;
- Having completed 16 h of training in palliative care;
- Having no physical or sensory disabilities [e.g., writing, hearing/speaking difficulties];
- Being found healthy after a comprehensive geriatric assessment;
- Being willing to participate in the study.

2.1. Data Collection Method

This study was conducted between November 2023 and May 2024 with individuals over the age of sixty at Ege U3A in İzmir. All the students who met the research criteria were included in the sample. The data for the study were collected using an individual information form and a semi-structured interview form. During the pre-test phase, the individual information form and close-ended questions regarding the concept of palliative care and their past volunteer experience were administered. Subsequently, 2-day (totaling 16 h) palliative care training was provided.

After the training, a consent form was signed, and the purpose of the study was explained. The students who agreed to participate underwent a comprehensive geriatric assessment, and those without health problems affecting their ability to listen to and understand the lessons were included in the study. Socio-demographic information was collected using the individual information form. In the open-ended interview form, the participants were asked to write in their own handwriting and of their own free will whether they would like to offer support in the field of palliative care and the areas in which they would be willing to volunteer. It was explained that there would be no sanctions, obligations, or requirements regarding what they wrote, and if they did not wish to volunteer, they were asked to clearly express that in writing as well.

2.2. *Data Collection Tools*

2.2.1. Individual Information Form

The participants were asked about their age, gender, marital status, family structure, how many years they have been a U3A student, what the concept of palliative care means to them, whether they had received palliative care training before, and their experience or intention to work as a volunteer.

2.2.2. Open-Ended Interview Form

The interview form included 1 open-ended question and 2 yes/no questions aimed at revealing the volunteering profiles of individuals. The questions from the interview form are provided below.

1. After receiving training in palliative care, would you consider working as a volunteer to support palliative care? Yes/No
2. If your answer to the above question is 'yes,' in which areas and what kind of support would you like to provide as a volunteer for patients after receiving training in palliative care?
3. Would you like to be part of the volunteer pool for supporting palliative care patients and stay in communication with the training team? Yes/No

2.3. *Data Analysis*

In the data analysis, a qualitative content analysis was conducted. After transcribing the open-ended responses, a thematic content analysis was performed using MAXQDA 2020.1, a qualitative data analysis program. The researchers identified the themes, participants [volunteers were coded as V1, V2, V3], and sub-themes that represented the codes through iterative discussions until a consensus was reached [12].

Ethical Considerations

Permission was obtained from the Medical Research Ethics Committee of Ege University, decision No. 23-9T/58, on 7 September 2023. The Ege U3A students who agreed to participate were informed about the study and their written consent was obtained. The participants were also informed that they could withdraw from the study at any stage.

3. Findings

The average age of the 70 students included in the study was 67.47 (60–89) years. A total of 85% of the participants were married, 40% lived with their spouse, and 37.14% had been students at the Ege U3A for 3 years. It was noted that none of the students knew the meaning of palliative care before their training, and none had previously received palliative care training. Prior to the training, it was found that 82.85% of the students had not previously provided volunteer services, and 72% had not considered working as a volunteer.

After the training, 90% of the students expressed a desire to work as volunteers in palliative care, and 87% indicated that they wished to stay in communication within the volunteer pool. The areas in which the older individuals indicated they could or would like to provide support, based on their written statements, were categorized into five dimensions. Three experts in the research evaluated the written statements separately and extracted themes. Then, the experts reviewed the themes created together, and as a result, six main themes were reached without any sub-theme groups. These were as follows: physical and social support, educational support, medical/clinical support, financial support, spiritual support, and caregiving for pediatric patients.

3.1. Social and Physical Support Dimension

The day should begin with a sweet smile, followed by approaching the patient with that warmth and assisting with their daily self-care. I help them with physical activities as desired [V1, V11, V18].

I would like to provide physical care if health professionals teach me how to do it [V18].

I can assist with personal care and help with exercise [V23], [V36], [V53].

I would take on patient care for specific time intervals, such as 1–2 h a day or one day a week [V45].

I can assist with the patient's nutrition and personal care [V46], [V47].

I would cut their hair and nails and ensure body hygiene [V55].

Then, I try to uplift their energy by engaging in conversations they enjoy, providing an environment that will be beneficial to them as much as possible. I make sure they feel and live in that room as if it were their home [V1].

I would play games, read books, take them outside depending on their condition, and listen to their memories [V3].

I would read books to patients for an hour or listen to them [I observed that older individuals have a great need to share their life experiences, and conversing always relaxes and calms them] [V4].

I would like to bring a meal to a palliative care patient and give their family member a day of rest, even if just for one day [V5].

I would try to distract my hospitalized friend or someone in need by discussing comforting topics [telling jokes, making humorous remarks] to help them shift their thoughts, even if just a little [V7].

At suitable times, I would try to help others in need by engaging in conversations, reading books, or doing their shopping [V10].

I would be present for tests and treatments to support the person and ensure their feelings are positive. If they are anxious or scared, I would find a topic or activity to distract them [e.g., reading a book] [V11, V31, V32, V33].

For a person who has lost their sight, you could describe the facial expressions and environment while watching a movie. I would like to be someone's eyes, ears, or hands and feet [V12].

I can assist with their shopping and any needs outside the hospital [V13].

I would like to read books and poems, find topics of interest to them to discuss, and help open up their inner world to relax them [V14], [V40].

I would like to solve puzzles, play chess, and teach Alzheimer's and dementia patients, sharing my knowledge to be helpful [V18].

Washing their clothes, boosting their spirituality and motivation, and providing psychological support are also very valuable [V19].

I would like to share that I can easily provide support on specific days and times for tasks related to the outside world that those in need of palliative care [in a home setting] might have difficulty managing, such as paying electricity and water bills, handling applications to official authorities, and other bank or tax office transactions that they cannot attend to themselves [V21].

I would communicate with the family and provide support to them. I would also interact with the patient. I can arrange appointments for the patients and take them to check-ups. I would facilitate visits with people the patient wants to see. Additionally, I can help with household chores [V23].

I can support individuals by staying with the patient for a couple of hours if they need to go to a health center or hospital to obtain supplies or see a doctor and cannot leave the house. If the patient and their family can go outside, I can take them for a drive to get fresh air and help them get away from their current environment [V24].

I can feed the patient, administer their medication, and measure their blood pressure. If the patient can speak, I can chat with them; if they enjoy reading, I can read books to them [V25].

I would like to contribute to the process by giving presentations on music and poetry for palliative patients [V26].

I would try to help older patients with walking, participating in their shared memories, and assisting with tasks like shopping and banking [V28].

Since I attend folk dance classes, I would also provide support in this area [V29].

I can help a conscious patient relax by deepening the conversation to express their current thoughts in words, feed them, and manage their medication [V30].

I can care for patients without family. I would sit by their side and listen to them. I would talk to them to make them feel that they are not alone and that there are people who care about them. I can provide emotional support, boost their spirits, and follow up on hospital procedures [V37].

As a man, although I may not be able to provide as much service as women, I would like to assist with technical matters. I would like to work on repairing and maintaining equipment such as chairs, beds, and other tools used by patients and staff [V44].

Physical health is just as important as mental and emotional well-being. I practice a sport that has a remarkable effect on individuals by integrating both. I can do simple Tai Chi with them, and face yoga is also included [V48].

Caregiver Burden I know that my late spouse, A, experienced a lot of difficulties due to dementia. For this reason, I want to help caregivers in the hospital [V2].

I would provide support to caregivers according to their needs [V3], [V35].

I had my parents and three siblings, but I felt alone and abandoned. I deeply experienced loneliness, helplessness, and social isolation. I would like to share and alleviate loneliness by talking with someone in an analogous situation [V6].

If possible, I would support caregivers by completely relieving them for a while so they can rest, relax, and clear their minds and spirits. I would ensure that their loved ones are fully cared for while the caregivers are away for a few hours or a few days, allowing them to rest and recuperate [V9].

I would assist with tasks such as cleaning and laundry for the caregivers of patients who are bedridden for long periods [V13].

During the caregiver's rest periods, I could accompany the patient myself [V15].

Volunteers' involvement with patients relieves the caregivers. Being away from the environment and taking a breather not only boosts their spirits but also provides hope for the future [V17].

I can provide psychological support to the patient's caregiver and assist them on certain nights. For example, I would ensure they get some rest and offer help through communication, as far as my abilities allow [V20].

I can visit the caregivers and listen to their concerns while chatting with them over sweet and salty homemade snacks [V22].

I can stay by the patient's side to give the caregiver a break, handle external errands such as pharmacy, market, and grocery shopping, and cook meals according to their preferences [V25].

I can give the caregivers a rest for 3–4 h and visit them [V27, V33, V38, V41, V34].

I can give him/her a break to rest his/her companion, allowing him/her to get away from the hospital environment and take a day for himself/herself by walking and getting fresh air [V30].

3.2. Educational Support Dimension

In the social volunteer project, I can support by taking courses or seminars for training if needed [V8].

I would like to work in education and consultancy services within palliative care [V42].

I can volunteer to provide information and suggestions for Alzheimer's patients [V43].

If I were to volunteer, I would encourage the widespread adoption of volunteering by motivating young students to participate in such activities, even if only for a short period [V55].

I could organize small-scale celebrations for patients on special occasions, as long as their health permits [V56].

When it comes to education and training, I would volunteer to work in every aspect. I would read and explain and use my training in drama and theater to dramatize various topics [V57].

3.3. Medical/Clinical Support Dimension

I would like to work as a physiotherapist in palliative care as a volunteer. Palliative care patients may need assistance with certain movements they are unable to perform [V67].

After retiring, I participated in various courses such as first aid and I want to contribute as well [V29].

I can measure the patient's blood pressure/temperature and provide massages [V39].

If the patient is bedridden and unable to turn themselves, I can apply medication recommended by the doctor to prevent bedsores [V41].

I think I can support all these tasks, such as maintaining proper nutrition, personal care, administering medications on time, and providing ongoing medical support at home or from healthcare institutions [V50].

I can share my knowledge and experiences with dialysis patients and their families. I can provide training on how to change fluids during peritoneal dialysis, apply hygiene rules, and care for catheters [V52].

3.4. Financial Support Dimension

I can provide all kinds of assistance to individuals facing financial difficulties. I believe it's important to buy them pajamas, nightgowns, and their favorite foods and fruits [V19].

Based on my observations, they often have significant financial needs [such as toilet paper, diapers, and paper towels]. I would like to cover these as much as my budget allows [V22].

I can provide financial assistance to patients in need. I can help with their shopping [V23].

I would buy small gifts for them [V49].

3.5. Spiritual Support Dimension

I would like to volunteer to support the fulfillment of patients' psychosocial and spiritual needs [V51].

I would like to communicate with patients who have not yet lost consciousness and provide them with spiritual support. At the same time, I would support the patients' relatives by talking about life and death as much as I can, giving them encouragement, and reflecting positively on the patient [V58].

3.6. Pediatric Palliative Care

I would like to tell stories to children using puppets because it is entertaining and motivating [V51, V56].

I would help children [V13].

I would play their favorite games with small children, read their favorite books, help with their lessons, and do arts and crafts with them. I would also buy gifts they would like and make treats such as cakes, cookies, candies, pastries, and börek [savory pastries] to bring to them [V28].

If our patient is a child, I would engage them in various games and entertainment activities to ensure they have a good time. If they have the opportunity to go outside, I would take them on outings, ensure they have an enjoyable experience, and assist in lightening the load for their parents [V44].

Since I understand and love children's world very well, I would try to address any gaps in their education if they are unable to attend school. I could engage in activities like drawing, paper covering, puzzles, and paper cutting with them. I would fulfill all the needs that a mother could provide [V53].

With the necessary training provided to me, I can offer spiritual and psychological support to hospitalized children, read books to them, and perform massage therapy [V65].

4. Discussion

The rising demand for health and social care is driven by rapid population aging, social exchange, and care workforce shrinkage, which requires innovative initiatives to harness the time and energy of older adults [13]. Many older people in their 60s and 70s remain capable of contributing to society. Productive engagement encompasses unpaid and paid activities that generate goods and services for society, such as volunteering. Late-life volunteering has gained increasing attention in health promotion, as volunteering contributes to better health, the prevention of depression, and an improved quality of life among older adults. Promoting volunteering can also facilitate mutual help and strengthen the community's caring capacity, potentially reducing the reliance on care professionals [14–16].

The average age of the Ege U3A students participating in the study was 67.47 (60–89) years. The approach of the older people towards voluntary services at U3A, where they actively engage in self-development and healthy aging, showed a significant change before and after the palliative care training we provided. Many older individuals who experience restrictions in their social lives frequently face issues such as social isolation, depression, and physical limitations. These health problems can partially reduce their potential for volunteering. With the training we provided, older individuals whose awareness of volunteering was strengthened and supported were encouraged to volunteer in specialized areas such as palliative care, despite their physical limitations. Their strength and motivation enabled them to contribute in meaningful ways. In a quantitative study conducted in Italy with a single-group pre-test/post-test design involving 19 older participants, it was reported that, after one year, there was an increase in the physical capacities, walking ability, and social participation of the participants [17]. Jenkinson and colleagues (2013) found in their review of forty experimental studies that older individuals who volunteer in their communities experience an improved quality of life and a reduction in depressive feelings and thoughts [18]. In our study, the U3A students expressed that social participation made them feel good, both psychologically and physiologically, and that helping others motivated them. The life experiences and instincts of U3A students to share their experiences in palliative care demonstrate that they can make the most significant contributions in the social support dimension.

Despite the increased participation rates of older adults in volunteer activities in developed countries in recent years, the advancements and research in this field remain insufficient [19,20]. In Türkiye, when examining volunteer activities, it was observed that sports organizations, religious groups, and social service charities dominate in terms of financial support, while rights-based organizations and support groups/NGOs make up a very small percentage. In Türkiye, volunteer activities often include charitable assistance to neighbors, families, and the poor; food aid during religious holidays and other special occasions; scholarships and educational support provided by foundations; assistance from organized civil society organizations; practices such as giving alms [zekat]. As a result, ongoing volunteer services often rely on financial support and are limited to a single type of activity [21]. Participation in sustained volunteer services is quite limited. The World Giving Index, published annually by the Charities Aid Foundation, periodically evaluates countries' levels of volunteering by considering metrics such as making monetary donations to charities, spending time volunteering with organizations, and helping those in need or strangers. According to the latest report from 2022, which includes Türkiye, the Charities Aid Foundation's World Giving Index ranked Türkiye 104th globally, with a participation rate of 11% in volunteer activities, including spending time or money on these activities [22]. This indicates that Türkiye is ranked quite low globally in terms of volunteer activities and is at an insufficient level [23].

For Turkish people, policymakers can encourage public awareness by preparing public service announcements, posters on public transportation, and short videos in subways, hospitals, and schools for recruiting volunteers. The need for volunteers increases as each day passes. Practices such as hiring people who are in an organization voluntarily could also be implemented, as is the case in European countries.

Older individuals have indicated that, when they are unable to provide physical assistance, they can offer financial support within their budget, prepare and deliver meals, and read books to others. The 2013 report "Volunteering and Older Adults" from Canada emphasizes similar support provided by volunteer seniors and highlights the importance of this support for both the country and the older person [24]. In our study, the older participants thoroughly grasped the need for social and psychological support for palliative care patients, as conveyed through the training content. In their written statements, they expressed a desire to assist with patients' shopping, handle bureaucratic tasks [such as banking and paying bills], and provide spiritual support and motivation by either accompanying patients in palliative care services or taking them out of the service for a day. In Denmark, which implements volunteer services at the highest standards globally [25], it is noted that volunteers involved in strengthening social support networks not only provide support to the older person but also create motivation for themselves. Similar results have been highlighted in other European countries as well [26–28].

Our study highlights that older individuals, in particular, show a notable interest in volunteering in the field of pediatric palliative care. Older individuals, having reached a state of spiritual fulfillment and experiencing an increased frequency of loss within their social circles, are navigating the grieving process and grief psychology in a more meaningful way. In Korea, it has been highlighted that older volunteers demonstrate better adaptation to the grieving process and are more adept at managing end-of-life symptoms compared to university students working as pediatric palliative care volunteers [29,30]. Utilizing this potential volunteer strength of older people in pediatric palliative care is highly valuable.

In Türkiye, there is no infrastructure where individuals wishing to volunteer in palliative care can register or receive training to join this system. The services provided are conducted within closed structures of associations, foundations, and non-governmental organizations. In this area, it is necessary to create a database moving from general to specific and to begin by adapting a method suitable for Türkiye's cultural structure from European countries that can successfully maintain this practice. In Turkish culture, although the extended family structure, which traditionally took care of older people at home with its own resources, has evolved into a nuclear family structure, there is still an understanding that families will try to take care of older people with their own means. Alongside the need to preserve this cultural structure, an urgent social support network should be developed for older people who are increasingly forced to live alone, and this network should be primarily provided by the state.

5. Conclusions

In our research, it was observed that older individuals with a high profile of volunteering are willing to work within their physical limitations and resources, and they recognize the need to support patients in this field. When older individuals receive conscious and systematic educational support based on their life experiences, it becomes more feasible and effective to harness this existing potential for volunteering. No previous pilot studies on older volunteers in palliative care have been conducted in Türkiye, according to our research, making this study a pioneering contribution to the volunteer database in this field. The next step of our research will be to train individuals who will volunteer in these areas and ensure their active participation in palliative care services. This will serve as an effective starting point and a motivating application for the development of a volunteer pool in Türkiye.

6. Limitations

Our study was conducted on a limited population of individuals aged 60 and above who had adopted a lifelong learning goal. A more extensive profile analysis on a broader population was not possible, which is a limitation of our research. A group with a high potential to demonstrate a willingness to volunteer was included in this research; therefore, the lack of inclusion of people with physical disabilities or those who see volunteering as an emotional burden is one of the limitations of this research. One of the limitations is that the research results were evaluated immediately after the training, and a similar volunteer motivation could not be evaluated in the long term.

Author Contributions: Conceptualization, G.D. and G.P.; methodology, Y.K.Ö.; software, S.Ş.; validation, G.D., G.P. and Y.K.Ö.; formal analysis, Y.K.Ö.; investigation, G.D. and G.P.; resources; G.D. and Y.K.Ö.; data curation, G.D. and G.P.; writing—original draft preparation, G.D. and G.P.; writing—review and editing, G.D. and G.P., Y.K.Ö. and S.Ş.; visualization, S.Ş.; supervision, S.Ş.; project administration, G.D.; funding acquisition, G.D., Y.K.Ö., S.Ş. and G.P. All authors have read and agreed to the published version of the manuscript.

Funding: This research was funded by Ege University Rectorate Scientific Research Projects Coordination Unit Coordination Office grant number 30796. https://bap.ege.edu.tr/ accessed on 7 September 2023.

Institutional Review Board Statement: The study was conducted in accordance with the Declaration of Helsinki and approved by the Ethics Committee of Ege University Medical Research Ethics Committee [protocol code 23-9T/58 and accessed on 7 September 2023].

Informed Consent Statement: Informed consent was obtained from all subjects involved in the study.

Data Availability Statement: Data are contained within the article.

Acknowledgments: We thank to University of the Third Age students for administrative and technical support.

Conflicts of Interest: The authors declare no conflicts of interest.

Abbreviations

U3A: Ege University of the Third Age; WHO: The World Health Organization.

References

1. Güntert, S.T.; Wehner, T.; Mieg, H.A. Definition of Volunteer Work and a Model of Volunteer Activity. In *Organizational, Motivational, and Cultural Contexts of Volunteering. SpringerBriefs in Psychology*; Springer: Cham, Switzerland, 2022. [CrossRef]
2. Sakar, Z.M. İstatistikler ışığında yaşlı bakım hizmetleri alanında ülkemizde uygulanan politikalar. *Sos. Polit. Çalışmaları Derg.* **2023**, *23*, 179–203. [CrossRef]
3. Kurtkapan, H. Aktif yaşlılık ve yerel yönetim uygulamaları: İstanbul örneği. *Senex Yaşlılık Çalışmaları Derg.* **2018**, *2*, 38–52.
4. Arbeit, B.F.; Konsumentenschutz, S.U. *Freiwilligenengagement Bevölkerungsbefragung 2016*; Archivnummer: 23.004.027; BMASK: Wien, Austria, 2016.
5. Palaz, F.S. Volunteering Among Adults Aged 50+ and their Motivations for Volunteering: The Case of Europe. *J. Econ. Cult. Soc.* **2021**, *64*, 163–182. [CrossRef]
6. Sahin, S.; Kocakoc, N.; Arayici, M.E.; Baybas, B.K.; Boyacioglu, H.; Akcicek, S.F. Evaluation of the quality of life in the university of third age students: A cross-sectional study. *Eur. Geriatr. Med.* **2023**, *14*, 389–396. [CrossRef]
7. Oğlak, S.; Canatan, A. Yaşam boyu öğrenme ve aktif yaşlanma bakış açısından Üçüncü Yaş Üniversiteleri: İyi uygulama örnekleri. *Yaşlı Sorunları Araştırma Derg. YSAD* **2020**, *13*, 131–141. [CrossRef]

8. Çölgeçen, Y.; Çölgeçen, H. Aktif yaşlanma açısından hayat boyu öğrenme: Üçüncü yaş üniversiteleri. *Turk. Stud. Educ.* **2020**, *15*, 2495–2511. [CrossRef]
9. Altun, F. *Ekonomik ve Sosyal Boyutlarıyla Yaşlılık (Içindeki; Aca, Z. Aktif Yaşlanma Kavramının Temel Çerçevesini Anlamak ve Türkiye'de Aktif Yaşlanmaya Yönelik Politikalar;* Gazi Kitapevi: Ankara, Türkiye, 2021.
10. Gesell, D.; Hodiamont, F.; Bausewein, C.; Koller, D. Accessibility to specialist palliative care services in Germany: A geographical network analysis. *BMC Health Serv. Res.* **2023**, *23*, 786. [CrossRef]
11. Aslan, Y. Türkiye'de ve Dünya'da palyatif bakım modellerine genel bakış. *Anadolu Güncel Tıp Derg* **2020**, *2*, 19–27. [CrossRef]
12. Tekindal, M.; Özden, A.S.; Gedik, T.E.; Ege, A.; Erim, F.; Tekindal, M.A. Nitel Araştırmaların Raporlanmasında Standartlar: SRQR Kontrol Listesinin Türkçe Uyarlaması. *OPUS Int. J. Soc. Res.* **2021**, *18*, 5425–5443. [CrossRef]
13. Organization for Economic Cooperation and Development. Old-Age Dependency Ratio (Indicator). 2023. Available online: https://data.oecd.org/pop/old-age-dependency-ratio.htm (accessed on 13 March 2023).
14. Lu, S.; Chui, C.; Lum, T.; Liu, T.; Wong, G.; Chan, W. Promoting Late-Life Volunteering with Timebanking: A Quasi-Experimental Mixed-Methods Study in Hong Kong. *Innov. Aging* **2024**, *8*, igae056. [CrossRef]
15. Chan, W.; Chui, C.H.K.; Cheung, J.C.S.; Lum, T.Y.S.; Lu, S. Associations between volunteering and mental health during COVID-19 among Chinese older adults. *J. Gerontol. Soc. Work.* **2021**, *64*, 599–612. [CrossRef]
16. Morawski, L.; Okulicz-Kozaryn, A.; Strzeleck, M. Older volunteering in Europe: The relationship between volunteering and quality of life depends on volunteering rates. *Voluntas* **2022**, *33*, 256–268. [CrossRef]
17. Cristina Gagliardi, C.; Pillemer, K.; Gambella, E.; Piccinini, F.; Fabbietti, P. Benefits for Older People Engaged in Environmental Volunteering and Socializing Activities in City Parks: Preliminary Results of a Program in Italy. *Int. J. Environ. Res. Public Health* **2020**, *17*, 3772. [CrossRef]
18. Jenkinson, C.E.; Dickens, A.P.; Jones, K.; Thompson-Coon, J.; Taylor, R.S.; Rogers, M.; Bambra, C.L.; Lang, I.; Richards, S.H. Is volunteering a public health intervention? A systematic review and meta-analysis of the health and survival of volunteers. *BMC Public Health* **2023**, *13*, 773. [CrossRef]
19. Alsehaimi, A. Impact of volunteer work on improving the quality of social life from the perspective of social work specialists. *Int. J. Soc. Work.* **2023**, *10*, 1. [CrossRef]
20. von Bonsdorff, M.B.; Rantanen, T. Benefits of formal voluntary work among older people. A review. *Aging Clin. Exp. Res.* **2011**, *23*, 162–169. [CrossRef]
21. Erdoğan, E.; Uyan-Semerci, P.; Yentürk, N.; Yurttagüler, L. *Türkiye'de Gönüllülük Deneyimler, Sınırlılıklar ve Yeni Açılımlar;* İstanbul Bilgi Üniversitesi Yayınları: Kasım, Türkiye, 2020; ISBN 978-605-399-567-8.
22. World Giving Index 2022. The Charities Aid Foundation 2022. Available online: https://www.cafonline.org/docs/default-source/about-us-research/caf_world_giving_index_2022_210922-final.pdf (accessed on 5 October 2024).
23. Kesgin, B. Türkiye'de Gönüllülük Çalışmaları Üzerine bir Değerlendirme. *MSGSÜ Sos. Bilim.* **2016**, *13*, 119–131. Available online: https://dergipark.org.tr/tr/download/article-file/757865 (accessed on 6 November 2024).
24. Cook, S.L.; Speevak Sladowski, P. Volunteering and Older Adults Final Report. 2013. Available online: https://volunteer.ca/wp-content/uploads/2024/06/Volunteering_and_Older_Adults_Final_Report_2013.pdf (accessed on 6 November 2024).
25. Ehlers, A.; Naegele, G.; Reichert, M. *Volunteering by Older People in the EU;* European Foundation for the Improvement of Living and Working Conditions: Dublin, Ireland, 2011; ISBN 978-92-897-1012-1. [CrossRef]
26. Steunenberg, B.; van der Mast, R.; Strijbos, M.J.; Inouye, S.K.; Schuurmans, M.J. How trained volunteers can improve the quality of hospital care for older patients. A qualitative evaluation within the hospital elder life program (HELP). *Geriatr. Nurs.* **2016**, *37*, 458–463. [CrossRef]
27. Blair, A.; Bateman, C.; Anderson, K. "They take a lot of pressure of us": Volunteers reducing staf and family care burden and contributing to quality of care for older patients with cognitive impairment in rural hospitals. *Australas J. Ageing* **2019**, *38*, 34–45. [CrossRef]
28. de Sandes-Guimarães, L.V.; Dos Santos, P.C.; Alves, C.P.G.P.; Cervato, C.J.; Silva, A.P.A.; Leão, E.R. The effect of volunteer-led activities on the quality of life of volunteers, residents, and employees of a long-term care institution: A cohort study. *BMC Geriatr.* **2023**, *23*, 151. [CrossRef]
29. Moon, Y.J. Volunteer Experiences of Pediatric Palliative Care among University Students: A Phenomenological Approach. *J. Hosp. Palliat. Care* **2022**, *25*, 121–132. [CrossRef] [PubMed] [PubMed Central]
30. Burbeck, R.; Low, J.; Sampson, E.L.; Scott, R.; Bravery, R.; Candy, B. Volunteer activity in specialist paediatric palliative care: A national survey. *BMJ Support Palliat Care.* **2015**, *5*, 287–293. [CrossRef] [PubMed]

healthcare

MDPI

Article

Preparedness for Caregiving Role and Telehealth Use to Provide Informal Palliative Home Care in Portugal: A Qualitative Study

Paula Caetano [1,2], Ana Querido [1,3,4] and Carlos Laranjeira [1,3,5,*]

1 School of Health Sciences, Polytechnic University of Leiria, Morro do Lena, Campus 2, Alto do Vieiro, Apartado 4137, 2411-901 Leiria, Portugal; pcaetano67@hotmail.com (P.C.); ana.querido@ipleiria.pt (A.Q.)
2 Centro de Saúde de Ourém, Unidade Local de Saúde da Região de Leiria, Rua Dr. Armando Henrique dos Reis Vieira, 2490-546 Ourém, Portugal
3 Centre for Innovative Care and Health Technology (ciTechCare), Polytechnic University of Leiria, Campus 5, Rua das Olhalvas, 2414-016 Leiria, Portugal
4 Center for Health Technology and Services Research (CINTESIS), NursID, University of Porto, 4200-450 Porto, Portugal
5 Comprehensive Health Research Centre (CHRC), University of Évora, 7000-801 Évora, Portugal
* Correspondence: carlos.laranjeira@ipleiria.pt

Abstract: Background/Objectives: Given the increasing occurrence of long-term illnesses, it is imperative to focus on adequately preparing and assisting those who assume the responsibility of caregiving. Our study aims to explore whether caregivers feel prepared to provide informal palliative home care, their experiences, and the usefulness of telehealth in managing daily activities. **Methods:** Using a descriptive qualitative research design and a purposeful sampling technique, thirteen primary family caregivers who provide informal palliative home care were recruited. Data collection was conducted through face-to-face individual interviews conducted from May 2023 to July 2023. Data were analyzed using Braun and Clarke's reflexive thematic analysis. **Results:** Caregivers were mainly female (n = 8) with a mean age of 59.5 years (SD = 9.42). Based on our findings, three overarching themes emerged: (1) becoming a caregiver, (2) support-from-home palliative care team, and (3) telehealth in palliative home care. The reasons that influence the preparedness of family caregivers include their own desires, health conditions, their range of responsibilities, and the consequences that arise from the situation's complexity. Telehealth helps fulfill the patient's wishes to be at home in EoL and provides caregivers with access to professional guidance and support. **Conclusions:** Specialized home-based palliative care teams must be aware of caregivers' self-assurance, knowledge, skills, and aptitudes in carrying out daily responsibilities and in managing emotions to improve preparedness for caregiving, loss, and its aftermath. The provision of professional PC services in the home along with a robust support system for informal caregivers is invaluable.

Keywords: caregivers; home care; palliative care; preparedness; telehealth; qualitative study; Portugal

1. Introduction

Palliative care (PC) plays a crucial role in enhancing the quality of life, particularly during the later stages of illness, and aims to alleviate the burden of the condition. The World Health Organization (WHO) has provided a definition of PC as a strategy that enhances the quality of life for patients and their families who are facing challenges associated with life-threatening illnesses [1]. It is delivered through the management, evaluation, and therapy of pain and other bodily, psychological, and spiritual issues. Since the release of the Quality of Death Index in 2021 [2], there has been a growing emphasis on enhancing the comfort and autonomy that individuals experience during their final stages of life. As highlighted in the Quality of Death Index, end-of-life (EoL) care preferences serve as an indicator of the standard of care provided by PC [2]. While several individual, structural, and contextual factors influence the place of death, a recent umbrella review found that most people preferred to die at home [3]. The crucial factor enabling death at home is the presence of family members or close individuals and their preparedness to assume the responsibility of delivering EoL care for those who desire to die in their own homes [4]. In the context of PC, the term "family" encompasses not just formal relationships but also those that are self-defined or identified by the patient as significant. In this vein, family caregivers (referred to henceforth as caregivers) include family members, friends, or other people who have emotional and social bonds with a patient. They are unpaid lay people with a close supportive role who share the patient's illness experience and who undertake vital care work and emotional management [5]. However, caregivers often lack adequate training to effectively carry out caring responsibilities, especially during the transition from hospital to home [6–8]. Consequently, caregivers frequently experience a sense of unpreparedness when it comes to caring for a person with palliative needs residing at home [9–11]. Several challenges were found during PC transitions from acute care to community-based care, including physical discomfort, medication-related disorientation, ambiguity regarding healthcare obligations, and emotional turmoil [12]. A lack of caregiver preparedness may lead to unforeseen hospital admissions, resulting in significant financial burdens on the healthcare system, potential health hazards for patients, and an augmented workload for caregivers [13]. Caregivers derive purpose from their responsibilities, which motivate them to effectively manage the difficulties associated with taking care of an individual in need [14]. To alleviate the burdens of caregiving and facilitate the ability to maintain a purposeful life both within and outside of their caregiving responsibilities, it is necessary to provide supplementary support [14,15]. Studies have found several important factors related to receiving PC at home, including healthcare accessibility, caregiver support, tailored person-centered care, multidisciplinary care provision, and quality improvement [16,17].

Several studies have demonstrated that specialized home PC teams who provide support for patients and their families at home can result in a higher proportion of individuals being able to die in their own homes, thereby reducing hospital admissions and hospital stays [18–20]. The model of PC organization in Portugal [21] includes palliative care units that offer in-patient care; Hospital Support Palliative Care Teams that provide PC advice and support to the entire hospital structure; and finally, Home Palliative Care Teams (HPCT) that care for patients in their homes, support their families and caregivers, and advise family doctors and nurses who provide care at home [21]. The model implemented in Portugal exemplifies the principles of accessibility and fairness. However, a need for expansion has become apparent, especially in the realm of home-based palliative intervention. Due to financial and structural barriers, as well as low political priority, there are inequalities in access to HPCT [22]. There is evidence of a lack of awareness and comprehension of PC among the Portuguese general population [23]. More exactly, there are misconceptions regarding the goals of palliative care that delay timely PC referrals and restrict informed decision-making.

Given the increasing occurrence of long-term illnesses, it is imperative to focus on adequately preparing and assisting persons who take on the responsibility of caregiving [24]. Caregiving has been linked to diverse outcomes, both positive (like personal development) and negative (like emotional fatigue) [25]. Prior studies have identified that those assuming the responsibility of a caretaker are more susceptible to experiencing injuries and illnesses, including anxiety and despair [26,27]. Some persons may experience caregiver burden due to the growing and intricate nature of some chronic diseases. Specifically, the shift to a demanding caregiving position, where individuals assist with the activities of daily living, was discovered to be linked to the deterioration of caregiver functionality [28]. Individuals may encounter varying levels of burden depending on the nature and regularity of their caregiving responsibilities, as well as their attitudes towards the activities and challenges associated with providing care.

A person-centered approach that prioritizes the intricate needs of the individual rather than the physical aspects of care has not yet been universally adopted in PC settings [29].

Evidence also revealed deficiencies in inter-professional communication, fragmentation of care, and coordination of care [30]. These challenges can be mitigated through digital health technology (DHT) using different telecommunication tools (i.e., a smartphone, tablet, or desktop) to provide healthcare remotely in an interactive or passive mode that could benefit caregivers and care recipients at home. For instance, evidence demonstrates the beneficial effects on caregivers' self-esteem, self-efficacy, mastery, and burden [31]. Given that various chronic ailments can provide distinct difficulties for caregivers, many studies have specifically examined individual chronic illnesses, such as dementia [32] or cancer [33]. Support in various domains may be required by caregivers, and the customization of digital devices has been proposed as a means to address individual caring needs [34]. Specifically, tailoring digital devices and promoting digital literacy could aid in addressing concerns related to the volume and accuracy of general health data, such as excessive information and subpar readability [35,36].

Although earlier studies have examined a wide range of DHT, there is a lack of literature on carers' perceptions of the usage of telehealth to assist in daily activity management [37]. Regarding caregivers who play a major role in caring for people with PC needs, studies that use a qualitative research approach and focus on their experiences are still scarce in the Portuguese context. Therefore, this study aims to explore how caregivers feel prepared to provide informal palliative home care, their experiences, and the usefulness of telehealth in managing daily activities. We hope to contribute a better understanding of their importance for caregivers wishing to support death at home.

2. Materials and Methods

2.1. Study Design

This qualitative descriptive study is part of a wider research project that aims "to co-design, develop, and test the feasibility of the Help2Care-PAL mHealth app that addresses the needs of caregivers of palliative patients cared for at home" [38]. Qualitative methodologies are valuable for examining the attitudes, values, and motivations that underlie individual decisions on health [39]. In this vein, the social constructivism theory underpins this study, and knowledge was co-created through the interaction between researchers and participants [39].

This study adheres to the consolidated standards for reporting qualitative research (COREQ) recommendations [40] (Supplementary Table S1).

2.2. Sample and Recruitment

Using a purposeful sampling technique [41], caregivers were invited to take part in this study if they fulfilled the following inclusion criteria: (a) Men or women aged at least 18 years with close bonds to the person receiving PC at home, i.e., based on the NECPAL tool; patients were included if they positively answered the question "*Would you be surprised if this patient dies in the next year?*" and if they also fulfilled at least one of clinical indicators in terms of disease severity and progression and the disease-specific indicators [42]. (b) Unpaid primary carers who provide informal palliative home care. (c) Primary carers residing with the patient or living near the patient. Participants were excluded if they provided care to family members residing in nursing homes, if they had cognitive impairment, or if they could not understand and speak Portuguese.

To determine the number of participants for this study, we used the criterion of data saturation. Recruitment stopped when including more people or data no longer contributed important information [43].

2.3. Data Collection

Data collection was conducted through face-to-face individual interviews conducted from May 2023 to July 2023. Suitable caregivers were preselected by the staff of a HPCT from the Alentejo region (Portugal). Subsequently, the first author (P.C.) contacted participants via telephone, providing them with detailed information about the study and scheduling initial interviews, including the time and location. Every caregiver supplied written consent after being fully briefed. The interviews were conducted in a private room within the participant's home. The risk of being perceived as intrusive was balanced against the benefits of establishing a safe environment and demonstrating sensitivity to requirements.

The semi-structured interview guide drew from the current research [38,44,45] and the authors' clinical expertise in the subject. It included the following topics: (a) perceived preparedness for different domains of caregiving, including communication with relatives and considerations about the caregivers' concerns; (b) caregivers' perspectives and challenges when caring at home and using telehealth in health-seeking behaviors.

We conducted a pilot interview and made some minor adjustments, which allowed for the incorporation of the pilot interview as part of our data. The first author (P.C.) carried out all individual face-to-face interviews. Interviews lasted between 40 and 60 min and were audio-recorded and transcribed verbatim. Each interview commenced as an open conversation when caregivers were encouraged to express their experiences and preferences regarding their role as caregivers and their requirements for home care support. The interview guide served as a prompt during the interview to guarantee that the aforementioned subjects were addressed. Open questions, such as inquiries about individuals, objects, or concepts, were posed to expand or refine the scope of interest. Interview notes were made after each interview, mainly to describe the atmosphere during the interviews. No repeat interviews were carried out. Further, all transcripts were returned to participants for comments and/or corrections.

Given that the interviews were conducted in European Portuguese, the interview extracts were translated and subsequently back-translated to ensure the preservation of the original meaning. Alpha-numeric codes (P1, P2, ...) were associated with data extracts to safeguard the anonymity of caregivers.

2.4. Data Analysis

Inspired by Braun and Clarke's reflexive thematic analysis, data were analyzed to define the conceptual framework of the main topics that emerged from the interviews [46]. Table 1 depicts the six-phase process as proposed by Braun and Clarke [47]. Every interview was carefully analyzed, and the process of coding commenced using phrases that were the length of a sentence from the text. The codes were categorized into themes and modified following each interview. After completing five interviews, the coding process transitioned to including lengthier phrases consisting of multiple sentences. An attempt was made to transition from descriptive codes to interpretive codes in order to discern the wider relationships among participants' experiences. Following the completion of each interview, the coding matrix underwent a thorough evaluation to identify the prominent elements in the participants' experiences [46]. Qualitative data analysis software WebQDA (Version 3.0, Universidade de Aveiro, Aveiro, Portugal) was used to facilitate data storage and management.

The research team used an inductive approach to generate thematic categories. Several research meetings were conducted to facilitate the sharing and comparison of the findings, as well as the identification of common themes. If there were differing perspectives, a decision was made by consensus. All researchers included in this study are registered nurses (RN) with diverse perspectives and firsthand experiences in the field of EoL care. The main researcher (P.C.) is a female mental health nurse specialist who works in community care and has practical experience with PC individuals. The second and third researchers possess expertise in working, teaching, and researching in the field of PC, as well as expertise in qualitative studies (A.Q. and C.L.). All researchers have experience as informal caregivers of their older loved ones and faced the difficulties of balancing their professional, familial, and caregiving roles. These diverse experiences enhanced the interpretation of the material and decreased potential biases.

Table 1. Six-phase process of reflexive thematic analysis [46,47].

Analytic Phases	Description
Phase one: familiarization with the data	Examining and reviewing the complete dataset to gain a deep understanding of the collected information.
Phase two: generating initial codes	Coding is the systematic procedure used to generate concise descriptive or interpretive labels for components of information that may be pertinent to the research question(s).
Phase three: generating themes	This phase commences once all pertinent data items have been encoded. The emphasis transitions from the analysis of individual data elements within the dataset to the analysis of the collective significance and relevance throughout the dataset.
Phase four: reviewing potential themes	Systematic examination of the candidate themes connected with the coded data items and the complete dataset.
Phase five: defining and naming theme	During this stage, the researcher produces a comprehensive examination of the thematic framework. Each distinct topic and sub-theme must be articulated with both the dataset and the research question(s).
Phase six: producing the report	Providing a succinct and captivating narrative of the data, both within and across themes.

2.5. *Trustworthiness*

We employed Guba and Lincoln's trustworthiness criteria [48]. Firstly, we established credibility by employing investigator triangulation and collecting qualitative data from multiple sources, such as interview transcripts, quotations, and researcher notes. Keeping an open-minded attitude, recognizing personal biases, and practicing self-reflection throughout the entire study process helped validate findings and enhanced their credibility. Secondly, we achieved transferability by providing comprehensive descriptions of the study design, participants, context, sampling, data collection, and analysis. Thirdly, we ensured dependability by subjecting our study to an external audit conducted by other researchers. Lastly, we attained confirmability by documenting reflexive reports during data collection and analysis. Peer debriefing and reflexive journaling enabled researchers to record their thoughts, biases, and reflections, promoting transparency and reducing subjectivity [48].

2.6. *Ethics*

This study was carried out in compliance with the Declaration of Helsinki and the European General Data Protection Regulation (GDPR2016/679). Permission was sought and granted by the Ethics Committee of Unidade Local de Saúde—Baixo Alentejo (code: 7.4.1. approved on 15 February 2023). Before harvesting data, participants were informed about this study's objectives and the possibility of terminating their participation without any consequences. Those who agreed to participate signed an informed consent form. There were no financial rewards associated with participation. The personal data of the participants was anonymized in the material, and only the authors had access to it. All participant data were compiled in a digital folder only accessible by the principal investigator. Archives are to be destroyed one year after completion of the study.

Participants were provided with follow-up contacts if they experienced distressing emotions or thoughts during the interviews. A follow-up contact was not requested by any of the participants.

3. Results

3.1. Sample Characteristics

In total, 13 individual interviews with family carers were conducted. Eight were female with a mean age of 59.5 ± 9.42 years (range of 44 to 82 years). The main participants in this study were primarily spouses (n = 5) or children (n = 7) who were responsible for providing care to their family members. The time in the caregiving role varied between 4 months and 15 years (average time = 40.5 months). Most care recipients had a cancer illness trajectory (n = 8). A sample description is provided in Table 2.

Table 2. Participants' background (n = 13).

Participant	Sex	Age	Illness Trajectory (Care Recipient)	Education Level	Relationship with Care Recipient	Time in the Caregiver Role
P1	Male	63	Heart failure	9th grade (3rd cycle of basic education)	Son	1.5 years
P2	Female	44	Cancer	Licentiate's degree	Granddaughter	1 year
P3	Female	57	Cancer	12th grade (secondary education)	Daughter	8 months
P4	Female	53	Cancer	Licentiate's degree	Daughter	1 year
P5	Female	66	Cancer	Licentiate's degree	Daughter	7 years
P6	Male	70	Cancer	4th grade (1st cycle of basic education)	Husband	4 months
P7	Male	48	Neurodegenerative disease	12th grade (secondary education)	Husband	2.5 years
P8	Female	62	Dementia	Licentiate's degree	Daughter	15 years
P9	Female	82	Dementia	4th grade (1st cycle of basic education)	Wife	4 years
P10	Female	56	Dementia	9th grade (3rd cycle of basic education)	Daughter	3.5 years
P11	Female	53	Cancer	12th grade (secondary education)	Wife	5 months
P12	Female	60	Cancer	4th grade (1st cycle of basic education)	Daughter	2 years
P13	Female	60	Cancer	4th grade (1st cycle of basic education)	Wife	5 years

3.2. Overview of Findings

The thematic analysis resulted in three themes and seven subthemes, as indicated in Table 3. The factors that influence the preparedness of caregivers include their own desires, health conditions, their range of responsibilities, and the consequences arising from the situation's complexity. Furthermore, telehealth helped caregivers in their daily activities at home, namely in symptom management and self-care promotion. However, participants indicated some drawbacks and challenges. These findings are discussed in more detail in the following sections.

Table 3. Main themes and subthemes.

Main Themes	Sub-Themes
Become a caregiver	Caregiving as a natural decision
	Imposed caregiving
Support from home palliative care team	Compassionate caring relationships
	Managing complex situations and emotional turmoil
	Participating in treatment decision-making
Telehealth in palliative home care	Symptom management and self-care promotion
	Drawbacks and challenges of telehealth

3.2.1. Became a Caregiver

This main category outlines the nature of becoming a caregiver either by personal choice or imposed circumstances.

(a) Caregiving as a natural decision

Participants demonstrated that they became caregivers by voluntary choice, either by their own decision or the influence of others. This was driven by cultural imperatives, leading to a strong desire to help as much as possible. P3's switch to caring was motivated by her desire to reciprocate the attention her father had provided her during his youth: *I don't want to give up my father, I don't see being at home or with him longer as a sacrifice. In fact, I take advantage of every moment I can to be with him.*

Similarly, P8's choice to engage in caregiving was motivated by a strong sense of filial reciprocity towards her mother:

> *I chose to be a caregiver. I do this with a lot of love and it was always something I wanted to do. It was taking care of my mother, because she was a caregiver and I absolutely didn't want anyone else to take care of her.*

Although family caregivers had no prior experience of caring for someone with PC needs, they expressed a desire to uphold the patient's overall health and comfort by enabling EoL care in a setting that was both comfortable and familiar to the patient.

> P7: *I had never taken care of anyone, and I needed to learn something. Even though it's different from what a physiotherapist does, I know that when she needs it and he can't, I can help her in some way with the exercises so that she feels more comfortable.*

> P5: *Yes, it's not only a benefit for me, but I think it's also a benefit for my mother. I always try to make sure she stays "alive", connected with us, even though sometimes that's difficult.*

Two participants also expressed their intention to safeguard and assist the patient, which influenced the families' choice to manage EoL care in their own home.

> P3: *Being focused essentially on the person's well-being or on transmitting tranquillity, love, and security to the people we are caring for, I think is fundamental.*

> P13: *I feel good about complying with his wishes. He's fine, after all he's home, in the place he always wanted to be.*

(b) Imposed caregiving

Some participants experienced a change in their circumstances that was not within their power or choice but was influenced by social expectations.

> P1: *We are three brothers and none of them showed interest in taking care of my mother. I ended up having to take over (. . .) I stopped having a life of my own, I had to give up a lot of things.*

P6: *I am married to her, and I have responsibilities towards my wife. I had no other option.*

Additionally, handling multiple roles and a feeling of duty to provide care and support also hindered the desire for marital independence.

P8: *Today, I recognize that the need for permanent care made me put my marriage on the back burner. My husband and I have given up several things on several occasions so that I can always be present.*

Being a caregiver intersects with different areas of life. Caregivers face difficulties when handling conflicting demands between caregiving and other important duties and obligations, which are described as "overwhelming" and "disruptive". Caregivers also grappled with caregiving demands imposed by others when sometimes they felt limited due health constraints.

P9: *With dementia, he (*husband*) sometimes becomes aggressive, which makes me feel extremely overwhelmed. I try not to value it, but it's very difficult. My daughter tells me to go ahead, because he is very sick. But it hurts to hear what he says, because I also have my health problems and I try very hard to give him the best.*

P12: *Despite trying to always be there to support my mother at this stage, I have to maintain another professional activity to cover expenses, which is very demanding.*

3.2.2. Support from Home Palliative Care Team

This theme reflects the person-centered care promoted by the PC team, whether through close communication or by supporting the management of complex situations and shared decision-making.

(a) Compassionate caring relationships

Caregivers believed that these interactions enhanced PC professionals' comprehension of their caregiving requirements and that a strong rapport with professionals fostered caregivers' sense of being appreciated as individuals and, to some degree, relieved feelings of isolation and disbelief.

P1: *I can't imagine what my mother would have become if it weren't for them (the team). We live in a remote village and contact with the team helped reduce the isolation we felt. She often has crises and whenever I need to, I contact the team who helps me deal with the uncontrolled symptoms.*

Despite P4's initial negative stereotype that associated PC with abandonment, over time, she reported having changed her perception.

P4: *I always thought that palliative care was used when there was nothing else to do. My daughter worked in palliative care and helped me change my mind. Furthermore, the community palliative care team has been a fundamental anchor in monitoring my mother. They are very kind, and we have built a relationship of trust.*

(b) Managing complex situations and emotional turmoil

Most of the participants expressed significant concerns over intense anxiety and worry associated with the uncertain fate of the patient's decline towards the EoL. They emphasized how this impacted their overall well-being. Further, participants highlighted the emotional challenge when they thought about impending death and future life.

P4: *The biggest concern is having to watch him suffer (father) and trying to understand what he is feeling. The anguish that is generated is the worst thing for those who care (...) When I see him worse, I think that death is near, and it makes me feel so sad.*

P2: *My concern is facing existential suffering and the human frailty when death is near. I talk openly about imminent death with the team, but it's so difficult though to talk about loss and its aftermath. What will it be like afterwards?*

Families must deal with abrupt fluctuations in the patient's well-being without sufficient understanding of what to anticipate and how to respond. Consequently, it is unsurprising that caregivers (as well as patients) experience distressing situations intertwined with the patient's emotional connection to their family. The complexity of daily care situations generates in caregivers a "merry-go-round of emotions".

> P11: *It's a mix of feelings. When there is a good day, I can get up and be filled with joy. But, on the other hand, when things get worse, there is sadness and frustration. Yesterday I cried with emotion when I saw him sitting. But then there's always a brake, something that doesn't let me live to the fullest... But the palliative care team helps me deal with these challenges.*

> P7: *When they come to the house, they are never there to clock in or do chores, everything they do is with love and care. Besides, they are always available. I have had to contact nurses by phone, and even if they don't answer right away, they return the call as soon as possible. For us caregivers, this is a comfort, especially when we are having a lot of difficulties. I give you the example of fan leaks (i.e., BIPAP) which sometimes leave me distressed.*

Occasionally, there were instances of discord between the desires of patients, the capabilities of caregivers, and the perception of what was appropriate for the patient. This could impact the standard of care delivered and the overall carer experience. The HPCT assists in resolving care conflicts, particularly when patients' nourishment or eating declines just a little.

> P12: *What we desire is not always the same as what others value. I realized this when my mother asked me to leave her in bed and I insisted on getting her up. After all, what I wanted was for her to get better. But my expectation was unrealistic. The nurse told me that I was doing a good job, after all I just wanted to do my best...*

> P6: *In addition to her physical limitations, the most difficult thing is being able to feed her. I've been told not to worry, but it's so hard to watch her waste away.*

Finally, one participant stated it was through the HPCT that he became aware of the existence of peer-support groups for caregivers that offer the possibility to openly discuss challenging events and gain insight into how others manage them.

> P7: *The team doctor told me about the APELA (Portuguese Association of Patients with Multiple Sclerosis) which offers support to caregivers. It was from there that I met other people experiencing identical processes, which is very important for exchanging experiences. After all, we are "not alone" in our experiences and emotions.*

(c) Participating in treatment decision-making

All participants expressed complete satisfaction with the services provided by HPCT and appeared mainly at ease in delivering patient care in a home setting. Many participants were inspired by a PC team in terms of their comprehension of palliation and the standard of caregiving. They expressed a desire for the patient to avoid being admitted to the hospital.

> P7: *There were several times when I was heard by the team about my wife's condition, the objective was to keep her comfortable, avoiding a trip to the emergency department.*

> P2: *Our goal as a family has always been to ensure the best for my grandmother, and when we were told that we could care for her at home with the support of the team, that was very important. It was the care we wanted, and our wishes were respected.*

Providing instruction to caregivers on medical interventions, such as administering subcutaneous injections and treating wounds, as well as ensuring that professionals are available around the clock for medical guidance, was deemed very important by caregivers. Receiving counseling for EoL and emotional support was also found to be beneficial.

P6: *I have the support of the team.... Her tumour was external and was bleeding a lot. She even had radiotherapy and the wound was very "ugly". It wasn't easy for me to treat, but I did it based on the guidance the team gave.*

P4: *When my mother had severe pain and would not give in to oral morphine, they switched the opioid to the subcutaneous route and taught me how to manage the therapy. At first it wasn't easy, but when I realized that she got better it made me feel valued.*

P5: *In moments when I am less well, the team understands this and tries to help me with guidance. They are always available when I need. I feel listened to, which is very important when we live in constant stress... sometimes we just need to be heard and have our concerns attended to.*

Interestingly, one participant reinforced the role of the caregiver in detecting changes in patients' behavior that are sometimes underestimated by professionals.

P4: *The fact that you are with her 24 h a day, 7 days, makes you more sensitive to identifying changes that when the nurses come to the house, they cannot perceive. So, I try to talk to them and participate in decisions about adjusting therapy.*

3.2.3. Telehealth in Palliative Home Care

Although there are limitations to telehealth use, this theme underlines that its use enhances and expands caregivers' ability to connect with PC professionals from the comfort of their homes.

(a) Symptom management and self-care promotion

Caregivers considered that telehealth provided them with more access to professionals in emergency situations (i.e., whenever they required immediate assistance), giving them a feeling of not being alone. They experienced a sense of relief during emergency situations when the staff would send them a text message containing the name of the medication to be administered, and thereafter provide a follow-up either on the same day or the next day.

P3: *Not long ago he (father) had a crisis bout of hiccups, and it was exasperating... and I asked the team to do a teleconsultation, which helped me understand what I could do immediately. They also sent me messages with information that supported care.*

The caregivers needed to be aware that professionals were accessible to them, providing care and monitoring them through telehealth. This fostered emotions of nurturance, attachment, alleviation, serenity, and heightened safety.

P5: *I have never used digital resources but knowing that they are available generates security and some relief.*

Monitoring symptoms at home allowed for the effective reporting of symptoms to the HPCT, and conducting follow-ups remotely was seen as less intrusive compared to a phone call. Participants in teleconsultations with HPCT experienced focused responsiveness and opportunities for direct consensus on the allocation of responsibilities for future actions.

P1: *I make a point of recording the frequency and intensity of symptoms, I use the Edmonton scale, and then I send it via WhatsApp to the team and they tell me what I should do.*

When PC needed to be increased, participants mentioned that telehealth may intensify face-to-face support as physical function worsens. P2 stated: *Telehealth enables me to discern those who necessitate additional in-person assistance. In my situation, as my husband's health continues to decline, professionals visit him more regularly since he is no longer able to utilize telehealth systems.*

Lastly, P10 mentioned that the professionals on the team recommended a free app with some mindfulness exercises to relax: *Since I started using it, I have felt greater peace of mind, I never thought it would work, but I feel good. These are moments of self-care that are very important for us caregivers.*

(b) Drawbacks and challenges of telehealth

However, some caregivers had a sense of insecurity when utilizing telehealth due to their limited digital literacy. While participants recognized the value of telehealth, limited knowledge, unfamiliarity with the technology, and misinformation posed barriers to the utilization of telehealth.

> P3: *Digital information has very good things, but we have to know how to filter… the information is not always the most appropriate.*
>
> P6: *I have difficulty using cell phones… they offered me a smartphone and I had to give it up because I couldn't get used to it and I always had to get help from my grandchildren. I'm from the time when these things didn't exist. They've already explained it to me, but I have difficulty handling it.*

4. Discussion

To the best of our knowledge, this is one of the first attempts to explore caregivers' preparedness to provide informal palliative home care, their experiences, and how helpful telehealth is to managing daily activities. The knowledge gained from this study is particularly intriguing as it provides a more profound comprehension of home-based PC interventions and their potential impact on caregivers.

Several reasons influence family members to offer home-based PC for their ill relatives. Among these factors, family values were identified as a significant driving force leading a family member to decide to provide care and assume the role of caregiver [45,49]. Family caregivers aimed to preserve the patient's well-being by enabling EoL care in a location the patient would perceive as pleasant and familiar [11,45,49,50]. Adult children who had cared for an ailing parent felt a sense of obligation to reciprocate the affection they had received from their parents, which was also a significant influence [51,52]. Despite challenging circumstances, a family's determination to safeguard and assist the patient formed the foundation for their choice to administer EoL care in the comfort of their own home [52]. The combination of these values enabled family members to maintain their dedication to their caregiving responsibilities and provided the necessary strength to navigate the intricate difficulties associated with caregiving [49]. As underlined by the evidence, the concept of reciprocity of care refers to the caregivers' sense of giving back to their loved ones [53]. This is strongly influenced by cultural and religious beliefs, as well as the assumption that family caregivers should receive assistance.

The findings emphasize that most caregivers had no prior experience in providing care for people with PC needs, which aligns with previous studies indicating that caregivers can acquire expertise and improve their skills over time through hands-on caring experiences or by studying the caregiving practices of others [54]. Our findings also suggest that some family members experienced a sense of obligation to assume the role of caregiver and a limited sense of autonomy due to societal norms that expect them to provide care for an ill family member [52]. Family members who possessed a strong inclination to safeguard the patient reported feeling more prepared for their position, but those who were affected by societal standards often expressed feelings of unease. Managing various duties can result in excessive strain, and it is crucial to maintain a balance between these conflicting responsibilities [55]. In our study, the importance of maintaining a balance was particularly notable, particularly when the responsibilities of being a caregiver were overshadowed by other familial obligations.

A significant number of caregivers reported obtaining assistance from PC services. Implementing home-based PC allowed family caregivers to feel better equipped and ready for the challenges ahead [45,49]. In practice, the involvement of PC professionals facilitated access to resources and education that helped caregivers manage the patient's illness [56]. Psychologically, family caregivers perceive healthcare professionals as a crucial support network that helps lessen the weight of their responsibilities and diminish their feelings of loneliness [51]. Unaided caregivers who provided care at home without assistance from healthcare providers frequently expressed feelings of being overwhelmed and encountered difficulties, such as misinterpreting the symptoms of the patients [52].

In this current study, caregivers emphasized the significance of compassionate and close relationships in establishing trust with PC professionals. This reassured them that they were valued members of a collaborative team focused on enhancing the patient's overall health and well-being [56]. Establishing a rapport involves dedicating time to patients, engaging in constructive encounters, and building trust through a combination of hope and honesty [57].

Previous evidence reinforces our findings, highlighting the advantages of home-based PC interventions for patients and caregivers. These interventions have positive effects on multiple aspects, including answering information needs, enhancing quality of life, decreasing hospital admissions, reducing patients' symptom burdens and resource utilization, increasing family satisfaction rates, and increasing the likelihood of patients achieving home deaths [19,54,58–60].

In home-based PC, it is common to observe a conflict between the dedication of family caregivers to the patient and their perception of the hardship associated with caregiving [60,61]. However, our participants expressed a strong desire to actively participate in decision-making and provide support to patients by advocating for them and respecting their autonomy [62–64]. Caregivers' awareness and their trust that health care professionals are watching over them may reduce feelings of being isolated and foster caregivers' preparedness for loss and bereavement [65,66]. Peer support can also help to reduce isolation and loneliness by decreasing caregiver burden and improving the carer's quality of life and bereavement adjustment [67]. It should be noted that inadequate readiness for death was linked to negative outcomes in the bereavement process, including complicated grief, anxiety, and sadness after loss [68]. Death unpreparedness may be seen as a risk factor for caregivers of patients with life-limiting illnesses [66,69].

Our study indicates that healthcare personnel possess a satisfactory level of awareness regarding the information and practical support required by family caregivers, particularly during the final phase. Furthermore, telehealth can ensure continuity of care [70] and enhance the bond between caregivers and healthcare practitioners [71]. Our findings demonstrate that the utilization of telehealth enhanced caregivers' ability to connect with healthcare professionals while still being able to remain in the comfort of their own homes. Telehealth facilitates a patient's desire to be at home in EoL and provides caregivers with access to professional guidance and support [72]. In parallel, monitoring symptoms at home enables the transmission of symptom information to HPCTs in order to prevent or manage pain and other symptoms [73]. Person-based factors, rather than organization constraints, were more commonly identified as obstacles in the delivery of PC via telehealth. This finding aligns with evidence in the prior literature [74,75], particularly, research emphasizing the significance of digital literacy for successfully delivering telemedicine care [76]. The findings also suggest that design flaws in digital advising systems have adverse effects on the usability and user-friendliness of certain caregivers, exacerbating their reliance on assistance [72].

Although telehealth allows for close interaction, the absence of in-person visits makes it challenging to evaluate social needs that extend beyond conventional health-related concerns such as pain management. However, the ability to see a patient's surroundings and intervene can greatly enhance their overall quality of life. An effective way of facilitating this comprehensive approach is to provide hybrid care, where telehealth is incorporated into patient care but is not the only method of service delivery. The inclusion of telehealth as an additional option to traditional in-person care aligns with the findings of our study. Telehealth has the potential to enhance early integrated PC by offering greater accessibility to patients in their own homes, provided that the equipment and connectivity are reliable and urgent needs are evaluated and resolved during in-person visits [72].

4.1. Strengths and Limitations

The implementation of an interview study facilitated the comprehension of the home-based care experience delivered by family members. The coding was performed by the first author (P.C.). This could have introduced a certain degree of bias, which is a potential constraint. To mitigate any potential bias, the research team pursued a rigorous methodology involving an iterative process, namely discussing the findings. Therefore, any assumptions or preexisting ideas concerning informal home care were identified and discussed. The decision to exclusively recruit participants from one HPCT was adopted for practical reasons. However, this choice imposed limits on this study's transferability. Nonetheless, we posit that the concerns expressed by participants may resemble those encountered in other regions of the country.

This was a purposive small study, only focused on qualitative analysis. The recruitment of family carers was challenging because of the time limitations given their many responsibilities. Further mixed method research use of large sample sizes is needed to better understand caregiving preparedness and telehealth use, as well as outcome measures for caregivers (i.e., burden, well-being, quality of life, perceived health, and digital literacy). Participating caregivers were mostly female and well-educated. All were white and spoke Portuguese fluently. Thus, the perspectives presented in this study may not reflect the experiences of caregivers with more diverse backgrounds. Future research should include additional sociodemographic variables in the sample selection process, such as income, employment type, dependency levels of care recipients, and the extent of formal and informal support. These factors can greatly impact a carer's capacity to deliver care. Additionally, future studies should triangulate the perspectives of caregivers, patients, and professionals to provide a comprehensive view of preparedness for caregiving and death. It might also be valuable to explore how telehealth can enhance training strategies to improve the psychological well-being of caregivers and provide them with better support.

Lastly, given the potential bias in the interpretation of the findings, the predominantly positive framing, and the research team's experience in PC, the researchers strived to mitigate biases and uphold impartiality throughout the study. For instance, during data collection, we employed accurate phrasing of our questions, built rapport with each participant, and ensured that data collection was concurrent with data analysis. Furthermore, researcher reflexivity and consensus coding ensured unbiased, reliable, and accurate data analysis.

4.2. Implications for Practice

Considering the essential role that caregivers play in delivering care at home, it is necessary to ensure a strong level of engagement and assistance for caregivers in PC. In this vein, the provision of professional PC services in the home, along with a robust support system for informal caregivers, is invaluable. The support system could be enhanced by collaborating with healthcare experts to implement the new public health approach to PC, known as compassionate communities [77]. Additional measures are required to enhance EoL care, specifically focusing on home-based family care, particularly in nations with limited resources.

This study also highlights the broad influence of family dynamics on decision-making process in PC and how the bond between the patient and family caregiver shapes their preferences. Healthcare professionals need to consider how the extended family influences the level of agreement or disagreement between patients and family caregivers, as well as the expectations of both parties regarding their roles within the family. Engaging in discussions about future care via advanced care planning can enable patients and family caregivers to adapt to changes in their care preferences [78].

Furthermore, enabling healthcare professionals to enhance and strengthen their expertise in PC—for example, using care navigators—would facilitate the provision of timely and comprehensive supportive care. In this sense, telehealth services should be considered to achieve the full potential of PC [79]. Telehealth, the practice of delivering virtual healthcare services using Internet platforms, is widely acknowledged as valuable, particularly for providing after-hours telephone assistance and facilitating video conferences for interactive case discussions [80]. The availability of online caregiving resources is contingent upon Internet connectivity. Consequently, in areas where certain groups have limited access to the Internet, a telehealth system that offers both online and offline services for family caregivers could prove beneficial. Further research should also focus on investigating the telehealth experiences among individuals with life-limiting illnesses and the oldest-old caregivers. It is crucial to examine the varying experiences of these individuals in terms of usability and knowledge related to telehealth. If family caregivers are provided with training and educational interventions, telehealth modalities can be effectively employed to deliver a diverse array of skills.

5. Conclusions

As far as we know, this is one of the first studies to investigate informal home-based PC in Portugal from the viewpoint of family caregivers. Three main themes emerged: (1) becoming a caregiver, (2) support-from-home palliative care team, and (3) telehealth in palliative home care. This study emphasizes the substantial advantages of home-based PC interventions, enhancing the caregiver's satisfaction rates and raising the probability of patients reaching death at home. Furthermore, they reduce the frequency of healthcare use, particularly hospital admissions and trips to the emergency department. Assistance by professionals and health services should be improved by developing a higher level of awareness and giving priority to the needs and readiness of carers, who have a unique position as both providers and recipients of care. Services and healthcare providers should improve their communication strategies, actively promote meaningful inclusion, tackle access difficulties, and enhance the support provided in their respective roles. This highlights the importance of a person-centered approach in EoL care and strengthens the long-term sustainability of the healthcare system through the valorization of informal care.

Supplementary Materials: The following supporting information can be downloaded at: https://www.mdpi.com/article/10.3390/healthcare12191915/s1, Table S1: Consolidated criteria for reporting qualitative studies (COREQ): 32-item checklist.

Author Contributions: Conceptualization, P.C., A.Q. and C.L.; methodology, P.C. and C.L.; software, P.C. and C.L.; validation, C.L.; formal analysis, P.C. and C.L.; investigation, P.C. and C.L.; resources, P.C. and A.Q.; data curation, P.C. and C.L.; writing—original draft preparation, P.C. and C.L.; writing—review and editing, P.C., A.Q. and C.L.; visualization, P.C. and C.L.; supervision, C.L.; project administration, C.L.; funding acquisition, C.L. All authors have read and agreed to the published version of the manuscript.

Funding: This study received funding under the project Help2Care-PAL: Support the caregiver in palliative care, funded by Fundação "LaCaixa" (IC21-00035). This work is also supported by national funds through FCT—Fundação para a Ciência e a Tecnologia, I.P. (UIDB/05704/2020 and UIDP/05704/2020)—and under the Scientific Employment Stimulus-Institutional Call (https://doi.org/10.54499/CEECINST/00051/2018/CP1566/CT0012, accessed on 20 August 2024).

Institutional Review Board Statement: This study was conducted in accordance with the Declaration of Helsinki and approved by the Ethics Committee of Unidade Local de Saúde—Baixo Alentejo (code: 7.4.1. approved on 15 February 2023).

Informed Consent Statement: Informed consent was obtained from all subjects involved in this study.

Data Availability Statement: All data generated or analyzed during this study are included in this article. This article is based on the first author's master's dissertation in Palliative Care at the School of Health Sciences—Polytechnic University of Leiria.

Acknowledgments: The authors express their profound gratitude to the caregivers who generously contributed and the staff that participated in the recruitment process.

Conflicts of Interest: The authors declare no conflicts of interest. The funders had no role in the design of the study; in the collection, analyses, or interpretation of data; in the writing of the manuscript; or in the decision to publish the results.

References

1. World Health Organisation. *Planning and Implementing Palliative Care Services: A Guide for Programme Managers*; World Health Organisation: Geneva, Switzerland, 2018.
2. Finkelstein, E.A.; Bhadelia, A.; Goh, C.; Baid, D.; Singh, R.; Bhatnagar, S.; Connor, S.R. Cross Country Comparison of Expert Assessments of the Quality of Death and Dying 2021. *J. Pain Symptom Manag.* **2022**, *63*, e419–e429. [CrossRef] [PubMed]
3. Pinto, S.; Lopes, S.; de Sousa, A.B.; Delalibera, M.; Gomes, B. Patient and Family Preferences About Place of End-of-Life Care and Death: An Umbrella Review. *J. Pain Symptom Manag.* **2024**, *67*, e439–e452. [CrossRef]
4. Morris, S.M.; King, C.; Turner, M.; Payne, S. Family carers providing support to a person dying in the home setting: A narrative literature review. *Palliat. Med.* **2015**, *29*, 487–495. [CrossRef]
5. Payne, S.; Hudson, P.; Grande, G.; Oliviere, D.; Tishelman, C.; Pleschberger, S.; Firth, P.; Ewing, G.; Hawker, S.; Kerr, C. White Paper on Improving Support for Family Carers in Palliative Care, Part 2. *Eur. J. Palliat. Care* **2010**, *17*, 286–290.
6. Allen, J.; Woolford, M.; Livingston, P.M.; Lobchuk, M.; Muldowney, A.; Hutchinson, A.M. Informal carer support needs, facilitators and barriers in transitional care for older adults from hospital to home: A scoping review. *J. Clin. Nurs.* **2023**, *32*, 6773–6795. [CrossRef] [PubMed]
7. Chen, L.; Xiao, L.D.; Chamberlain, D.; Newman, P. Enablers and barriers in hospital-to-home transitional care for stroke survivors and caregivers: A systematic review. *J. Clin. Nurs.* **2021**, *30*, 2786–2807. [CrossRef] [PubMed]
8. Kraun, L.; De Vliegher, K.; Vandamme, M.; Holtzheimer, E.; Ellen, M.; van Achterberg, T. Older peoples' and informal caregivers' experiences, views, and needs in transitional care decision-making: A systematic review. *Int. J. Nurs. Stud.* **2022**, *134*, 104303. [CrossRef]
9. Guo, P.; Pinto, C.; Edwards, B.; Pask, S.; Firth, A.; O'bRien, S.; Murtagh, F.E. Experiences of transitioning between settings of care from the perspectives of patients with advanced illness receiving specialist palliative care and their family caregivers: A qualitative interview study. *Palliat. Med.* **2022**, *36*, 124–134. [CrossRef]
10. Morey, T.; Scott, M.; Saunders, S.; Varenbut, J.; Howard, M.; Tanuseputro, P.; Webber, C.; Killackey, T.; Wentlandt, K.; Zimmermann, C.; et al. Transitioning from Hospital to Palliative Care at Home: Patient and Caregiver Perceptions of Continuity of Care. *J. Pain Symptom Manag.* **2021**, *62*, 233–241. [CrossRef]
11. Prado, E.; Marcon, S.; Kalinke, L.; da Silva, M.; Barreto, M.; Takemoto, A.; Birolim, M.; Laranjeira, C. Meanings and Experiences of End-of-Life Patients and Their Family Caregivers in Hospital-to-Home Transitions: A Constructivist Grounded Theory Study. *Int. J. Environ. Res. Public Health* **2022**, *19*, 12987. [CrossRef]
12. Saunders, S.; Weiss, M.E.; Meaney, C.; Killackey, T.; Varenbut, J.; Lovrics, E.; Ernecoff, N.; Hsu, A.T.; Stern, M.; Mahtani, R.; et al. Examining the course of transitions from hospital to home-based palliative care: A mixed methods study. *Palliat. Med.* **2021**, *35*, 1590–1601. [CrossRef] [PubMed]
13. Nikbakht-Nasrabadi, A.; Mardanian-Dehkordi, L.; Taleghani, F. Abandonment at the Transition from Hospital to Home: Family Caregivers' Experiences. *Ethiop. J. Health Sci.* **2021**, *31*, 525–532. [CrossRef] [PubMed]
14. Chan, C.K.; Vickers, T.; Barnard, A. Meaning through caregiving: A qualitative study of the experiences of informal carers. *Br. J. Soc. Work* **2021**, *50*, 682–700. [CrossRef]
15. Beach, B.; Bélanger-Hardy, L.; Harding, S.; Perracini, M.R.; Garcia, L.; Tripathi, I.; Gillis, M.; Dow, B. Caring for the caregiver: Why policy must shift from addressing needs to enabling caregivers to flourish. *Front. Public Health* **2022**, *10*, 997981. [CrossRef] [PubMed]
16. Bhadelia, A.; Oldfield, L.E.; Cruz, J.L.; Singh, R.; Finkelstein, E.A. Identifying Core Domains to Assess the "Quality of Death": A Scoping Review. *J. Pain Symptom Manag.* **2022**, *63*, e365–e386. [CrossRef]
17. Hofmeister, M.; Memedovich, A.; Dowsett, L.E.; Sevick, L.; McCarron, T.; Spackman, E.; Stafinski, T.; Menon, D.; Noseworthy, T.; Clement, F. Palliative care in the home: A scoping review of study quality, primary outcomes, and thematic component analysis. *BMC Palliat. Care* **2018**, *17*, 41. [CrossRef]
18. Roberts, B.; Robertson, M.; Ojukwu, E.I.; Wu, D.S. Home Based Palliative Care: Known Benefits and Future Directions. *Curr. Geriatr. Rep.* **2021**, *10*, 141–147. [CrossRef]
19. Feliciano, D.R.; Reis-Pina, P. Enhancing End-of-Life Care with Home-Based Palliative Interventions: A Systematic Review. *J. Pain Symptom Manag.* **2024**, *in press*. [CrossRef]
20. Shepperd, S.; Gonçalves-Bradley, D.C.; Straus, S.E.; Wee, B. Hospital at home: Home-based end-of-life care. *Cochrane Database Syst. Rev.* **2021**, CD009231. [CrossRef]
21. da Cruz, M.B.; Nunes, R. Palliative care and the Portuguese health system. *Porto Biomed. J.* **2016**, *1*, 72–76. [CrossRef]
22. Marques, P.; Rêgo, F.; Nunes, R. Palliative Care in Portugal—From Intention to Reality, What Is Yet to Be Accomplished. *Nurs. Rep.* **2023**, *13*, 1477–1485. [CrossRef]
23. Dixe, M.D.A.; Santo, I.D.D.O.; Lopes, S.; Catarino, H.; Duarte, S.; Querido, A.; Laranjeira, C. Knowledge and Myths about Palliative Care among the General Public and Health Care Professionals in Portugal. *Int. J. Environ. Res. Public Health* **2020**, *17*, 4630. [CrossRef] [PubMed]

24. Tibell, L.H.; Årestedt, K.; Holm, M.; Wallin, V.; Steineck, G.; Hudson, P.; Kreicbergs, U.; Alvariza, A. Preparedness for caregiving and preparedness for death: Associations and modifiable thereafter factors among family caregivers of patients with advanced cancer in specialized home care. *Death Stud.* **2024**, *48*, 407–416. [CrossRef]
25. Gérain, P.; Zech, E. Informal Caregiver Burnout? Development of a Theoretical Framework to Understand the Impact of Caregiving. *Front. Psychol.* **2019**, *10*, 1748. [CrossRef] [PubMed]
26. Szabo, S.; Lakzadeh, P.; Cline, S.; Dos Reis, R.P.; Petrella, R. The clinical and economic burden among caregivers of patients with Alzheimer's disease in Canada. *Int. J. Geriatr. Psychiatry* **2019**, *34*, 1677–1688. [CrossRef]
27. Cejalvo, E.; Martí-Vilar, M.; Merino-Soto, C.; Aguirre-Morales, M.T. Caregiving Role and Psychosocial and Individual Factors: A Systematic Review. *Healthcare* **2021**, *9*, 1690. [CrossRef] [PubMed]
28. Liu, H.; Lou, V.W.Q. Transitioning into spousal caregiving: Contribution of caregiving intensity and caregivers' multiple chronic conditions to functional health. *Age Ageing* **2019**, *48*, 108–114. [CrossRef]
29. Kirtania, M.; Katta, A. Essential Elements of Home-based Palliative Care Model: A Rapid Review. *Indian J. Palliat. Care* **2023**, *29*, 359–367. [CrossRef]
30. Mertens, F.; Vanderstichelen, S.; Deveugele, M.; Deliens, L.; Pype, P. Family carers' experiences regarding patient transfers between care settings in palliative care: An interview study. *Ann. Palliat. Med.* **2023**, *12*, 767–782. [CrossRef]
31. Zhai, S.; Chu, F.; Tan, M.; Chi, N.C.; Ward, T.; Yuwen, W. Digital health interventions to support family caregivers: An updated systematic review. *Digit. Health* **2023**, *9*, 20552076231171967. [CrossRef]
32. Carter, G.; Monaghan, C.; Santin, O. What is known from the existing literature about peer support interventions for carers of individuals living with dementia: A scoping review. *Health Soc. Care Community* **2020**, *28*, 1134–1151. [CrossRef] [PubMed]
33. Shin, J.Y.; Choi, S.W. Online interventions geared toward increasing resilience and reducing distress in family caregivers. *Curr. Opin. Support. Palliat. Care* **2020**, *14*, 60–66. [CrossRef]
34. Ruggiano, N.; Brown, E.L.; Shaw, S.; Geldmacher, D.; Clarke, P.; Hristidis, V.; Bertram, J. The Potential of Information Technology to Navigate Caregiving Systems: Perspectives from Dementia Caregivers. *J. Gerontol. Soc. Work* **2019**, *62*, 432–450. [CrossRef] [PubMed]
35. Daraz, L.; Morrow, A.S.; Ponce, O.J.; Farah, W.; Katabi, A.; Majzoub, A.; Seisa, M.O.; Benkhadra, R.; Alsawas, M.; Larry, P.; et al. Readability of Online Health Information: A Meta-Narrative Systematic Review. *Am. J. Med. Qual.* **2018**, *33*, 487–492. [CrossRef]
36. Khaleel, I.; Wimmer, B.C.; Peterson, G.M.; Zaidi, S.T.R.; Roehrer, E.; Cummings, E.; Lee, K. Health information overload among health consumers: A scoping review. *Patient Educ. Couns.* **2020**, *103*, 15–32. [CrossRef] [PubMed]
37. Margarido, M.G.; Shah, A.; Seto, E. Smartphone applications for informal caregivers of chronically ill patients: A scoping review. *NPJ Digit. Med.* **2022**, *5*, 33. [CrossRef]
38. Laranjeira, C.; Dixe, M.A.; Martinho, R.; Rijo, R.; Querido, A. Building Bridges for "Palliative Care-in-Place": Development of a mHealth Intervention for Informal Home Care. *Front. Psychol.* **2022**, *13*, 862347. [CrossRef]
39. Creswell, J.W. *Research Design: Qualitative, Quantitative, and Mixed Methods Approaches*; Sage Publications: Thousand Oaks, CA, USA, 2014.
40. Tong, A.; Sainsbury, P.; Craig, J. Consolidated criteria for reporting qualitative research (COREQ): A 32-item checklist for interviews and focus groups. *Int. J. Qual. Health Care* **2007**, *19*, 349–357. [CrossRef]
41. Patton, M.Q. *Qualitative Research & Evaluation Methods: Integrating Theory and Practice*, 4th ed.; Sage Publications Inc.: Thousand Oaks, CA, USA, 2015.
42. André, P.; Pina, P. Prevalência e Características das Pessoas Com Necessidades Paliativas Internadas em Serviços Hospitalares Generalizados: Contributo Para a Tradução e Validação da Ferramenta NECPAL-CCOMS-ICO© Para a População Portuguesa. Tese de Mestrado, Faculdade de Medicina da Universidade de Lisboa. 2018. Available online: https://repositorio.ul.pt/handle/10451/37857?locale=en (accessed on 28 April 2024).
43. Moser, A.; Korstjens, I. Series: Practical guidance to qualitative research. Part 3: Sampling, data collection and analysis. *Eur. J. Gen. Pract.* **2018**, *24*, 9–18. [CrossRef]
44. de Siqueira Silva, Í.; de Araújo, A.J.; Lopes, R.H.; Silva, C.R.D.V.; Xavier, P.B.; de Figueirêdo, R.C.; Brito, E.W.G.; Lapão, L.V.; Martiniano, C.S.; de Araújo Nunes, V.M.; et al. Digital home care interventions and quality of primary care for older adults: A scoping review. *BMC Geriatr.* **2024**, *24*, 507. [CrossRef]
45. Barlund, A.S.; André, B.; Sand, K.; Brenne, A.T. A qualitative study of bereaved family caregivers: Feeling of security, facilitators and barriers for rural home care and death for persons with advanced cancer. *BMC Palliat. Care* **2021**, *20*, 7. [CrossRef] [PubMed]
46. Braun, V.; Clarke, V. Using thematic analysis in psychology. *Qual. Res. Psychol.* **2006**, *3*, 77–101. [CrossRef]
47. Braun, V.; Clarke, V. Reflecting on reflexive thematic analysis. *Qual. Res. Sport Exerc. Health* **2019**, *11*, 589–597. [CrossRef]
48. Korstjens, I.; Moser, A. Series: Practical guidance to qualitative research. Part 4: Trustworthiness and publishing. *Eur. J. Gen. Pract.* **2018**, *24*, 120–124. [CrossRef]
49. Zarzycki, M.; Morrison, V.; Bei, E.; Seddon, D. Cultural and societal motivations for being informal caregivers: A qualitative systematic review and meta-synthesis. *Health Psychol. Rev.* **2023**, *17*, 247–276. [CrossRef]
50. Nysaeter, T.M.; Olsson, C.; Sandsdalen, T.; Hov, R.; Larsson, M. Family caregivers' preferences for support when caring for a family member with cancer in late palliative phase who wish to die at home—A grounded theory study. *BMC Palliat. Care.* **2024**, *23*, 15. [CrossRef]

51. Leow, M.Q.; Chan, S.W. The Challenges, Emotions, Coping, and Gains of Family Caregivers Caring for Patients with Advanced Cancer in Singapore: A Qualitative Study. *Cancer Nurs.* **2017**, *40*, 22–30. [CrossRef]
52. Salifu, Y.; Almack, K.; Caswell, G. 'My wife is my doctor at home': A qualitative study exploring the challenges of home-based palliative care in a resource-poor setting. *Palliat. Med.* **2021**, *35*, 97–108. [CrossRef]
53. Choo, P.Y.; Tan-Ho, G.; Dutta, O.; Patinadan, P.V.; Ho, A.H.Y. Reciprocal Dynamics of Dignity in End-of-Life Care: A Multiperspective Systematic Review of Qualitative and Mixed Methods Research. *Am. J. Hosp. Palliat. Care* **2020**, *37*, 385–398. [CrossRef]
54. Sarmento, V.P.; Gysels, M.; Higginson, I.J.; Gomes, B. Home palliative care works: But how? A meta-ethnography of the experiences of patients and family caregivers. *BMJ Support. Palliat. Care* **2017**, *7*, 390–403. [CrossRef]
55. Fringer, A.; Hechinger, M.; Schnepp, W. Transitions as experienced by persons in palliative care circumstances and their families—A qualitative meta-synthesis. *BMC Palliat. Care* **2018**, *17*, 22. [CrossRef] [PubMed]
56. Klarare, A.; Rasmussen, B.H.; Fossum, B.; Hansson, J.; Fürst, C.J.; Hagelin, C.L. Actions helping expressed or anticipated needs: Patients with advanced cancer and their family caregivers' experiences of specialist palliative home care teams. *Eur. J. Cancer Care* **2018**, *27*, e12948. [CrossRef] [PubMed]
57. Beng, T.S.; Xin, C.A.; Ying, Y.K.; Khuen, L.P.; Yee, A.; Zainuddin, S.I.; Chin, L.E.; Loong, L.C. Hope in Palliative Care: A Thematic Analysis. *J. Palliat. Care* **2022**, *37*, 177–182. [CrossRef]
58. Hamano, J.; Takeuchi, A.; Mori, M.; Saitou, Y.; Yamaguchi, T.; Miyata, N.; Shimizu, M.; Yamamoto, R.; Kimura, Y.; Kamiyama, Y.; et al. Comparison of survival times of advanced cancer patients with palliative care at home and in hospital. *PLoS ONE* **2023**, *18*, e0284147. [CrossRef] [PubMed]
59. Currow, D.C.; Agar, M.R.; Phillips, J.L. Role of Hospice Care at the End of Life for People with Cancer. *J. Clin. Oncol.* **2020**, *38*, 937–943. [CrossRef] [PubMed]
60. Wicaksono, R.B.; Muhaimin, A.; Willems, D.L.; Pols, J. Family Perspectives on Key Elements of Good Home Palliative Care in South and Southeast Asia: A Scoping Review. *Home Health Care Manag. Pract.* **2024**, 10848223231224779. [CrossRef]
61. Cheung, J.T.K.; Au, D.; Ip, A.H.F.; Chan, J.; Ng, K.; Cheung, L.; Yuen, J.; Hui, E.; Lee, J.; Lo, R.; et al. Barriers to advance care planning: A qualitative study of seriously ill Chinese patients and their families. *BMC Palliat. Care* **2020**, *19*, 80. [CrossRef]
62. Gerber, K.; Lemmon, C.; Williams, S.; Watt, J.; Panayiotou, A.; Batchelor, F.; Hayes, B.; Brijnath, B. 'There for me': A qualitative study of family communication and decision-making in end-of-life care for older people. *Prog. Palliat. Care* **2020**, *28*, 354–361. [CrossRef]
63. Symmons, S.M.; Ryan, K.; Aoun, S.M.; Selman, L.E.; Davies, A.N.; Cornally, N.; Lombard, J.; McQuilllan, R.; Guerin, S.; O'LEary, N.; et al. Decision-making in palliative care: Patient and family caregiver concordance and discordance-systematic review and narrative synthesis. *BMJ Support. Palliat. Care* **2023**, *13*, 374–385. [CrossRef]
64. Lin, C.P.; Evans, C.J.; Koffman, J.; Armes, J.; Murtagh, F.E.M.; Harding, R. The conceptual models and mechanisms of action that underpin advance care planning for cancer patients: A systematic review of randomised controlled trials. *Palliat. Med.* **2019**, *33*, 5–23. [CrossRef]
65. Caserta, M.; Utz, R.; Lund, D.; Supiano, K.; Donaldson, G. Cancer Caregivers' Preparedness for Loss and Bereavement Outcomes: Do Preloss Caregiver Attributes Matter? *Omega* **2019**, *80*, 224–244. [CrossRef]
66. Nielsen, M.K.; Neergaard, M.A.; Jensen, A.B.; Bro, F.; Guldin, M.B. Do we need to change our understanding of anticipatory grief in caregivers? A systematic review of caregiver studies during end-of-life caregiving and bereavement. *Clin. Psychol. Rev.* **2016**, *44*, 75–93. [CrossRef] [PubMed]
67. Trail, T.; Friedman, E.; Rutter, C.M.; Tanielian, T. The Relationship between Engagement in Online Support Groups and Social Isolation among Military Caregivers: Longitudinal Questionnaire Study. *J. Med. Internet Res.* **2020**, *22*, e16423. [CrossRef] [PubMed]
68. Szuhany, K.L.; Malgaroli, M.; Miron, C.D.; Simon, N.M. Prolonged Grief Disorder: Course, Diagnosis, Assessment, and Treatment. *Focus* **2021**, *19*, 161–172. [CrossRef] [PubMed]
69. Mateus, M.J.; Simões, L.; Ali, A.M.; Laranjeira, C. Family Experiences of Loss and Bereavement in Palliative Care Units during the COVID-19 Pandemic: An Interpretative Phenomenological Study. *Healthcare* **2024**, *12*, 1763. [CrossRef]
70. Sadang, K.G.; Centracchio, J.A.; Turk, Y.; Park, E.; Feliciano, J.L.; Chua, I.S.; Blackhall, L.; Silveira, M.J.; Fischer, S.M.; Rabow, M.; et al. Clinician Perceptions of Barriers and Facilitators for Delivering Early Integrated Palliative Care via Telehealth. *Cancers* **2023**, *15*, 5340. [CrossRef]
71. Bandini, J.I.; Scherling, A.; Farmer, C.; Fratkin, M.; Mistler, B.; Ast, K.; Ahluwalia, S.C. Experiences with Telehealth for Outpatient Palliative Care: Findings from a Mixed-Methods Study of Patients and Providers across the United States. *J. Palliat. Med.* **2022**, *25*, 1079–1087. [CrossRef]
72. Hughes, M.C.; Vernon, E.; Kowalczyk, M.; Zhou, H. Experiences of caregivers and hospice leaders with telehealth for palliative care: A mixed methods study. *Ann. Palliat. Med.* **2022**, *11*, 2302–2313. [CrossRef]
73. Gordon, B.; Mason, B.; Smith, S.L.H. Leveraging Telehealth for Delivery of Palliative Care to Remote Communities: A Rapid Review. *J. Palliat. Care* **2022**, *37*, 213–225. [CrossRef]
74. Almathami, H.K.Y.; Win, K.T.; Vlahu-Gjorgievska, E. Barriers and Facilitators That Influence Telemedicine-Based, Real-Time, Online Consultation at Patients' Homes: Systematic Literature Review. *J. Med. Internet Res.* **2020**, *22*, e16407. [CrossRef]

75. Chua, I.S.; Zachariah, F.; Dale, W.; Feliciano, J.; Hanson, L.; Blackhall, L.; Quest, T.; Curseen, K.; Grey, C.; Rhodes, R.; et al. Early Integrated Telehealth versus In-Person Palliative Care for Patients with Advanced Lung Cancer: A Study Protocol. *J. Palliat. Med.* **2019**, *22*, 7–19. [CrossRef] [PubMed]
76. Campanozzi, L.L.; Gibelli, F.; Bailo, P.; Nittari, G.; Sirignano, A.; Ricci, G. The role of digital literacy in achieving health equity in the third millennium society: A literature review. *Front. Public Health* **2023**, *11*, 1109323. [CrossRef] [PubMed]
77. Abel, J. Compassionate communities and end-of-life care. *Clin. Med.* **2018**, *18*, 6–8. [CrossRef] [PubMed]
78. Timóteo, C.; Vitorino, J.; Ali, A.M.; Laranjeira, C. Legacy in End-of-Life Care: A Concept Analysis. *Nurs. Rep.* **2024**, *14*, 2385–2397. [CrossRef]
79. Nwosu, A.C. Telehealth requires improved evidence to achieve its full potential in palliative care. *Palliat. Med.* **2023**, *37*, 896–897. [CrossRef]
80. Steindal, S.A.; Nes, A.A.G.; Godskesen, T.E.; Dihle, A.; Lind, S.; Winger, A.; Klarare, A. Patients' Experiences of Telehealth in Palliative Home Care: Scoping Review. *J. Med. Internet Res.* **2020**, *22*, e16218. [CrossRef]

healthcare

MDPI

Article

"What Do You Get? Nothing": A Qualitative Analysis of the Financial Impact of Family Caregiving for a Dying Relative at Home in Germany

Sally Pieper [1,*,†], Alina Kasdorf [1,†], Raymond Voltz [1,2,3] and Julia Strupp [1]

1 Department of Palliative Medicine, Faculty of Medicine and University Hospital, University of Cologne, Kerpener Str. 62, 50937 Cologne, Germany; alina.kasdorf@uk-koeln.de (A.K.); raymond.voltz@uk-koeln.de (R.V.); julia.strupp@uk-koeln.de (J.S.)

2 Center for Integrated Oncology Aachen Bonn Cologne Duesseldorf (CIO ABCD), Faculty of Medicine and University Hospital, University of Cologne, Eupener Str. 129, 50933 Cologne, Germany

3 Center for Health Services Research, Faculty of Medicine and University Hospital, University of Cologne, Kerpener Str. 62, 50937 Cologne, Germany

* Correspondence: sally.pieper@uk-koeln.de

† These authors contributed equally to this work.

Abstract: Background/Objectives: As a result of demographic change in Germany, the number of people in need of care is steadily increasing, with a correspondingly larger proportion of care being provided by family members at home. Family caregivers face significant challenges in providing such care, particularly when balancing work responsibilities. Many experience a loss of income due to reduced working hours or the necessity of leaving the labor market. Additional caregiving costs, such as medical expenses, transportation, and home modifications, further exacerbate their financial burden. **Methods**: This study consists of an online survey, which included the German version of the Carer Support Needs Assessment Tool (CSNAT), designed to assess the support needs of family caregivers. Respondents were asked to describe their support needs in open-text responses. To illustrate their experiences, a qualitative content analysis was conducted. **Results**: Out of the 320 questionnaires, 304 of them contained open-text responses that could be analyzed. Important themes included the need for support in the workplace, financial security, and assistance with administrative barriers. In addition to more flexible working hours and greater understanding from employers, the need for financial compensation for loss of working time was expressed. **Conclusions**: Despite a growing awareness of the gaps in support, the needs of family caregivers remain inadequately addressed, leaving them financially burdened and unsupported. Ultimately, this study calls for a re-evaluation of societal attitudes toward caring, arguing for greater recognition of the economic contributions of family caregivers and the implementation of supportive policies.

Keywords: dying at home; family caregivers; financial loss; caregiver burden; end of life

1. Introduction

The global health care landscape is facing significant challenges due to demographic shifts, particularly aging populations and increasing chronic diseases [1,2]. This trend is straining health care systems worldwide, necessitating structural adaptations and a shift towards home-based care [3].

The number of people in need of care in Germany has risen sharply in recent years due to demographic change. In December 2023, 5.69 million people needed care, of whom around 86% (4.49 million) were cared for at home—mainly by relatives (67%) [4]. Indeed, care provided by family caregivers plays a central role in the German health care system: It is estimated that around 5 million people in Germany provide care to relatives at home [5], with women more likely to provide care [6]. Overall, between 5% and 6% of adults provide care on a regular basis [7].

One of the main contributors to home care are the terminally ill, as many people prefer to spend the last days and hours of their lives at home and to die there [8], which means that end-of-life care tasks are shifting from medical care institutions to family members. This development poses considerable challenges for family caregivers [9,10]. In particular, reconciling care and work is becoming increasingly problematic [11], as the proportion of working family caregivers under the age of 65 has risen from 53% to 66% [7]. This is particularly significant when accounting for the length of care, as 64% of care situations last longer than a year [12]. The baby boomer generation's retirement will exacerbate this situation, leaving fewer working age individuals to support a growing number of care-dependent people [13,14]. This combination of care recipients 'desire to be cared for and die at home and family caregivers' work commitments creates additional burdens that require extensive support [15].

The financing of home-based end-of-life care in Germany relies primarily on statutory long-term care insurance, supplemented by health insurance and out-of-pocket expenses. Depending on their level of dependency, people in need of long-term care receive cash allowances ("Pflegegeld") for caregiving or in-kind benefits ("Pflegesachleistungen") for professional home care [16,17]. However, gaps in coverage persist, often leaving families with additional costs for home adaptations or extended care [18]. Fewer than 10% of people in need of home care do not have family caregivers involved in their care [19]. This means that family caregivers provide the majority of all care services today, making them a crucial social and economic resource for the health care system [19–21]. Among those who provide familial care, financial difficulties are widespread, with 38% of family caregivers reporting moderate to high financial stress and 45% experiencing at least one financial impact, such as reduced savings or increased debt [22]. In addition, recent studies have shown that family caregivers are often forced to reduce their working hours or take short-term sick leaves [23].

In Germany, there is limited research from the perspective of family members regarding their burdens, especially concerning their financial strains. Therefore, our study aimed to investigate the financial impact of caring for a seriously ill and dying family member in Germany by using a panel. Our study is part of a larger project called "Dying at Home". The results of the interviews and a large online survey have been published elsewhere [23,24].

2. Materials and Methods

2.1. Study Design, Population, and Data Collection

The online observational panel survey was designed to be completed via a computer or mobile device with open-text options.

The survey consisted of three parts: (i) items generated from a qualitative multi-method study combining the results of semi-structured interviews and focus group discussions to explore the support needs of family caregivers of patients wishing to die at home; (ii) a German version of the Carer Support Needs Assessment Tool (CSNAT) (called KOMMA in German (The KOMMA assessment form (communication with relatives) was used in this study (Copyright 2019 University of Cambridge/The University of Manchester, all rights reserved). The KOMMA was translated by Sabine Pleschberger, Johannes Bükki, and Christiane Kreyer from the original version, and the CSNAT was developed by Dr.

Gail Ewing and Prof. Gunn Grande (Copyright @ 2009 University of Cambridge/The University of Manchester, all rights reserved)) [25,26], and (iii) socio-demographic and patient characteristics. This publication focuses on the exploratory analysis of open-text comments, while the remaining data and results of the survey, including a detailed description of the survey methods, have been analyzed and published elsewhere [23].

This study was prospectively registered in the German Clinical Trials Register (DRKS00026229) on 25 November 2021. Ethical approval was granted by the Ethics Committee of the Medical Faculty of Cologne (#21-1466). Family caregivers were included in this study if they were older than 18 years and had given written consent to participate in this study. Deaths before 2016 were excluded to minimize recall bias. The survey was open from 19 September 2022 to 13 November 2022.

The survey was conducted anonymously, with the first section providing detailed information on data protection and obtaining informed consent from participants. After consent was given, no data sensitive to privacy were collected. Participants were assigned an ID, ensuring that the dataset contained no names or personally identifiable information.

The 14 questions of the CSNAT, which were used retrospectively, asked about the family members' need for support in different areas of life, such as knowledge about the disease, time for themselves, resources, legal and professional issues, caregiving, and day and night help. Participants in the online survey were able to choose between the response options "No", "A little more", "Much more", and "Significantly more". The research team (AK, JS) added an open-text option to each of the items. The optional open-text provided an opportunity to specify the type of support the person would have liked, allowing for a more precise consideration and, if necessary, the addition of individual needs. This procedure was agreed upon with the KOMMA team prior to the start of the survey.

2.2. Analysis

As part of the qualitative analysis, all open-text comments on support needs collected in the questionnaires were entered into MAXQDA 2024 in order to carry out systematic coding. Using content analysis, we analyzed the open-text content and developed a category system with main and subcategories in a multi-step process [27,28]. The open-texts were coded and analyzed by SP in consultation with AK. S.P. and A.K. reviewed and discussed the codes and categories to reach consensus, making adjustments as needed. First, relevant text passages were identified based on their connection to the research question. By analyzing these passages, preliminary codes were formed inductively. It became clear that some participants expressed a similar need for additional support in several areas.

As part of the inductive coding process, item 31, which deals with professional, legal, and financial support, was examined in more detail. After coding all text passages, they were sorted thematically. Main and subcategories were created for a higher level of abstraction. SP and AK repeatedly consulted each other to discuss the codes critically. The analysis made it possible to develop specific codes within each main category in order to capture more precisely the different ways in which support needs were expressed. The team selected exemplary open-text quotations based on representativeness and expressiveness of their content.

3. Results

3.1. Survey Sample

From a total of 320 questionnaires collected in this study, the open-text data of the informants could be analyzed in 304 cases, which means that 95% of the informants added comments to at least one of the available open-text fields in their questionnaires [23]. Women made up the majority of the sample, representing 70.7% of participants (Table 1).

Table 1. Demographics and characteristics of study population (subgroup n = 304/320).

Characteristics	Total	
	n	%
Family caregivers		
Age		
Mean (SD, Min—Max)	50.5 (13.7, 18–82)	
Gender		
Male	86	28.3
Female	215	70.7
Diverse	3	1.0
Relationship		
Spouse/Partner	33	10.9
Son/Daughter	125	41.1
Brother/Sister	9	3.0
Son/Daughter-in-law	20	6.6
Grandson/-daughter	47	15.5
Friend	18	5.9
Neighbor	20	6.6
Volunteer	11	3.6
Other	21	7.0
Employment status *		
Was employed in the last 3 months	197	67.7
Was not employed in the last 3 months	94	32.3
Deceased		
Age		
Mean (SD, Min–Max)	77.5 (13.8, 19–105)	
Gender		
Male	156	51.3
Female	147	48.4
Diverse	1	0.3
Diagnosis **		
Cancer	111	36.5
Neurological disease	95	31.3
Cardiovascular disease	104	34.2
Respiratory disease	42	13.8

* Total n = 291, missing or not applicable n = 13 ** Multiple response possible.

3.2. Open-Text Analysis

A total of 133 respondents expressed a great need for support in the areas of financial, legal, and professional matters. Of these, 40% stated that they needed much more support, and 21% needed significantly more support. The open-text comments were organized into three major categories with subcategories (Table 2).

Table 2. Overview of categories and subcategories.

Category	Subcategory
Employer support	Employer flexibility Sick leave/leave of absence for care Understanding of the employer Financial compensation due to loss of work

Table 2. *Cont.*

Category	Subcategory
Employer support	Employer flexibility Sick leave/leave of absence for care Understanding of the employer Financial compensation due to loss of work
Financial support	More care allowance Financial security Information and advice
Administrative barriers	Bureaucratic barriers Difficulties with care levels Assistance with documents

3.2.1. Employer Support

Participants expressed specific wishes and needs for their employers in terms of support that would enable them to better reconcile their work commitments with their caregiving responsibilities. This category was divided into the following sub-categories:

- Employer flexibility: One of the participants' requests was to be able to organize their working hours more flexibly in order to make it easier to combine work and caring responsibilities. Reflecting this wish, one participant noted, "*Less working hours, more flexible working hours*" (Respondent-ID: 254).
- Sick leave/leave of absence for care: In order to fulfill caring responsibilities at home, participants emphasized that they sometimes have to take sick leave. One of the respondents commented on this: "*For example, I took sick leave to be there for my grandmother. I'm sure there are other ways*" (Respondent-ID: 210). This quote emphasizes the lack of options for time off, forcing participants to rely on other options, such as sick leave.
- Understanding of the employer: This sub-category highlighted the need for more understanding from participants' employers. Specifically, respondents often described employers showing little consideration for their caring responsibilities: "*If my employer had also accepted family caregiving leave. Unfortunately, I work in a care home and was called in during my free time*" (Respondent-ID: 108).
- Financial compensation due to loss of work: A key issue was the financial loss suffered by participants who worked while caring for a seriously ill relative. One family carer said, "*Unable to work because of caring (24-h on-call duty)! Financial support for family caregivers too!!!*" (Respondent-ID: 42). Another participant wrote, "*Financial compensation for family caregivers who give up years of their lives and are unable to go to work*" (Respondent-ID: 57).

3.2.2. Financial Support

Two sub-categories were identified in this area, focusing on the financial security of participants:

- More care allowance: With regard to the carer's allowance, there was a need for comprehensive cost coverage by the care insurance funds. One respondent said, "*That the care insurance fund covers everything you need*" (Respondent-ID: 175).
- Financial security: A key aspect in the area of financial support is financial security. The following quote from a caring relative underlines that financial pressure also had an impact on their own health: "*What do you get? NOTHING. Caring relatives should be financially and socially secure so that they have a clear head for caring. Maybe then fewer of them will fall ill themselves, because they are carrying a double and triple burden*" (Respondent-ID: 63). The challenge of organizing professional care without sufficient financial resources was also discussed: "*but we were too poor to pay for night care or personal care through a care service*" (Respondent-ID: 88).

3.2.3. Administrative Barriers

This area represented two overarching aspects that were reflected in both the professional and financial contexts. Many participants reported a high level of bureaucracy and a lack of adequate advice, which was an additional burden.

- Information and advice: A key aspect of this category was the lack of knowledge and advice, particularly in relation to the types of support available, whether financial or care-related. Participants emphasized the importance of being informed about possible support: "*Providing knowledge, help with applications, etc. What is possible at all—financial support, care support*, etc.". (Respondent-ID: 256).
- Bureaucratic barriers: The need for better support in overcoming bureaucratic barriers was repeatedly emphasized by family caregivers. In particular, lengthy and often frustrating dealings with authorities were described as a significant burden: "*Battles with authorities, social applications, many hours invested that you don't really have*" (Respondent-ID: 184).
- Difficulties with care levels: Dissatisfaction with the classification into care levels was another issue raised by participants. They reported discrepancies between their relative's actual care needs and the care categorization they were given, which they felt did not reflect their individual needs: "*The carer who did the categorization for care was probably blind and deaf. Or just completely idiotic. My father couldn't walk five steps without gasping for breath, he couldn't wash himself or prepare his medication, let alone take it. He was totally dependent on help. And what did he get? With a lot of hanging and asking, just level 1. That kind of thing is a cheek [meaning ridiculous]*" (In Germany, the previous levels of care were replaced by five levels of care as of 1 January 2017. This categorization reflects a person's level of independence and determines the corresponding care benefits. The categorization is carried out by the care insurance company on the basis of an expert opinion that determines the individual's need for support [29]) (Respondent-ID: 119).
- Assistance with documents: Dealing with the amount of paperwork was a significant challenge for family caregivers. Filling in forms and applications was perceived as very stressful. Many respondents said that more support was needed in this area to reduce the bureaucratic burden: "*Support in dealing with the mountain of paperwork, applications, etc.*" (Respondent-ID: 58).

These subcategories helped us better recognize specific differences within the overarching area of "financial, legal, or professional matters" and illustrate the complexity of needs.

4. Discussion

This study aimed to explore the financial impact of caring for a seriously ill and dying family member at home. The findings highlight the significant challenges faced by family caregivers and the need for comprehensive support, particularly in the areas of workplace policies and financial security.

One noteworthy aspect of this care dynamic concerns gender disparities, as our findings are in line with wider research on the persistence of gender inequalities in the assumption of care work [30]. Women of working age are more likely to provide care and spend more time providing care than men, often while maintaining their employment [31]. This "gender care gap" leads to restrictions on women's life choices and earning potential [30].

The age of panel participants in this study appears to be younger than in other studies. This difference suggests that the unique focus on balancing work and caring for a dying relative may have attracted family caregivers with a demographic less represented in traditional self-selected samples, highlighting a critical but often overlooked perspective on intergenerational care dynamics.

Our findings show that family caregivers face several critical barriers, including balancing work commitments, financial insecurity, and bureaucratic barriers. These factors not only impede their ability to provide care but also affect their overall well-being [32]. It is essential to recognize and address these issues through appropriate resources and support systems [33,34].

The health care reform in Denmark in 2007 shows that systematic changes are possible. Focusing on specialization, centralization, and digitalization, the reform has attracted international attention [35]. It significantly restructured the health sector, with the specific aim of improving the transparency and quality of home care [36,37]. The Danish system stands out among European countries for its comprehensive coverage: 59% of those in need of care receive state-provided care [38]. As a result, Denmark is among the countries with the lowest rates of daily care, similar to other Nordic countries, where individuals requiring such care benefit from the well-developed formal long-term care sector and better paid coverage [39]. While some countries, particularly in Northern Europe, have developed robust policies and services for caregivers [40], others, particularly in the Global South, lack comprehensive support systems [41]. Cross-country studies highlight differences in caregiver experiences, with those in countries offering more developed formal support generally reporting lower burden and higher well-being [42]. Workplace policies to support caregiving vary internationally, with some countries implementing innovative approaches such as shared paid leave systems [43].

In particular, family caregivers of terminally ill patients often face significant out-of-pocket expenses, including medical supplies, medications, and transportation costs for medical visits. According to a recent study by Hastert et al. [44], logistical costs were the most common out-of-pocket expenses (58%), followed by medication costs (35%) and medical bills (17%). Furthermore, severe financial hardship was reported by 38% of family caregivers. Such financial burdens can lead to increased debt and reduced savings, resulting in long-term economic hardship.

Family caregivers are an important social and economic resource for the health care system [19–21], and caring should not negatively affect the economic future of family caregivers. Many family caregivers who work are forced to reduce their working hours or interrupt their careers to provide care, with both short- and long-term financial consequences [45]. A recent study by Kasdorf et al. [23] found that 28% of respondents had to take sick leave to care for a relative. In addition, 40.4% reported having to use their savings to pay for care, and 36.9% reported that their net monthly income was insufficient to cover the cost of care [23]. Long-term effects may include difficulties returning to work or loss of pension benefits. To mitigate these effects, frameworks need to be implemented that allow family caregivers to maintain both their caring responsibilities and their professional and financial futures [45]. These caregivers should be able to combine work and care by benefitting from financial support, flexible working hours, and the opportunity to work from home [46]. Instead, the lack of support in the workplace emerged as a key concern for many family caregivers. Participants expressed a strong desire for more adaptable working hours to balance caring and work responsibilities, a finding that is consistent with the wider research [47,48]. In addition, the need for leave options and greater employer understanding was highlighted, underlining a gap in employer support. Policies such as carer's leave could help family caregivers take the time they need without fear of losing their jobs or income. In order to facilitate a sensitive approach to serious illness, death, and bereavement and to promote communication and emotional support among colleagues at work, training programs in bereavement support, such as those offered by the LAUT project in Germany ("Letzthelfer:innen am Arbeitsplatz-für einen sensiblen Umgang mit Sterben, Tod und Trauer (LAUT)," available at https://letzthelferamarbeitsplatz.com/ (accessed 3 February 2025)), should be implemented [49].

Additionally, participants in our study expressed a strong need for a more comprehensive financial safety net, as many face significant economic hardship due to reduced working hours or an inability to work. Financial stress, in turn, can have a negative impact on the physical and mental health of family caregivers [22,50]. In addition, many participants reported that they could not afford professional care services, highlighting the financial barriers to accessing adequate support [51].

Bureaucratic barriers and a lack of information about available financial resources compound the stress family caregivers face [52]. The time-consuming and often confusing application processes for financial and care-related support contribute to family carer burnout and feelings of helplessness [53]. Research suggests that proactive support is essential to meet the needs of family caregivers. A "buddy" system, where knowledgeable individuals link families to health and social care services, could bridge the gap between family caregivers' needs and available support [54]. Raising awareness of family caregiving in both social and professional settings is also essential, especially as demographic changes increase the need for care [21]. Policy makers should prioritize the inclusion of these recommendations in their policy considerations [32].

In sum, our findings highlight several areas where improvements are urgently needed. Changes in workplace policies, financial support systems, and bureaucratic processes are required to better support family caregivers. Policies that promote flexibility in the workplace, ensure adequate financial compensation, and reduce bureaucratic barriers are crucial to reducing the burden on family caregivers. In addition, clearer information and guidance on available services and benefits will help family caregivers navigate the complexities of caregiving and ultimately improve the quality of care for their loved ones.

Strengths and Limitations

To our knowledge, this is the first study in which the German version of the CSNAT has been used retrospectively in a questionnaire and expanded to include open-text comments, which enables a more precise analysis of family caregivers' needs. The large sample size permitted a meaningful assessment of family caregivers' needs in addition to the quantitative data collection, which has been published elsewhere [23]. The qualitative analysis provided a detailed analysis of individual statements, giving family caregivers a voice. The use of a panel achieved a high response rate, ensuring the representativeness of the results across different conditions and regions of Germany. There is, though, a potential risk of self-selection, as 65% of survey participants were panel members. Furthermore, as the survey was conducted online, participants' digital competences may have influenced the results differently depending on their age, with older participants potentially having less experience with online surveys. This may partly explain the differences in the age distribution of our sample compared to other studies. Although our retrospective research design, which asked bereaved family caregivers to report on their experiences of end-of-life care, may have limitations, such as possible recall bias and the influence of emotion, studies have shown that brief events are often accurately recalled [8].

The validity of the CSNAT for family caregivers in palliative care has been demonstrated internationally [55]. The domains of the CSNAT comprehensively cover the different areas of support needs, and it serves as a tool in research and everyday palliative care [25].

5. Conclusions

Although the gaps in support for family caregivers have long been recognized, the individual needs of family caregivers and the needs-based implementation of effective interventions have not been sufficiently explored. The burden on family caregivers remains high, and families carry much of the burden with seemingly no financial support. As home care becomes more prevalent, financial support for family caregivers is essential to meet the increasing demands of end-of-life care at home. Key measures include the introduction of income replacement benefits, similar to parental leave, to mitigate income loss during caregiving periods. In addition, the recognition of caregiving time for pension purposes can help prevent long-term financial disadvantages. A more flexible and less bureaucratic use of respite care services, such as short-term care and relief care, is also crucial to provide family caregivers with the breaks they need. Widening access to these services and increasing the availability of community-based and digital support, complemented by better advice on existing support services through practical helpers, such as a "Buddy in the last year of life" or "Last-Aiders at work", can further improve family caregivers' access to practical, emotional, social, and financial support.

Author Contributions: Conceptualization, J.S., A.K. and R.V.; methodology, J.S., A.K. and S.P.; validation, J.S., A.K. and R.V.; formal analysis, S.P. and A.K.; investigation, J.S. and A.K.; resources, J.S. and A.K.; data curation, J.S., A.K. and S.P.; writing—original draft preparation, S.P.; writing—review and editing, J.S., A.K. and R.V.; visualization, S.P.; supervision, J.S. and A.K.; project administration, J.S. and A.K.; funding acquisition, J.S., R.V., and A.K. All authors have read and agreed to the published version of the manuscript.

Funding: This project was funded by the Federal Ministry for Family Affairs, Senior Citizens, Women and Youth (BMFSFJ, grant number #ZMI8-2521BAP369).

Institutional Review Board Statement: This study was conducted in accordance with the Declaration of Helsinki and approved by the Ethics Commission of the Faculty of Medicine in Cologne (protocol code #21-1466, approval date: 25 November 2021). This study was prospectively registered in the German Clinical Trials Register (DRKS00026229).

Informed Consent Statement: Informed consent was obtained from all subjects involved in this study.

Data Availability Statement: Selected parts from the original contributions presented in this study are included in the article. Further inquiries can be addressed to the corresponding author.

Acknowledgments: The authors would like to express their thanks to all participants, families, and project partners supporting us with the recruitment and performance of this study. We extend our thanks to the Federal Ministry for Family Affairs, Senior Citizens, Women and Youth for funding this study.

Conflicts of Interest: The authors declare no conflicts of interest.

References

1. Ogugua, J.O.; Muonde, M.; Maduka, C.P.; Olorunsogo, T.O.; Omotayo, O. Demographic Shifts and Healthcare: A Review of Aging Populations and Systemic Challenges. *Int. J. Sci. Res. Arch.* **2024**, *11*, 383–395. [CrossRef]
2. Dawson, W.D.; Bangerter, L.R.; Splaine, M. The Politics of Caregiving: Taking Stock of State-Level Policies to Support Family Caregivers. *Public Policy Aging Rep.* **2020**, *30*, 62–66. [CrossRef]
3. Wheatley, M.C. Adapting Health Systems for an Aging World: Policy Innovations and Global Strategies. *Prem. J. Public Health* **2024**, *24*, 362. [CrossRef]
4. Mehr Pflegebedürftige—Statistisches Bundesamt. Available online: https://www.destatis.de/DE/Themen/Querschnitt/Demografischer-Wandel/Hintergruende-Auswirkungen/demografie-pflege.html (accessed on 8 February 2025).
5. Schnitzer, S.; Kuhlmey, A.; Engelmann, F.; Budnick, A. Informal Caregivers and How Primary Care Physicians Can Support Them. *Dtsch. Ärztebl. Int.* **2021**, *118*, 507–508. [CrossRef]
6. Fuchs, J.; Gaertner, B.; Rommel, A.; Starker, A. Informal Caregivers in Germany—Who Are They and Which Risks and Resources Do They Have? *Front. Public Health* **2023**, *11*, 1058517. [CrossRef]
7. Geyer, J.; Schulz, E. Who Cares? Die Bedeutung Der Informellen Pflege Durch Erwerbstätige in Deutschland. 2014. Available online: https://www.semanticscholar.org/paper/Who-cares-Die-Bedeutung-der-informellen-Pflege-in-Geyer-Schulz/b3234081b8dcbf51f01fe464198a1fbb6d827e77#citing-papers (accessed on 15 October 2024).
8. Voltz, R.; Dust, G.; Schippel, N.; Hamacher, S.; Payne, S.; Scholten, N.; Pfaff, H.; Rietz, C.; Strupp, J. Improving Regional Care in the Last Year of Life by Setting up a Pragmatic Evidence-Based Plan–Do–Study–Act Cycle: Results from a Cross-Sectional Survey. *BMJ Open* **2020**, *10*, e035988. [CrossRef]
9. Michaels, J.; Chen, C.; Ann Meeker, M. Navigating the Caregiving Abyss: A Metasynthesis of How Family Caregivers Manage End-of-Life Care for Older Adults at Home. *Palliat. Med.* **2022**, *36*, 81–94. [CrossRef]
10. Hackmann, T.; Moog, S. Pflege Im Spannungsfeld von Angebot Und Nachfrage. *Z. Für Sozialreform* **2010**, *56*, 113–138. [CrossRef]
11. Xiang, E.; Guzman, P.; Mims, M.; Badr, H. Balancing Work and Cancer Care: Challenges Faced by Employed Informal Caregivers. *Cancers* **2022**, *14*, 4146. [CrossRef]
12. Jenull, B.; Frate, N. Wie schaffen wir den Spagat zwischen Pflege und Erwerbsarbeit?: Eine Studie zur Vereinbarkeit von Pflege und Erwerbsarbeit an der Alpen-Adria-Universität. *Z. Für Gerontol. Geriatr.* **2019**, *52*, 761–766. [CrossRef]
13. Knecht, S.; Reiners, H.; Siebler, M.; Platz, T.; Flöel, A.; Busse, R. Schleichender demografischer Wandel und neurologische Rehabilitation—Teil 1: Situationsbeschreibung. *Nervenarzt* **2023**, *94*, 708–717. [CrossRef] [PubMed]
14. Eisenreich, T. Pflegenotstand—Die Doppelte Demografische Lücke. *Sozialwirtschaft Aktuell* **2023**, *33*, 1–3. [CrossRef]
15. Bijnsdorp, F.M.; Van Der Beek, A.J.; Pasman, H.R.W.; Boot, C.R.L.; De Boer, A.H.; Plaisier, I.; Onwuteaka-Philipsen, B.D. Home Care for Terminally Ill Patients: The Experiences of Family Caregivers with and without Paid Work. *BMJ Support. Palliat. Care* **2022**, *12*, e226–e235. [CrossRef] [PubMed]
16. Theobald, H. Home-Based Care Provision within the German Welfare Mix: Home-Based Care Provision. *Health Soc. Care Community* **2012**, *20*, 274–282. [CrossRef]
17. SGB XI—Sozialgesetzbuch Elftes Buch—Soziale Pflegeversicherung. 1995. Available online: https://www.gesetze-im-internet.de/sgb_11/__36.html (accessed on 10 January 2025).
18. Geyer, J.; Börsch-Supan, A.; Haan, P.; Perdrix, E. *Long-Term Care in Germany*; National Bureau of Economic Research: Cambridge, MA, USA, 2023; p. w31870.
19. Wetzstein, M.; Rommel, A.; Lange, C. Robert Koch-Institut Pflegende Angehörige—Deutschlands größter Pflegedienst. 2016. Available online: https://edoc.rki.de/handle/176904/3137 (accessed on 20 February 2025).
20. Reinhard, S. Valuing and supporting the invisible workforce of family caregivers. *Innov. Aging* **2023**, *7*, 241. [CrossRef]
21. Van Den Berg, B.; Brouwer, W.B.F.; Koopmanschap, M.A. Economic Valuation of Informal Care. *Eur. J. Health Econ.* **2004**, *5*, 36–45. [CrossRef]
22. Reinhard, S.; Feinberg, L. Caregiver Health and Well-Being, and Financial Strain. *Innov. Aging* **2020**, *4*, 681–682. [CrossRef]
23. Kasdorf, A.; Voltz, R.; Strupp, J. Dying at Home: What Is Needed? Findings from a Nationwide Retrospective Cross-Sectional Online Survey of Bereaved People in Germany. *Palliat. Support. Care* **2024**, *ahead of print*. [CrossRef]
24. Kasdorf, A.; Voltz, R.; Strupp, J. The Buddy Intervention: Designing an Additional Support System for the Last Year of Life. Qualitative Insights from Triangulated Interviews and Focus Group Discussions. *J. Public Health* **2024**, *32*, 2001–2013. [CrossRef]
25. Ewing, G.; Brundle, C.; Payne, S.; Grande, G. The Carer Support Needs Assessment Tool (CSNAT) for Use in Palliative and End-of-Life Care at Home: A Validation Study. *J. Pain Symptom Manag.* **2013**, *46*, 395–405. [CrossRef] [PubMed]
26. Kreyer, C.; Bükki, J.; Pleschberger, S. Development of a German Version of the Carer Support Needs Assessment Tool (CSNAT): The Process of Translation and Cultural Adaptation. *Palliat. Support. Care* **2020**, *18*, 193–198. [CrossRef] [PubMed]
27. Pohontsch, N.J. Die Qualitative Inhaltsanalyse. *Die Rehabil.* **2019**, *58*, 413–418. [CrossRef]

28. Mayring, P. Qualitative Content Analysis: Theoretical Background and Procedures. In *Approaches to Qualitative Research in Mathematics Education*; Bikner-Ahsbahs, A., Knipping, C., Presmeg, N., Eds.; Advances in Mathematics Education; Springer: Dordrecht, The Netherlands, 2015; pp. 365–380, ISBN 978-94-017-9180-9.
29. Pflegegrad—Statistisches Bundesamt. Available online: https://www.destatis.de/DE/Themen/Gesellschaft-Umwelt/Gesundheit/Glossar/Pflegegrad.html (accessed on 16 February 2025).
30. Häußler, A. Who cares? Sorgearbeit als individuelle Aufgabe und gesellschaftliche Herausforderung. *Haushalt Bild. Forsch.* **2019**, *8*, 41–53. [CrossRef]
31. Kochskämper, S.; Neumeister, S.; Stockhausen, M. Wer pflegt wann und wie viel? Eine Bestandsaufnahme zur häuslichen Pflege in Deutschland. *IW Trends* **2020**, *47*, 67–83. [CrossRef]
32. Kuhlmey, A.; Budnick, A. Pflegende Angehörige in Deutschland: Vereinbarkeit von Pflege und Erwerbstätigkeit. *Bundesgesundheitsblatt-Gesundheitsforschung-Gesundheitsschutz* **2023**, *66*, 550–556. [CrossRef]
33. Hastert, T.A.; Ruterbusch, J.J.; Nair, M.; Noor, M.I.; Beebe-Dimmer, J.L.; Schwartz, K.; Baird, T.E.; Harper, F.W.K.; Thompson, H.; Schwartz, A.G. Employment Outcomes, Financial Burden, Anxiety, and Depression Among Caregivers of African American Cancer Survivors. *JCO Oncol. Pract.* **2020**, *16*, e221–e233. [CrossRef]
34. Hebdon, M.C.T.; Xu, J.; Reblin, M.; Clayton, M.F.; Mooney, K.; Ellington, L. Balancing Work and Hospice Caregiving—A Closer Look at Burden, Preparedness, and Mental Health. *J. Pain Symptom Manag.* **2022**, *63*, 283–292. [CrossRef]
35. Kretzler, M.; Berger, E.; Reichebner, C.; Offermanns, M.; Heber, R.; Krause, C.; Schulz, M.; Busse, R. Deutschland Und Dänemark—Verschiedene Welten? Ein Umfassender Vergleich Der Gesundheitssysteme. *Gesundh.-Sozialpolitik* **2020**, *74*, 13–20. [CrossRef]
36. Andersen, P.T.; Jensen, J.-J. Healthcare Reform in Denmark. *Scand. J. Public Health* **2010**, *38*, 246–252. [CrossRef]
37. Rostgaard, T. Quality Reforms in Danish Home Care—Balancing between Standardisation and Individualisation: Balancing between Standardisation and Individualisation. *Health Soc. Care Community* **2012**, *20*, 247–254. [CrossRef] [PubMed]
38. Schulz, E.; Geyer, J. Pflegebedarfe Und Pflegesettings—Ein Vergleich Formeller Und Informeller Pflege in Ausgewählten Europäischen Ländern. *Vierteljahrsh. Zur Wirtsch.* **2014**, *83*, 137–157. [CrossRef]
39. Maia, A.C.; Nogueira, P.; Henriques, M.A.; Farinha, C.; Costa, A. Ageing and Long-Term Informal Care: The Reality of Two Countries in Europe: Denmark and Portugal. *Int. J. Environ. Res. Public Health* **2022**, *19*, 10859. [CrossRef]
40. Cahill, S.; Bielsten, T.; Zarit, S.H. Developing a Framework for the Support of Informal Caregivers: Experiences from Sweden, Ireland, and the United States. *Res. Aging* **2023**, *45*, 385–395. [CrossRef]
41. Bourissi, H.; Mellas, S. Government Recognition and Support for Family Caregivers: A Comparative Review of Policies in Northern and Southern Countries With a Focus on Oncology Caregivers. *Cureus* **2024**, *16*, e63085. [CrossRef]
42. Zarzycki, M.; Vilchinsky, N.; Bei, E.; Ferraris, G.; Seddon, D.; Morrison, V. Cross-Country Variations in the Caregiver Role: Evidence from the ENTWINE-iCohort Study. *BMC Public Health* **2024**, *24*, 898. [CrossRef]
43. Kanda, K.; Sakurazawa, H.; Yoshida, T. International Comparison of Social Support Policies on Long-Term Care in Workplaces in Aging Societies. *Int. J. Environ. Res. Public Health* **2022**, *19*, 3284. [CrossRef]
44. Hastert, T.A.; Kyko, J.M.; Ruterbusch, J.J.; Robinson, J.R.M.; Kamen, C.S.; Beebe-Dimmer, J.L.; Nair, M.; Thompson, H.S.; Schwartz, A.G. Caregiver Costs and Financial Burden in Caregivers of African American Cancer Survivors. *J. Cancer Surviv.* **2024**, *18*, 565–574. [CrossRef]
45. Heger, D.; Korfhage, T. Short- and Medium-Term Effects of Informal Eldercare on Labor Market Outcomes. *Fem. Econ.* **2020**, *26*, 205–227. [CrossRef]
46. Fischer, B.; Müller, K.-U. Bessere Vereinbarkeit von Beruf Und Pflege Kann Zielkonflikt Zwischen Renten- Und Pflegepolitik Lösen. *DIW Wochenber.* **2020**, *87*, 853–860. [CrossRef]
47. Scheuermann, J.-S.; Gräßel, E.; Pendergrass, A. Vereinbarkeit von Erwerbstätigkeit und häuslicher Pflege: Einflussfaktoren auf eine pflegebedingte Erwerbstätigkeitsreduktion und arbeitsbezogene Wünsche pflegender Angehöriger. *Gesundheitswesen* **2024**, *86*, S45–S53. [CrossRef] [PubMed]
48. Plöthner, M.; Schmidt, K.; De Jong, L.; Zeidler, J.; Damm, K. Needs and Preferences of Informal Caregivers Regarding Outpatient Care for the Elderly: A Systematic Literature Review. *BMC Geriatr.* **2019**, *19*, 82. [CrossRef] [PubMed]
49. Voltz, R.; Strupp, J.; Bollig, G. Last Aid at the Workplace | Palliativzentrum | Uniklinik Köln. Available online: https://palliativzentrum.uk-koeln.de/forschung/letzte-lebenszeit/last-aid-at-the-workplace/ (accessed on 3 February 2025).
50. Vitaliano, P.P.; Young, H.M.; Zhang, J. Is Caregiving a Risk Factor for Illness? *Curr. Dir. Psychol. Sci.* **2004**, *13*, 13–16. [CrossRef]
51. Pinquart, M.; Sorensen, S. Correlates of Physical Health of Informal Caregivers: A Meta-Analysis. *J. Gerontol. Ser. B Psychol. Sci. Soc. Sci.* **2007**, *62*, P126–P137. [CrossRef]
52. Strommen, J.; Fuller, H.; Sanders, G.F.; Elliott, D.M. Challenges Faced by Family Caregivers: Multiple Perspectives on Eldercare. *J. Appl. Gerontol.* **2020**, *39*, 347–356. [CrossRef]
53. Kingsberry, S.Q.; Mindler, P. Misperceptions of Medicaid Ineligibility Persist among African American Caregivers of Alzheimer's Dementia Care Recipients. *Popul. Health Manag.* **2012**, *15*, 174–180. [CrossRef]

54. Berry, L.L.; Dalwadi, S.M.; Jacobson, J.O. Supporting the Supporters: What Family Caregivers Need to Care for a Loved One With Cancer. *J. Oncol. Pract.* **2017**, *13*, 35–41. [CrossRef]
55. Alvariza, A.; Holm, M.; Benkel, I.; Norinder, M.; Ewing, G.; Grande, G.; Håkanson, C.; Öhlen, J.; Årestedt, K. A Person-Centred Approach in Nursing: Validity and Reliability of the Carer Support Needs Assessment Tool. *Eur. J. Oncol. Nurs.* **2018**, *35*, 1–8. [CrossRef]

healthcare

MDPI

Article

Exploring End-of-Life Care for Patients with Breast Cancer, Dementia or Heart Failure: A Register-Based Study of Individual and Institutional Factors

Terje P. Hagen [1,*] and Erika Zelko [2,3]

1 Department of Health Management and Health Economics, University of Oslo, Blindern, P.O. Box 1072, 0316 Oslo, Norway
2 Institute of General Medicine, Johannes Kepler University, Altenberger Straße 69, 4040 Linz, Austria; erika.zelko@jku.au
3 Institute of Palliative Medicine, Medical Faculty, University Maribor, Slomskov trg 15, 2000 Maribor, Slovenia
* Correspondence: t.p.hagen@medisin.uio.no

Abstract: Objective: To examine variations in end-of-life care for breast cancer, heart failure, and dementia patients. Data and methods: Data from four Norwegian health registries were linked using a personal identification number. Longitudinal trends over 365 days and the type of care on the final day of life were analyzed using descriptive techniques and logistic regression analysis. Results: Patients with dementia were more commonly placed in nursing homes than patients in the two other groups, while patients with heart failure and breast cancer were more frequently hospitalized than the dementia patients. Breast cancer and heart failure patients had a higher likelihood of dying at home than dementia patients. The higher the number of general practitioners, the higher was the probability of home-based end-of-life care for cancer patients, while an increasing non-physician healthcare workers increased the likelihood of home-based care for the other patient groups. Conclusions: Diagnoses, individual characteristics, and service availability are all associated with the place of death in end-of-life care. The higher the availability of health care services, the higher also is the probability of ending the life at home.

Keywords: end-of-life care; palliative care; social and long-term care; Norway

1. Introduction

End-of-life (EoL) care, though lacking a precise definition, generally refers to healthcare provided to individuals approaching death. This care encompasses ongoing treatment for the underlying disease, and palliative measures to manage symptoms and enhance the quality of life (QoL) [1]. The provision of EoL care typically involves a collaborative decision-making process, often supported by an established advanced care plan [1]. Emerging evidence from multiple studies suggests that initiating EoL care in a timely manner can bring about numerous benefits [2–4]. These include enhancing patients' QoL, alleviating symptoms, and potentially reducing the unnecessary utilization of acute care services—which extends beyond just cancer patients [2–4]. Despite the beneficial effects of EoL and palliative care, global statistics indicate that only around 14% of patients in need receive palliative care [5]. Even in high-income countries, the results are comparable [6].

In Norway, where healthcare services are predominantly public and free, municipalities oversee primary health care, including primary palliative care and local emergency rooms (emergency primary healthcare clinics), while specialist healthcare is provided by four state-driven health regions, typically upon referral from primary care [7,8]. Palliative care is integrated into public health services, with specialist palliative care centers in hospitals staffed by at least one palliative care physician and one oncology nurse (ON). These specialists are available for consultation within hospitals and by primary care clinicians (general practitioners and ONs), who can also refer patients to them [8].

The geographical location of individuals at end-of-life has wide-ranging implications for healthcare delivery, costs, and, notably, for individuals' preferences regarding care, particularly the realizations of desires to spend their final days at home [6,8]. Despite the widespread preference for home-based care at the end of life, the opportunity to do so is only available to a relatively small percentage of individuals, typically ranging from 10% to 30% in most countries [6,9–14], also including Norway [15].

Gomes and her team identified several essential conditions that are almost prerequisites for patients to have the option of spending their final days at home. These conditions include the patient's own preference, the family's preference, access to home palliative care, and the availability of district or community nursing [16]. In order to fulfill more individuals' desires to receive end-of-life care at home and to comprehensively address their needs, Kellehear stresses that "end-of-life care is everyone's business," thereby extending responsibility beyond just families and healthcare services to encompass communities [17].

Research has consistently demonstrated a rise in healthcare service utilization during the final months of life [18–21]. However, there remains a need to fully understand the key variables that affect service utilization, including types of care at end-of-life. Our study endeavors to bridge this gap by examining disparities in service utilization during the twelve months prior to death among patients with breast cancer, dementia, and heart failure. Additionally, we aim to identify individual and institutional factors that influence the likelihood of patients dying at home. Of particular interest are potential associations between the supply of services at the local level such as GPs and other types of health personnel, and the odds of spending the last day of life at home.

2. Material and Methods

2.1. Inclusion Criteria and Data Sources

Utilizing data from the Norwegian Causes of Death Registry (NCDR), our analysis includes all patients who passed away in 2019 with underlying diagnoses of breast cancer (ICD-10 D05), dementia (ICD-10 F00–F03), or heart failure (ICD-10 I60, I61, I63, I64). By employing personal identification numbers obtained from the NCDR, we combined data from various registers, including the National Patient Register (a discharge register), the Municipal Patient and User Register, the Education Register, and KOSTRA—a register that describes municipal use of resources. The Directorate of Health oversees the first two registers, while Statistics Norway manages the latter two.

Data were collected for the period covering the last 365 days before the date of death for each patient, except for variables describing the patients' co-morbidities where we collected data from the National Patent Register and the Municipal Patient and User Register for up to two years before the death date. All data were anonymized for the researchers.

2.2. Outcomes

The main outcomes were health service use the last 365 days before the death day (D0), including GP visits, home nursing, short- and long-term stays in municipal institutions (mainly nursing homes), as well as outpatient and inpatient stays in hospitals. Additionally, our analysis specifically investigated a binary variable indicating whether patients were at home (1) or in institutions (0), i.e., nursing home or hospital, on the day before their death (D-1). The reason for using D-1 as the time of measurement for 'Dying at home' was that services were not registered consistently on the death day.

2.3. Statistical Analyses

The characteristics of the cohorts were described by frequencies for categorical variables and by median for continuous variables.

To identify variables associated with 'dying at home' we performed a multivariate logistic regression analysis to estimate odds ratios (OR) and 96% confidence intervals (CI). We made separate analyses for the three cohorts that were defined by the causes of death with two groups of variables included, variables on patient and variables on municipal level. Variables on the individual level included gender, age categorized in 10-year age bands from 50 to 89 years and with patients below 50 and above 90 years in separate groups, marital status (indicator of informal care), education (primary, secondary, and higher education) and the number of comorbidities (0, 1–2, 3–4, 5 and above). The variables on the municipal level included the person years of GPs and caring personnel in total, both normalized by 10,000 inhabitants.

We registered data on 15 comorbidities (see Appendix A) from up to two years before the death day. Comorbidities were generated from the registration of both primary and secondary diagnoses and from both hospital inpatient and outpatient stays as well as consultations with GPs registered in the Municipal Patient and User Register.

Data management and analyses were conducted in SAS Studio 5.1 (SAS Institute Inc., Cary, NC, USA).

3. Results

3.1. Patient Population

In 2019, 606 patients succumbed to breast cancer, 2900 to dementia and 1415 to heart failure. Among breast cancer patients, the median age was 73.0 years, while for dementia patients it was 88.4 years and for heart failure patients it was 86.2 years (Table 1). When classified using 10-year age bands, the highest number of deaths occurred in the 70–79 age group, with 147 cases (24.3%) for the breast cancer patients. In the two other patient groups the highest numbers of death were in the age group 90 years and above.

Table 1. Patient characteristics.

		Breast Cancer	Dementia	Heart Failure
Total		N (%) 606 (100)	N (%) 2900	N (%) 1415
Gender	Female	600 (99.0)	1972 (84.4)	837 (59.2)
	Male	6 (1.0)	452 (15.6)	578 (40.9)
Age	<50 years	44 (7.3)	0 (0.0)	11 (0.8)
	50–59 years	98 (16.2)	2 (0.0)	19 (1.4)
	60–69 years	115 (19.0	35 (1.2)	50 (3.6)
	70–79 years	147 (24.3)	287 (9.9)	186 (13.2)
	80–89 years	129 (21.3)	1175 (40.5)	460 (32.7)
	90 years≤	73 (12.1)	1402 (48.3)	683 (48.5)
	Median	73.0	88.4	86.2
Education	Primary	177 (29.2)	1279 (44.4)	635 (45.5)
	Secondary	271 (44.7)	1209 (42.0)	612 (43.8)
	Higher	152 (25.1)	390 (13.55)	150 (10.7)
	Missing	6	22	12
Marital status	Others *	358 (59.1)	2110 (72.8)	1030 (73.1)
	Married	248 (40.9)	790 (27.2)	379 (26.9)
Comorbidities	0	305 (50.3)	298 (10.3)	133 (9.4)
	1–2	196 (32.3)	1318 (45.5)	443 (31.4)
	3–4	74 (12.2)	871 (30.0)	442 (31.4)
	5 or more	31 (5.1)	413 (14.2)	391 (27.8)
General Practitioners (GPs) per 10,000 inhabitants	<10.1	154 (24.8)	643 (22.2)	346 (24.6)
	10.2–10.9	155 (25.6)	794 (27.4)	312 (22.1)
	11.0–12.1	156 (24.1)	682 (23.5)	322 (22.9)
	12.2<	145 (23.9)	781 (26.9)	429 (30.5)
Non-physician healthcare personnel years per 10,000 inhabitants	<213.9	144 (23.8)	583 (20.1)	275 (19.5)
	213.9–258.97	157 (25.9)	681 (23.5)	287 (20.4)
	258.97–311.82	155 (25.6	867 (29.9)	404 (28.7)
	311.82	150 (24.8	769 (26.5)	443 (31.4)
Size of municipality	<5000 inhabitamts	73 (12.1)	310 (10.7)	223 (15.8)
	5000–15,000 inh	116 (19.4)	623 (21.5)	353 (25.1)
	15,000≤ inh	417 (68.8)	1967 (67.8)	833 (58.1)

* Others include unmarried, widowers, divorced or separated and others.

The breast cancer patients also deviate from the two other groups, with a higher share being married, having fewer comorbidities, and higher education levels—naturally reflecting these patients' younger age.

3.2. Service Use at End-of-Life

In the year leading up to their death, a significant proportion of breast cancer patients (64.0%) experienced at least one hospital admission, with 388 patients affected (Table 2). Furthermore, 556 patients (91.7%) received hospital treatments either as outpatients or during day stays. In contrast, the utilization of hospitals among patients with dementia in the year preceding death was notably lower, with only 10% admitted to hospitals and 33% receiving outpatient consultations or day stays. Dementia patients, however, were frequent users of nursing homes.

Table 2. Patients use of health service last 365 days of life (number of patients with at least one visit).

Type of Services	Breast Cancer N (% of Total)	Dementia N (% of Total)	Heart Failure N (% of Total)
Hospital admission	388 (64.0)	292 (10.0)	448 (31.8)
Hospital—outpatient or day stays	556 (91.7)	977 (33.7)	870 (61.7)
Nursing homes—long-term stays	102 (16.8)	2453 (84.6)	592 (42.0)
Nursing homes—short term stays	289 (47.7)	547 (18.9)	579 (41.1)
General practise (GP) visits	535 (88.2)	1167 (40.2)	923 (65.5)
Emergency room (local)	296 (48.8)	1322 (45.6)	709 (50.3)
Home nursing	403 (66.5)	741 (25.5)	818 (58.1)

Breast cancer patients were found to make an extensive use of general practitioner (GP) services and frequently visited local emergency rooms (emergency primary healthcare clinics). Conversely, dementia patients had a different utilization pattern, with fewer individuals visiting GPs. It is important to note that while in nursing homes, patients receive medical services from an attending physician who is not part of the GP list patient system.

In terms of care profile, heart failure patients fell somewhere between the utilization patterns observed in cancer and dementia patients.

The dynamic changes in service utilization are further illustrated in Figure 1a–c, highlighting the use of services during each of the final 365 days before death among the patient groups. For all three patient groups, hospital stays remained relatively low but gradually increased during the last two months of life. Long-term stays in nursing homes were frequent and steadily increased among dementia patients, while they remained at a lower level among breast cancer patients. Notably, there was a significant increase in short-term stays in nursing homes among breast cancer patients during the last 2–3 months of life. Furthermore, for the breast cancer patients, a progressive increase in home nursing was observed until the last 4–6 weeks, followed by a decline in the number of recipients. This decrease was primarily due to patients being transferred to nursing homes, especially for short-term stays.

The proportion of patients residing at home without any of the aforementioned services gradually diminished, particularly for the breast cancer patients. This trend corresponded to the increasing number of patients receiving care in hospitals, nursing homes, and through home nursing services.

3.3. Factors Associated with Home Care at End-of-Life

The vast majority of patients (84%) who passed away from dementia did so in municipal institutions, mainly in nursing homes (Figure 2). Similarly, 57% of heart failure patients passed away in institutions. In contrast, for breast cancer patients, the distribution is almost equal, with 52% passing away in institutions and 48% at home.

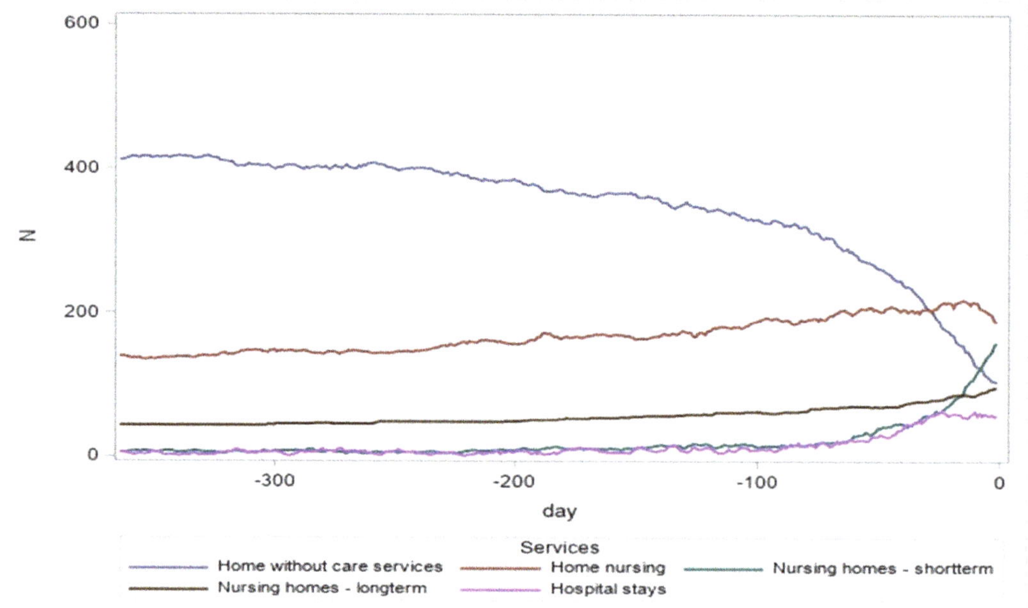

(a)

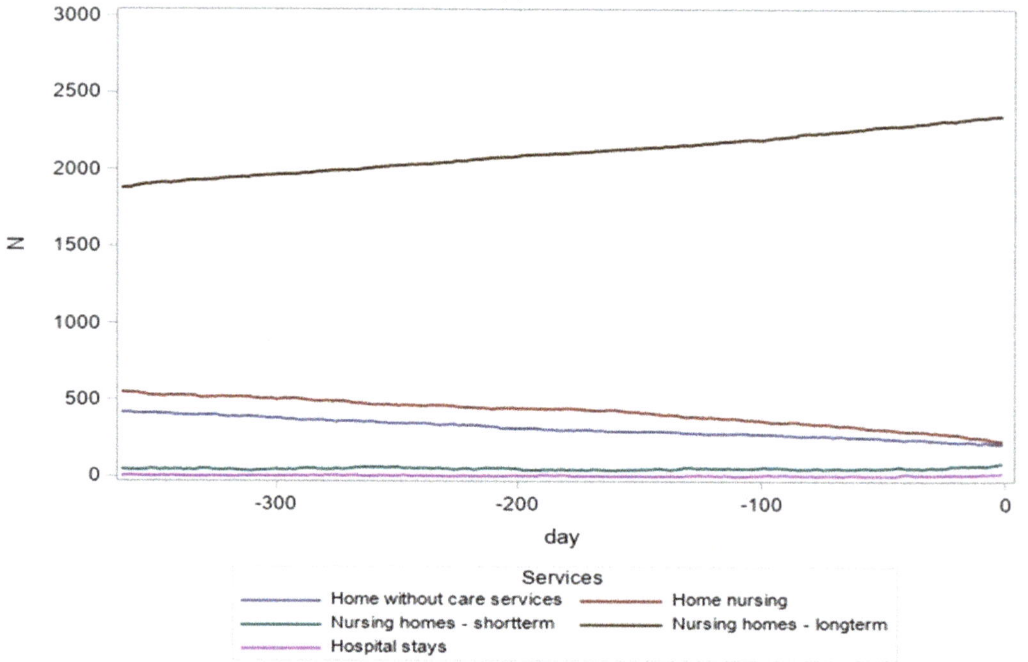

(b)

Figure 1. *Cont.*

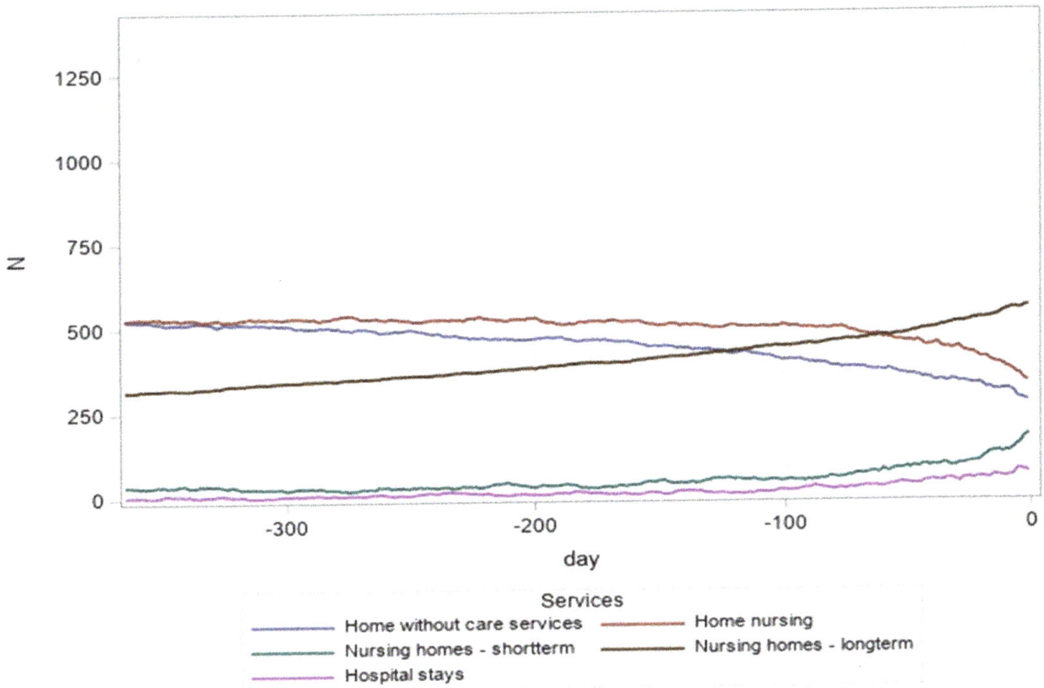

(c)

Figure 1. (**a**) Service use by day, last 365 days of life, breast cancer patients (N = 606); (**b**) service use by day, last 365 days of life, dementia patients (N = 2900); (**c**) service use by day, last 365 days of life, heart failure patients (N = 1415).

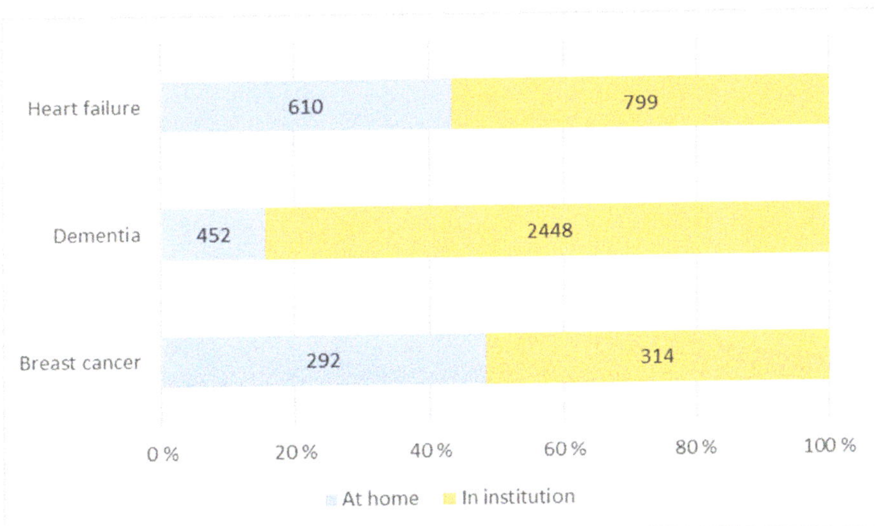

Figure 2. Number of patients at home or in institutions during the last day of life.

The associations between patient characteristics and place of care during the last day before death are presented in Table 3. It is evident that, except for the dementia patients, strong associations exist between the variable describing age groups and staying at home on the last day of life, with the lowest age groups demonstrating significantly higher odds of staying at home compared to older age groups. While there are indications that the odds of staying at home on the last day of life increase with educational level, the relationship is only significant for the heart failure patients. Moreover, an increase in the number of comorbidities decreased the odds of staying at home, with significant effects observed for the heart failure patients.

Table 3. Associations between patent characteristics, supply side variables and staying at home the last day before death. Odds ratio (95% Wald Confidence Limits).

		Breast Cancer	Dementia	Heart Failure
Gender	Male	Ref.	Ref.	Ref.
	Female	2.37 (0.41–13.79)	0.91 (0.72–1.17)	0.76 (0.59–0.98)
Age	80–89 years	Ref.	Ref.	Ref.
	<50 years	2.28 (1.06–4.90)	-	6.94 (0.85–56.34)
	50–59 years	2.23 (1.25–3.99)	-	3.62 (1.15–11.40)
	60–69 years	2.94 (1.69–5.11)	0.92 (0.32–2.68)	4.95 (2.32–10.53)
	70–79 years	1.78 (1.07–2.97)	0.84 (0.57–1.23)	1.87 (1.31–2.68)
	90 years≤	1.07 (0.56–2.02)	1.06 (0.85–1.33)	0.63 (0.51–0.86)
Education	Primary	Ref.	Ref.	Ref.
	Secondary	0.83 (0.56–1.25)	1.14 (0.91–1.43)	1.20 (0.94–1.52)
	Higher	1.01 (0.62–1.22)	1.02 (0.73–1.44)	1.43 (0.97–2.12)
Marital status	Others	Ref.	Ref.	Ref.
	Married	1.22 (0.85–1.76)	1.19 (0.92–1.53)	1.12 (0.85–1.48)
Comorbidities	0	Ref.	Ref.	Ref.
	1–2	0.95 (0.64–1.41)	0.84 (0.59–1.20)	0.59 (0.38–0.90)
	3–4	0.69 (0.38–1.22)	0.94 (0.65–1.36)	0.54 (0.35–0.82)
	5 or more	0.78 (0.34–1.80)	1.20 (0.80–1.80)	0.40 (0.26–0.63)
General Practisioners (GPS)s per 10,000 inhabitants	<10.1	Ref.	Ref.	Ref.
	10.2–10.9	1.51 (0.93–2.44)	0.57 (0.41–0.78)	0.97 (0.70–1.36)
	11.0–12.1	1.68 (1.00–2.80)	0.85 (0.64–1.14)	0.84 (0.60–1.18)
	12.2<	2.13 (1.17–2.28)	0.54 (0.38–0.75)	1.04 (0.71–1.51)
Non-physician healthcare personnel years per 10,000 inhabitants	<213.9	Ref.	Ref.	Ref.
	213.9–258.97	0.52 (0.32–0.86)	1.95 (1.36–2.78)	1.08 (0.75–1.55)
	258.97–311.82	0.77 (0.45–1.32)	1.96 (1.37–2.81)	1.37 (0.96–1.97)
	311.82	0.69 (0.38–1.28)	1.48 (0.98–2.23)	1.13 (0.74–1.72)
Population size	<5000	Ref.	Ref.	Ref.
	5000–14,900	1.16 (0.59–2.28)	1.31 (0.89–1.94)	1.16 (0.79–1.70)
	15,000<	1.49 (0.74–3.03)	0.55 (0.36–0.84)	1.12 (0.74–1.70)
N		600	2878	1397
Somer's D		0.33	0.27	0.32
Percent concordant		66.7	63.4	66.0

The likelihood of cancer patients receiving end-of-life care at home is higher when there are more general practitioners available, while the likelihood of the other two patient groups receiving home care increases with the availability of non-physician healthcare workers. It is important to highlight that the notable disparities are observed between the group that has the least access to municipal care services and the other three categories. This implies that when access to home care is severely restricted, patients are more inclined to spend their remaining days away from home.

4. Discussion

We evaluated the utilization of healthcare services over the last twelve months of life among patients with breast cancer, dementia, and heart failure. The most significant differences were observed in hospitalizations and long-term care in nursing homes. Among the three patient groups, patients with dementia were most frequently placed in nursing homes, while the rate of hospitalization was highest among patients with heart failure and breast cancer. The breast cancer and heart failure patients had a higher likelihood of dying at home than the dementia patients. Furthermore, the availability of general practitioners increased the probability of end-of-life care at home for cancer patients, while the availability of non-physician healthcare workers increased the likelihood of staying at home at end-of-life for the other two patient groups.

Our research findings aligned with those of other authors [6,22,23]. Several studies note that dementia patients are less frequently hospitalized at EoL. The frequency of hospitalizations also decreases for other elderly patients with chronic conditions and those where palliative needs were recognized in a timely manner [24–30]. Diernberger and colleagues furthermore highlight the importance of the geographical environment, as they found that the frequency of hospitalization during the final stages of life among older adults living in rural areas was generally lower than for those living in urban areas. However, when hospitalization did occur, it tended to be of a longer duration [25]. Another important factor influencing the rate of hospitalization was the availability of beds in nursing homes [26,31]. This was further studied by Chu and colleagues, who found that the accessibility of care in nursing homes significantly reduced rehospitalizations, particularly for individuals in the advanced stage of dementia [26].

The utilization of healthcare services is influenced by numerous factors as analyzed by Williamson et al. [31]. We observed a lower utilization of healthcare services among higher-educated patients with heart failure but not for the other two groups of patients. Except for dementia patients, we observed that higher age increased the use of health care services, firmed by numerous other researchers [24,28,29,32–37]. Comorbidity had a weak negative impact on the utilization of healthcare services in our study, a finding echoed by other authors [29,38–41]. However, it might be that the effect of comorbidities interacts with age. The conclusion of a French study was that being younger and having comorbidities were identified as key factors associated with more intensive care and more frequent hospitalizations in the final stages of life [40].

Some researchers emphasize the need to consider care pathways of patients when assessing factors influencing the utilization of healthcare services in the final months of life [42]. As Norwegian researchers ascertain, age and access to informal care (marital status) are strong indicators of patients' living arrangements and care [42]. The existence of local home-based palliative care and support are also associated with a greater likelihood of dying at home [43–45], a desire often expressed by many patients and their families [46–49]. Quinn and colleagues found that patients who received regionally organized, collaborative, home-based palliative care experienced a 48% reduced risk of hospital death compared to those receiving standard care. Noteworthy advantages of this approach included increased clinician home visits, postponed initial hospital admissions, shorter hospital stays, and more time spent at home [45]. Our study echoes this by finding that better access to formal care, be it either GPs or other health care workers, increased the odds of ending the life at home. Unfortunately, the frequency of palliative care for patients is lower than would be necessarily for enabling dying at home, especially for non-cancer patients [39,50,51].

A strength of our analysis is the use of data registries that cover the whole Norwegian population. Our sample could have been larger by including a longer time period, for example from 2019 to 2021. However, as the COVID-19 pandemic affected health care use from 2020, we decided not to do so.

5. Conclusions

Diagnoses, individual characteristics, and service availability are all associated with the place of death. The higher the availability of health care services, the higher also is the probability of ending life at home.

Author Contributions: Conceptualization, E.Z.; methodology, T.P.H.; data curation, T.P.H.; writing—original draft, T.P.H. and E.Z.; writing—review and editing, T.P.H. and E.Z. All authors have read and agreed to the published version of the manuscript.

Funding: This research was funded by Norwegian Research Council, grant number 296114.

Institutional Review Board Statement: DPIA for the NORCHER project was granted 30 March 2020, and ethical approval granted by the South-Eastern Regional Ethics Committee of Norway (ref. 170128 and date of approval 25 October 2020).

Informed Consent Statement: Patient consent was waived due to use of register data only.

Data Availability Statement: Data from the Norwegian Patient Registry, the Norwegian Registry for Primary Health Care and Statistics Norway have been used in this publication. The interpretation and reporting of these data are the sole responsibility of the authors, and no endorsement by the registry owners is intended nor should be inferred.

Acknowledgments: TPHs was partly funded by the Norwegian Research Council (NRC) through the Norwegian Centre for Health Services Research (NORCHER), NRC-grant number 296114. Both authors received internal university funding.

Conflicts of Interest: The authors have no competing interests to declare.

Appendix A

Table A1. Comorbidities.

Comorbidity	ICD-10 Codes
Stroke	I60–I66, I68–I69, G45
Dementia	F00–F03, G30
Hypertension	I10–I15
Coronary artery disease	I20–I25
Atrial fibrillation	I48
Cardiac insufficiency	I50
Diabetes mellitus	E10–E14
Atherosclerosis	I70
Cancer	C, D0
COPD and asthma	J44–J46
Depression	F32–F34
Parkinson's disease	G20
Mental disorders	F2, F30–F31
Renal insufficiency	N18
Alcoholism	F10–F19

References

1. Lee, J.-H.; Hwang, K.-K. End-of-Life Care for End-stage Heart Failure Patients. *Korean Circ. J.* **2022**, *52*, 659–679. [CrossRef] [PubMed]
2. Hill, L.; Geller, T.P.; Baruah, R.; Beattie, J.M.; Boyne, J.; de Stoutz, N.; Di Stolfo, G.; Lambrinou, E.; Skibelund, A.K.; Uchmanowicz, I.; et al. Integration of a palliative approach into heart failure care: A European Society of Cardiology Heart Failure Association position paper. *Eur. J. Heart Fail.* **2020**, *22*, 2327–2339. [CrossRef] [PubMed]
3. Huo, B.; Song, Y.; Chang, L.; Tan, B. Effects of early palliative care on patients with incurable cancer: A meta-analysis and systematic review. *Eur. J. Cancer Care* **2022**, *31*, e13620. [CrossRef] [PubMed]
4. McDermott, C.L.; Engelberg, R.A.; Khandelwal, N.; Steiner, J.M.; Feemster, L.C.; Sibley, J.; Lober, W.B.; Curtis, J.R. The Association of Advance Care Planning Documentation and End-of-Life Healthcare Use Among Patients with Multimorbidity. *Am. J. Hosp. Palliat. Med.* **2021**, *38*, 954–962. [CrossRef]
5. Palliative Care. Available online: https://www.who.int/health-topics/palliative-care (accessed on 14 April 2024).
6. Depoorter, V.; Vanschoenbeek, K.; Decoster, L.; Silversmit, G.; Debruyne, P.R.; De Groof, I.; Bron, D.; Cornélis, F.; Luce, S.; Focan, C.; et al. End-of-Life Care in the Last Three Months before Death in Older Patients with Cancer in Belgium: A Large Retrospective Cohort Study Using Data Linkage. *Cancers* **2023**, *15*, 3349. [CrossRef] [PubMed]
7. Sperre Saunes, I.; Karanikolos, M.; Sagan, A.; World Health Organization. Norway: Health System Review. *Health Syst. Transit.* **2020**, *22*, 1–163.

8. Johansen, M.-L.; Ervik, B. Talking together in rural palliative care: A qualitative study of interprofessional collaboration in Norway. *BMC Health Serv. Res.* **2022**, *22*, 314. [CrossRef] [PubMed]
9. KAGes, S. Koordination, Palliativbetreuung, Steiermark. Sterbeorte Österreich. 2020. Available online: https://www.hospiz.at/hospiz-palliative-care/sterben-in-oesterreich-zahlen-und-fakten/ (accessed on 26 January 2024).
10. Croatian Bureau of Statistics. Natural Change in Population. 2022. Available online: https://podaci.dzs.hr/en/statistics/population/natural-change-in-population/ (accessed on 29 January 2024).
11. Slovenian Registry on Mortality. Available online: https://www.healthinformationportal.eu/health-information-sources/mortality-data-1 (accessed on 20 March 2024).
12. Abba, K.; Lloyd-Williams, M.; Horton, S. Discussing end of life wishes—The impact of community interventions? *BMC Palliat. Care* **2019**, *18*, 26. [CrossRef] [PubMed]
13. Rainsford, S.; Glasgow, N.J.; MacLeod, R.D.; Neeman, T.; Phillips, C.B.; Wiles, R.B. Place of death in the Snowy Monaro region of New South Wales: A study of residents who died of a condition amenable to palliative care. *Aust. J. Rural Health* **2018**, *26*, 126–133. [CrossRef] [PubMed]
14. Cohen, J.; Houttekier, D.; Onwuteaka-Philipsen, B.; Miccinesi, G.; Addington-Hall, J.; Kaasa, S.; Bilsen, J.; Deliens, L. Which patients with cancer die at home? A study of six European countries using death certificate data. *J. Clin. Oncol.* **2010**, *28*, 2267–2273. [CrossRef] [PubMed]
15. Kjellstadli, C.; Allore, H.; Husebo, B.S.; Flo, E.; Sandvik, H.; Hunskaar, S. General practitioners' provision of end-of-life care and associations with dying at home: A registry-based longitudinal study. *Fam. Pract.* **2020**, *37*, 340–347. [CrossRef] [PubMed]
16. Gomes, B.; Calanzani, N.; Koffman, J.; Higginson, I.J. Is dying in hospital better than home in incurable cancer and what factors influence this? A population-based study. *BMC Med.* **2015**, *13*, 235. [CrossRef] [PubMed]
17. Kellehear, A. Compassionate communities: End-of-life care as everyone's responsibility. *QJM Int. J. Med.* **2013**, *106*, 1071–1075. [CrossRef] [PubMed]
18. Koroukian, S.M.; Douglas, S.L.; Vu, L.; Fein, H.L.; Gairola, R.; Warner, D.F.; Schiltz, N.K.; Cullen, J.; Owusu, C.; Sajatovic, M.; et al. Incidence of Aggressive End-of-Life Care Among Older Adults with Metastatic Cancer Living in Nursing Homes and Community Settings. *JAMA Netw. Open* **2023**, *6*, e230394. [CrossRef] [PubMed]
19. Luta, X.; Diernberger, K.; Bowden, J.; Droney, J.; Hall, P.; Marti, J. Intensity of care in cancer patients in the last year of life: A retrospective data linkage study. *Br. J. Cancer* **2022**, *127*, 712–719. [CrossRef]
20. Weng, X.; Shen, C.; Van Scoy, L.J.; Boltz, M.; Joshi, M.; Wang, L. End-of-Life Costs of Cancer Patients with Alzheimer's Disease and Related Dementias in the U.S. *J. Pain Symptom Manag.* **2022**, *64*, 449–460. [CrossRef] [PubMed]
21. Leniz, J.; Yi, D.; Yorganci, E.; Williamson, L.E.; Suji, T.; Cripps, R.; Higginson, I.J.; Sleeman, K.E. Exploring costs, cost components, and associated factors among people with dementia approaching the end of life: A systematic review. *Alzheimer's Dement. Transl. Res. Clin. Interv.* **2021**, *7*, e12198. [CrossRef] [PubMed]
22. O'connor, N.; Fox, S.; Kernohan, W.G.; Drennan, J.; Guerin, S.; Murphy, A.; Timmons, S. A scoping review of the evidence for community-based dementia palliative care services and their related service activities. *BMC Palliat. Care* **2022**, *21*, 32. [CrossRef] [PubMed]
23. van der Steen, J.T.; Dekker, N.L.; Gijsberts, M.-J.H.E.; Vermeulen, L.H.; Mahler, M.M.; The, B.A.-M. Palliative care for people with dementia in the terminal phase: A mixed-methods qualitative study to inform service development. *BMC Palliat. Care* **2017**, *16*, 28. [CrossRef] [PubMed]
24. Nothelle, S.; Kelley, A.S.; Zhang, T.; Roth, D.L.; Wolff, J.L.; Boyd, C. Fragmentation of care in the last year of life: Does dementia status matter? *J. Am. Geriatr. Soc.* **2022**, *70*, 2320–2329. [CrossRef] [PubMed]
25. Diernberger, K.; Luta, X.; Bowden, J.; Fallon, M.; Droney, J.; Lemmon, E.; Gray, E.; Marti, J.; Hall, P. Healthcare use and costs in the last year of life: A national population data linkage study. *BMJ Support. Palliat. Care* **2024**. [CrossRef]
26. Chu, C.-P.; Huang, C.-Y.; Kuo, C.-J.; Chen, Y.-Y.; Chen, C.-T.; Yang, T.-W.; Liu, H.-C. Palliative care for nursing home patients with dementia: Service evaluation and risk factors of mortality. *BMC Palliat. Care* **2020**, *19*, 122. [CrossRef] [PubMed]
27. Leniz, J.; Higginson, I.J.; Yi, D.; Ul-Haq, Z.; Lucas, A.; e Sleeman, K. Identification of palliative care needs among people with dementia and its association with acute hospital care and community service use at the end-of-life: A retrospective cohort study using linked primary, community and secondary care data. *Palliat. Med.* **2021**, *35*, 1691–1700. [CrossRef] [PubMed]
28. Ní Chróinín, D.; Goldsbury, D.E.; Beveridge, A.; Davidson, P.M.; Girgis, A.; Ingham, N.; Phillips, J.L.; Wilkinson, A.M.; Ingham, J.M.; O'Connell, D.M. Health-services utilisation amongst older persons during the last year of life: A population-based study. *BMC Geriatr.* **2018**, *18*, 317. [CrossRef] [PubMed]
29. Ho, V.; Chen, C.; Ho, S.; Hooi, B.; Chin, L.S.; Merchant, R. A Healthcare utilisation in the last year of life in internal medicine, young-old versus old-old. *BMC Geriatr.* **2020**, *20*, 495. [CrossRef]
30. Ossima, A.N.; Szfetel, D.; Denoyel, B.; Beloucif, O.; Texereau, J.; Champion, L.M.; Vié, J.F.P.; Durand-Zaleski, I. End-of life medical spending and care pathways in the last 12 months of life: A comprehensive analysis of the national claims database in France. *Medicine* **2023**, *102*, e34555. [CrossRef]
31. Williamson, L.E.; Leniz, J.; Chukwusa, E.; Evans, C.J.; ESleeman, K. A population-based retrospective cohort study of end-of-life emergency department visits by people with dementia: Multilevel modelling of individual- and service-level factors using linked data. *Age Ageing* **2023**, *52*, afac332. [CrossRef] [PubMed]

32. Ma, J.E.; Olsen, M.K.; McDermott, C.L.; Bowling, C.B.; Hastings, S.N.; White, T.; Casarett, D. Factors Associated with Hospital Admission in the Last Month: A Retrospective Single Center Analysis. *J. Pain Symptom Manag.* **2024**, *in press*. [CrossRef] [PubMed]
33. Amado-Tineo, J.P.; Oscanoa-Espinoza, T.; Vásquez-Alva, R.; Huari-Pastrana, R.; Delgado-Guay, M.O. Emergency Department Use by Terminally Ill Patients: A Systematic Review. *J. Pain Symptom Manag.* **2021**, *61*, 531–543. [CrossRef]
34. RReeve, R.; Srasuebkul, P.; Langton, J.M.; Haas, M.; Viney, R.; Pearson, S.A.; EOL-CC Study Authors. Health care use and costs at the end of life: A comparison of elderly Australian decedents with and without a cancer history. *BMC Palliat. Care* **2017**, *17*, 1–10. [CrossRef]
35. Langton, J.M.; Reeve, R.; Srasuebkul, P.; Haas, M.; Viney, R.; Currow, D.; Pearson, S.-A. Health service use and costs in the last 6 months of life in elderly decedents with a history of cancer: A comprehensive analysis from a health payer perspective. *Br. J. Cancer* **2016**, *114*, 1293–1302. [CrossRef] [PubMed]
36. Dunlay, S.M.; Redfield, M.M.; Jiang, R.; Weston, S.A.; Roger, V.L. Care in the last year of life for community patients with heart failure. *Circ. Heart Fail.* **2015**, *8*, 489–496. [CrossRef] [PubMed]
37. May, P.; Roe, L.; McGarrigle, C.A.; Kenny, R.A.; Normand, C. End-of-life experience for older adults in Ireland: Results from the Irish longitudinal study on ageing (TILDA). *BMC Health Serv. Res.* **2020**, *20*, 118. [CrossRef] [PubMed]
38. May, P.; Normand, C.; Cassel, J.B.; Del Fabbro, E.; Fine, R.L.; Menz, R.; Morrison, C.A.; Penrod, J.D.; Robinson, C.; Morrison, R.S. Economics of Palliative Care for Hospitalized Adults with Serious Illness: A Meta-analysis. *JAMA Intern. Med.* **2018**, *178*, 820–829. [CrossRef] [PubMed]
39. Evans, N.; Pasman, H.R.W.; A Donker, G.; Deliens, L.; Block, L.V.D.; Onwuteaka-Philipsen, B.; De Groote, Z.; Brearley, S.; Caraceni, A.; Cohen, J.; et al. End-of-life care in general practice: A cross-sectional, retrospective survey of 'cancer', 'organ failure' and 'old-age/dementia' patients. *Palliat. Med.* **2014**, *28*, 965–975. [CrossRef] [PubMed]
40. Salas, S.; Pauly, V.; Damge, M.; Orleans, V.; Fond, G.; Costello, R.; Boyer, L.; Baumstarck, K. Intensive end-of-life care in acute leukemia from a French national hospital database study (2017–2018). *BMC Palliat. Care* **2022**, *21*, 45. [CrossRef] [PubMed]
41. Aamodt, W.W.; Dahodwala, N.; Bilker, W.B.; Farrar, J.T.; Willis, A.W. Unique characteristics of end-of-life hospitalizations in Parkinson disease. *Front. Aging Neurosci.* **2023**, *15*, 1254969. [CrossRef] [PubMed]
42. Bjørnelv, G.; Hagen, T.P.; Forma, L.; Aas, E. Care pathways at end-of-life for cancer decedents: Registry based analyses of the living situation, healthcare utilization and costs for all cancer decedents in Norway in 2009–2013 during their last 6 months of life. *BMC Health Serv. Res.* **2022**, *22*, 1221. [CrossRef] [PubMed]
43. Quinn, K.L.; Hsu, A.T.; Smith, G.; Stall, N.; Detsky, A.S.; Kavalieratos, D.; Lee, D.S.; Bell, C.M.; Tanuseputro, P. Association between palliative care and death at home in adults with heart failure. *J. Am. Heart Assoc.* **2020**, *9*, e013844. [CrossRef] [PubMed]
44. Van Der Plas, A.G.; Oosterveld-Vlug, M.G.; Pasman, H.R.W.; Onwuteaka-Philipsen, B.D. Relating cause of death with place of care and healthcare costs in the last year of life for patients who died from cancer, chronic obstructive pulmonary disease, heart failure and dementia: A descriptive study using registry data. *Palliat. Med.* **2017**, *31*, 338–345. [CrossRef] [PubMed]
45. Quinn, K.L.; Stukel, T.A.; Campos, E.; Graham, C.; Kavalieratos, D.; Mak, S.; Steinberg, L.; Tanuseputro, P.; Tuna, M.; Isenberg, S.R. Regional col-laborative home-based palliative care and health care outcomes among adults with heart failure. *CMAJ* **2022**, *194*, E1274–E1282. [CrossRef] [PubMed]
46. Spary-Kainz, U.; Posch, N.; Paier-Abuzahra, M.; Lieb, M.; Avian, A.; Zelko, E.; Siebenhofer, A. Palliative Care Survey: Awareness, Knowledge and Views of the Styrian Population in Austria. *Healthcare* **2023**, *11*, 2611. [CrossRef] [PubMed]
47. Zelko, E.; Pajk, J.R.; Škvarč, N.K. An Innovative Approach for Improving Information Exchange between Palliative Care Providers in Slovenian Primary Health—A Qualitative Analysis of Testing a New Tool. *Healthcare* **2022**, *10*, 216. [CrossRef] [PubMed]
48. Benini, F.; Fabris, M.; Pace, D.S.; Verno, V.; Negro, V.; De Conno, F.; Orzalesi, M.M. Awareness, understanding and attitudes of Italians regarding palliative care. *Ann. Ist. Super. Sanita* **2011**, *47*, 253–259. [CrossRef] [PubMed]
49. Westerlund, C.; Tishelman, C.; Benkel, I.; Fürst, C.J.; Molander, U.; Rasmussen, B.H.; Sauter, S.; Lindqvist, O. Public awareness of palliative care in Sweden. *Scand. J. Public Health* **2018**, *46*, 478–487. [CrossRef] [PubMed]
50. Gomes, B.; Calanzani, N.; Curiale, V.; McCrone, P.; Higginson, I.J.; de Brito, M. Effectiveness and cost-effectiveness of home palliative care services for adults with advanced illness and their caregivers. *Cochrane Database Syst. Rev.* **2013**, *2013*, CD007760. [CrossRef] [PubMed]
51. Ikezaki, S.; Ikegami, N. Predictors of dying at home for patients receiving nursing services in Japan: A retrospective study comparing cancer and non-cancer deaths. *BMC Palliat. Care* **2011**, *10*, 3. [CrossRef] [PubMed]

healthcare

MDPI

Article

Dementia Education for Workforce Excellence: Evaluation of a Novel Bichronous Approach

Leah Macaden [1,2,*] and Kevin Muirhead [1,2]

1 Nursing Studies, School of Health in Social Science, University of Edinburgh, Edinburgh EH8 9AG, UK
2 Department of Nursing & Midwifery, University of the Highlands and Islands, Inverness IV2 3JH, UK
* Correspondence: leah.macaden@ed.ac.uk

Abstract: Dementia education and training for workforce development is becoming increasingly important in bridging knowledge gaps among health and social care practitioners in the UK and internationally. Dementia Education for Workforce Excellence (DEWE) was developed during the COVID-19 pandemic, blending both synchronous and asynchronous instruction and delivered across three different contexts: care homes, home care, and nurse education within the UK and India. This study aimed to evaluate DEWE using mixed methods with online survey data analyzed descriptively and interview data analyzed thematically. Integration of survey and interview data aimed toward a comprehensive evaluation of this novel approach for dementia workforce development. Thirty-four social care practitioners and nurse educators completed the online survey demonstrating high-level learner satisfaction, learning gains, behavioral change, and motivation to share new knowledge. Four key themes developed from the analysis of interviews (n = 9) around participants' pursuit of new knowledge; delivery modes in DEWE; learning gains and impact of DEWE; and adaptations for future program implementation. Findings suggest DEWE is an innovative resource that promotes person- and relationship-centered dementia care across all stages of one's dementia journey. Cultural adaptations are recommended for international delivery to ensure contextual alignment and maximum impact.

Keywords: dementia education; blended learning; online learning; bichronous learning; mixed methods; evaluation; workforce

1. Introduction

There are concerns internationally around the knowledge, skills, and attitudes of health and social care practitioners who provide care for people living with dementia [1]. Globally, the prevalence of dementia is 55 million with projections indicating an increase to 139 million by 2050 [2,3]. Notably, most of these people, approximately 75%, are anticipated to be concentrated in low- and middle-income countries [4].

In India, dementia prevalence for people aged 60 years and older is estimated to be 7.4% and increasing due to demographic transition [5]. Despite this, there is limited awareness and stigma associated with the condition [1]. Dementia symptoms can be considered as non-pathological deviations from normal ageing and supported within systems of family care with limited input from professionals [6]. The Indian Government has recognized the challenges with special provision for people with dementia included in national health programs and policy [1]. The Dementia India Report [7] highlighted health professional education as a critical component when developing national dementia services. Key areas for change included the development of in-service training for health professionals and Train the Trainer programs for carers and community health workers.

In the UK, dementia workforce development through education has been articulated in several government reports and strategies [8–14]. Dementia education in adult social care is a priority to meet the needs of practitioners who are increasingly providing specialist dementia care. Evidence suggests that asynchronous online courses can benefit social care practitioners in terms of knowledge and skills development [15,16]; however, social distancing requirements during the COVID-19 pandemic highlighted the value of integrating both asynchronous and synchronous delivery methods [17]. No studies are known to have combined asynchronous and synchronous online dementia education for social care practitioners, nor are there any studies known to have evaluated technology-enabled dementia education in India.

1.1. The Intervention

Dementia Education for Workforce Excellence (DEWE) was developed during the COVID-19 pandemic to equip health and social care practitioners to work in increasingly digitalized and ageing societies with growing numbers of people with dementia. DEWE integrates the philosophy of care within the Standards of Dementia Care in Scotland [11] that are underpinned by three National Dementia Strategies [10,12,13]. Program development was informed by Scotland's national dementia workforce development framework (Promoting Excellence: A framework for all health and social services staff working with people with dementia, their families, and carers) [14]. This framework prioritizes the rights of individuals living with dementia and integrates their dementia journey in its framework, structured at four practice levels: Informed, Skilled, Enhanced, and Expert. The levels correspond to the frequency and intensity of interactions that practitioners engage with people affected by dementia within their unique practice settings. DEWE was aligned to the skilled level of Promoting Excellence which outlines the knowledge and skills required by practitioners who have direct and/or substantial contact with people living with dementia.

The project lead previously developed two innovative and comprehensive dementia curricula for pre-registration nurse education in Scotland: Being Dementia Smart [18] and Dementia Enhanced Education to Promote Excellence (DEEPE), both mapped at the enhanced level of the Promoting Excellence Framework. DEWE was developed adopting a similar approach with input and consensus from an expert group that consisted of academics, clinicians, educational technologists, and experts with lived experience of dementia or dementia care giving.

DEWE lends itself to bichronous online learning—a blend of both asynchronous and synchronous delivery methods [17] where participants can participate flexibly during the asynchronous parts of the course alongside real-time participation for the synchronous sessions. For the asynchronous component, participants had free access to three online workbooks (Dementia Care Essentials; Dementia Care Priorities; & Dementia Care Enablers) with content mapped along the stages of the dementia journey. The key narrative was based on 'Barbara's Story' [19], a filmed ethnodrama that demonstrates the various stages and associated complexities of the dementia journey supported by learning activities and opportunities for reflective discussions. Learning resources also included short videos created by a general practitioner as an expert with lived experience of dementia [20] providing an emic perspective with insights into the higher needs of people with dementia including social activity, sense of belonging, self-esteem, and meaning in life [21]. Furthermore, a relationship-centered approach to dementia care was embedded to emphasize the importance of support for the wellbeing of both formal and informal carers to ensure high-quality person-centered dementia care [22]. Synchronous sessions (n = 16), via the Cisco Webex Platform, were spread over 6 weeks and facilitated by experts (with lived experience of dementia care giving and professionals). Live sessions embraced the philosophy of person-centered dementia care regularly interspersed with opportunities for reflective learning on dementia care from pre-diagnosis to end-of-life (Table 1).

Table 1. Themed content in DEWE.

Asynchronous Workbook		Session	Synchronous Duration	Facilitator
	Introduction to DEWE and Workbooks	1	30 min	1
1. Dementia Care Essentials	The Human Brain	2	1 h	1
	Dementia: What it is and what it is not	3	1 h	1
	Memory Changes in Dementia	4	30 min	1
	Sensory Changes in Dementia	5	30 min	1
2. Dementia Care Priorities	Living with Dementia: Person-centered approaches	6	1 h	1
	Stages of the Dementia Journey (Barbara's Story [a])	7	3 h	2
	Carer's Perspectives in Dementia	8	1 h	3
	Stress & Distress in Dementia	9	1 h	1, 4
	Dementia, Delirium and Depression	10	2 h	2
3. Dementia Care Enablers	Staff: Self-care and wellbeing during COVID-19 [b]	11	-	-
	Dementia & COVID-19 in Care Homes	12	1.5 h	5
	Implementing Change and Improvement	13	1.5 h	5
	Dementia Inclusive and Enabling Environments	14	2 h	1, 6
	End-of-life care in Dementia	15	2 h	1
	Relationship-centered Approaches to Dementia Care using the Six Senses Framework	16	2 h	1

[a] Included five principles of the Adults with Incapacity Act, Scotland, 2000 [23]; [b] Self-directed learning using NES staff wellbeing resources [24]; Facilitator: (1) Senior Lecturer—Nursing (Dementia Expertise); (2) Dementia Nurse Consultant; (3) Person with lived experience of dementia (Family Carer); (4) Clinical Psychologist; (5) Senior Lecturer—Nursing (Quality Improvement Expertise); (6) Dementia Link Worker.

1.2. Participants in DEWE

DEWE training was provided to nurse educators and social care practitioners (including care home and home care practitioners) to cascade the training for nursing capacity building in dementia care. The training was conducted in two cohorts during the pandemic—one from the UK and another from India. The inclusion of participants from India aimed to address the considerable resource gap for dementia workforce development within the Indian context despite the increasing prevalence of dementia.

1.3. Aim and Objectives

The overarching aim of the study was to evaluate DEWE training delivered using a bichronous approach with practitioners and educators from three different contexts.

1. To explore participants' perceptions on the content and quality of the dementia training.
2. To explore participants' perceptions and experiences of accessing the dementia training using a bichronous approach.

2. Materials and Methods

The evaluation was underpinned by Kirkpatrick's Model [25] using a mixed methods approach combining quantitative and free-text survey response data with qualitative data from interviews.

2.1. Sampling and Recruitment

All DEWE participants (n = 55) were invited to join the study via email, which included participant information and the contact details of the research team. Additionally, they were provided with a secure link to access and complete an online survey. Those who completed the survey had the opportunity to express an interest in participating in a one-to-one interview through a separate survey link. Interested participants were subsequently contacted by a member of the research team to schedule interviews.

2.2. Data Collection

Quantitative and free-text response data were collected via the online survey platform [26] six months after participation in DEWE using a variety of Likert scale, rating scale, and open-ended questions. The survey was structured according to Kirkpatrick's model which consists of four levels: (1) reactions to the training; (2) learning gains (knowledge, skills, and attitudes) due to the training; (3) behavioral changes due to the training; and (4) the results achieved due to the training. Consent was gained from all participants using the online survey platform.

Semi-structured interviews were conducted virtually via the Cisco Webex platform between January and February 2023 (within 18 months of participation in DEWE). The interview guide is available as Supplementary Material. Consent for interviews was obtained electronically from all participants using email. The average interview duration was 33 min.

The evaluation was structured at two time points primarily to assess the effectiveness of the intervention both in terms of knowledge and the application of learning in practice. Questionnaire completion was at six months to avoid any immediate recall bias and interviews were scheduled at 18 months to allow time and space for participants to report on how their learning had informed their practice or not.

2.3. Data Analysis

Quantitative survey data were analyzed using descriptive statistics in Microsoft Excel 2019 version 2108 and reported as either frequencies, percentages, or median values. Free-text responses were analyzed in Microsoft Excel using a deductive approach for alignment with Kirkpatrick's model and displayed alongside related quantitative data as participant quotations or in frequency tables.

Interview data were subject to reflexive thematic analysis [27] using an inductive approach. Analysis comprised six phases: (1) interview recordings were transcribed verbatim by a member of the research team (KM) and then transcripts were reviewed multiple times for data familiarization; (2) data were coded by one member of the research team (KM) using NVivo; (3) initial codes were clustered into provisional candidate themes through a process of development, revision, and refinement; (4) candidate themes were reviewed in relation to codes and the entire data set to consider alternative options for pattern development; (5) a detailed thematic framework was produced with descriptions of themes and subthemes; and (6) an analytic narrative was created including data extracts to tell the story of the data. Analytical processes were discussed regularly by KM & LM and an audit trail maintained to enhance trustworthiness [28].

Findings from both the survey and interviews were reviewed, and the most salient points were extracted. These findings were then converged with equal priority given to survey and interview findings. The integration resulted in two overarching themes: strengths of DEWE and areas for development. The mixed methods results were tabulated and categorized according to Kirkpatrick's model to facilitate the interpretation of the main study findings.

3. Results: Survey Findings

3.1. Demographics

Participants were 34 nurse educators and social care practitioners from the UK and India who completed DEWE between July 2021 and March 2022. Educators were either professors (n = 3) or associate/assistant professors in nursing (n = 8), nursing lecturers (n = 3), or nursing tutors (n = 3). Practitioners were carers (n = 7) or service managers (n = 2). Eight participants reported their role as being 'other' but did not provide any further details on their role.

3.2. Experience of Dementia Care and Education

Twelve educators (70.6%) taught on BSc Nursing programs, two (11.8%) taught on general nursing programs, whilst one (5.9%) taught on postgraduate programs. The remaining educators (11.8%) taught on a combination of programs. Five practitioners (55.6%) provided care to more than 15 people with dementia on a typical workday, whilst two (22.2%) provided care to between 11 and 15 people. Two practitioners (22.2%) did not provide dementia care at work.

3.3. Access to DEWE

A combination of personal computers and smartphones were most frequently used to access DEWE. Figure 1 demonstrates the devices used to access the training. Note the total does not tally to 34 (most likely as some participants have used multiple devices to access DEWE).

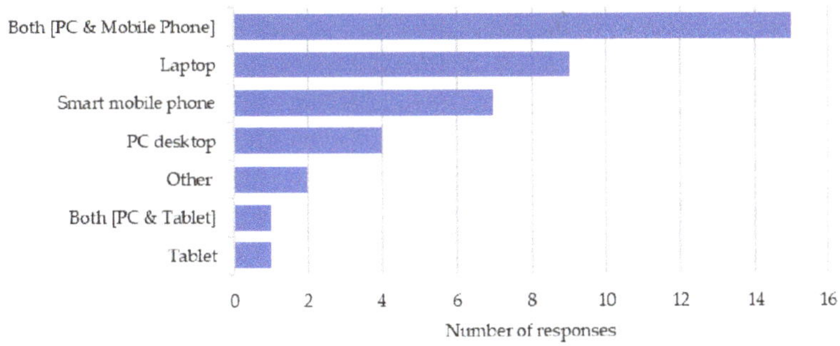

Figure 1. Devices used to access DEWE.

3.4. Level 1: Reaction to Asynchronous Resources

The presentation of the workbooks was highly rated among participants with most indicating the color scheme, font style, font size, icons, and illustrations being very good or excellent (Figure 2). There were high levels of agreement that the online workbooks were intuitive; however, some participants suggested that the workbooks were not easy to navigate (Figure 3). One participant suggested that the content could be more streamlined as *'a few videos were mixed up'* [80908493, Practitioner].

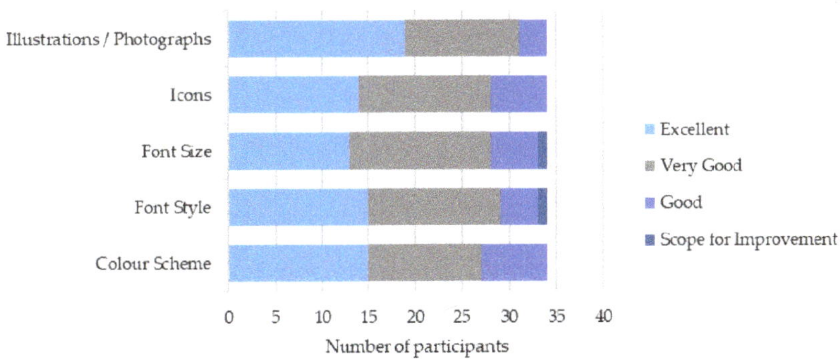

Figure 2. Presentation of the workbooks.

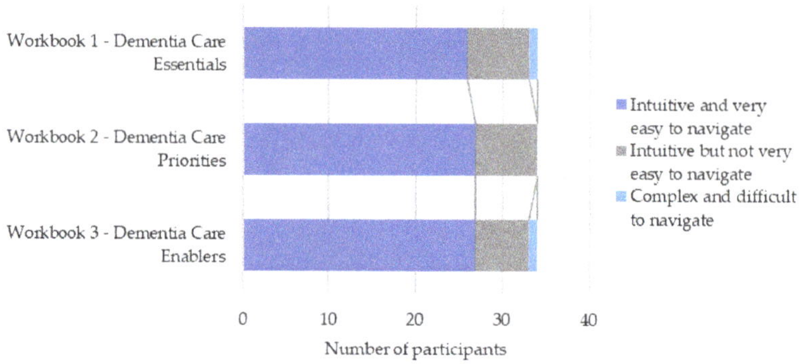

Figure 3. Ease of workbook navigation.

The workbooks were thought to work well but *'did not translate to hard copy which some staff without IT skills preferred to use'* [92124189, Other]. Another participant suggested that *'ease of use PDF copies would be useful'* [81022848, Practitioner].

Twenty-four participants rated the overall quality of the workbooks on a scale of 1–10 (1 being poor and 10 being excellent). The median scores (with interquartile range) for the three workbooks were: 9 (9, 10), 10 (9, 10), and 9 (9, 10) for Workbooks 1, 2, and 3 respectfully. The participants' reaction to the training was also measured as levels of agreement to various aspects of the training content (Figure 4).

3.5. Level 1: Reaction to Synchronous Resources

Feedback on the duration of the interactive sessions was mixed with some participants recommending a shorter duration whilst others recommended a longer duration. Alternative suggestions were to reduce the duration of interactive sessions and increase the frequency of sessions provided. Some participants were not satisfied with the delivery platform and recommended that this be changed for future delivery. Other suggestions to improve synchronous sessions included implementation of interactive icebreaker sessions, improved orientation to workbooks, and follow-up sessions.

3.6. Level 1: Reaction to Bichronous Learning

Participants described the aspects most and least enjoyed about blended learning in DEWE (Table 2).

Table 2. The aspects of DEWE most and least enjoyed by participants.

Enjoyed Most	Enjoyed Least
1. Group discussion and interactivity	1. Technical issues/videoconferencing platform
2. Course presentation/expert facilitation	2. Difficulty coordinating attendance
3. Reflective activities	3. Duration of interactive sessions (too long)
4. Workbooks	4. Duration of interactive sessions (too short)
5. Use of real-life stories and examples	5. Lack of participant interaction in break out rooms
6. Videos	6. Reflective activities
7. Structure and content (general)	7. Overall course duration (too short)
8. New knowledge	8. Digital skill requirements
9. Technology-enabled/blended approach	9. Technology-enabled delivery mode
10. Convenience	

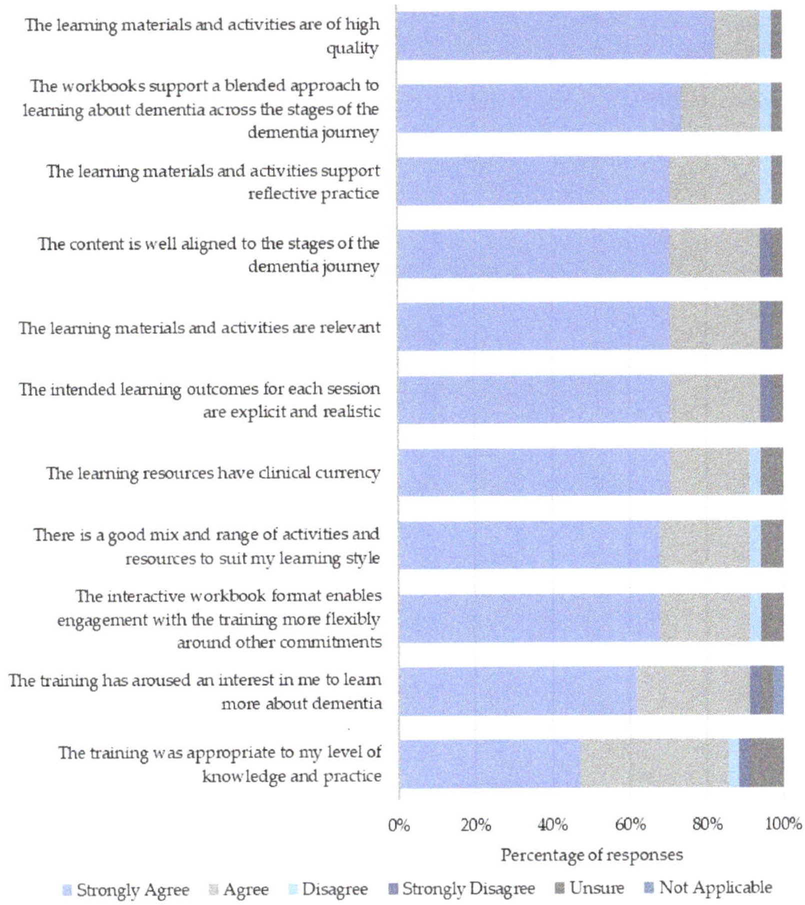

Figure 4. Reaction to the training content.

3.7. Preferred Mode of Learning

Twenty-four participants rated their preferred modes of dementia training on a scale of 1–5 (5 being most preferred and 1 being least preferred). Figure 5 shows the median scores for each training modality with high levels of preference for a blended approach.

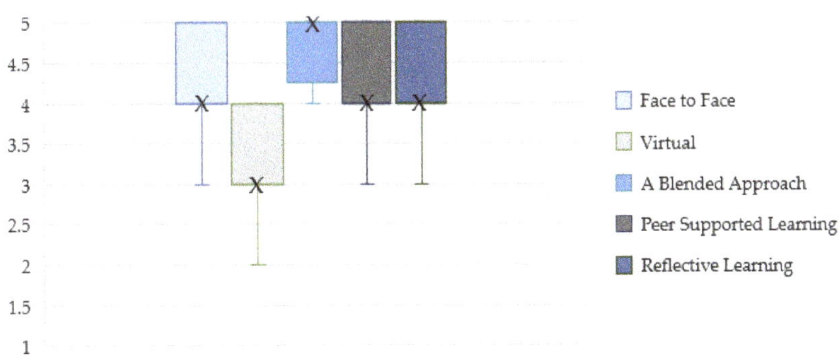

Figure 5. Preferred modes of dementia training. X denotes the median score.

3.8. Level 2: Learning Gains

Participants rated the relevance of the learning outcomes to their professional practice on a scale of 1 to 5. The median score for each outcome was 5, indicating high levels of relevance. Additionally, there was strong consensus that DEWE had enhanced various aspects of dementia care knowledge (Figure 6). Moreover, an overwhelming majority of participants (91.2%) reported that DEWE had equipped them with relevant skills transferable beyond the dementia care context (Figure 7).

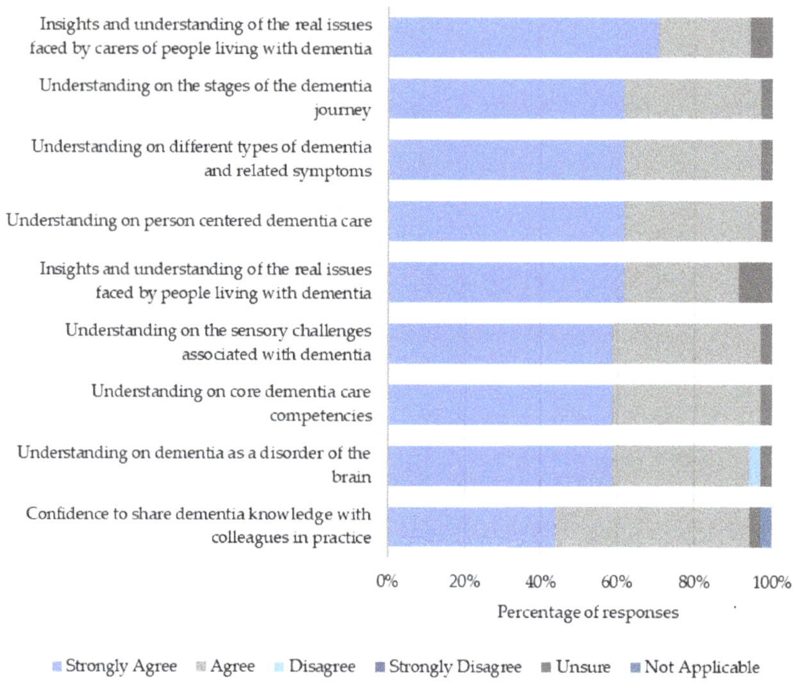

Figure 6. Learning gains following DEWE.

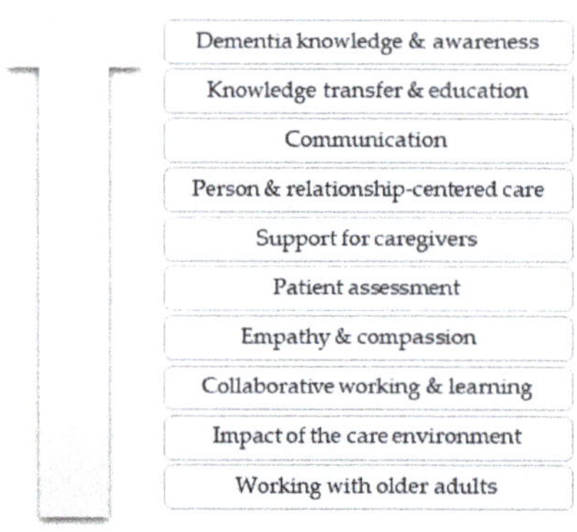

Figure 7. Transferable skills gained following DEWE.

3.9. Level 3: Practice-Based Behavioral Change

There were high levels of agreement that learning in DEWE had resulted in positive behaviors in practice (Figure 8).

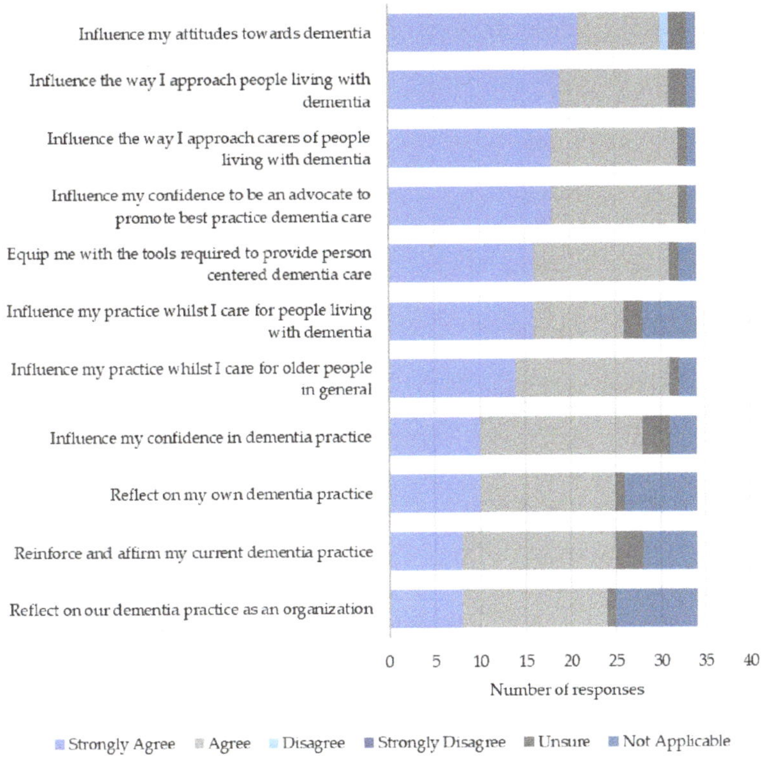

Figure 8. Practice-based behaviors following DEWE.

3.10. Level 4: Results

Following DEWE, participants were motivated to lead or influence dementia practice. Several were interested in leading dementia education through teaching and the development of educational initiatives:

> *"I would like to influence the way nurses learn and practice dementia care"*. [93011072, Educator]

Participants were also motivated to share knowledge gained and improve awareness and attitudes towards the condition:

> *"I would like to help change the attitudes of some carers and give them a confidence boost and help them with their knowledge"*. [81126963, Practitioner]

The training motivated participants to lead improvements in person-centered dementia care, communication with people living with dementia, and support for family members and carers affected by dementia. Specific areas of dementia practice that participants sought to change included dementia assessment, delirium awareness, management of stress and distress, implementation of dementia inclusive environments, pain management, and palliative care.

4. Results: Interview Findings

4.1. Demographics

The participants were six nurse educators (lecturers/tutors and coordinators of nursing programs) and three practitioners with experience of health and/or social care from India (n = 7) and the UK (n = 2). Participants were issued a code reflecting their demographic profile. The first part of the code was an arbitrary number of participation; the second reflected the participants' areas of practice (Educator = 01; Practitioner = 02); and the third related to participants' location (India = 01; UK = 02).

4.2. Themes

Four themes developed from the data analysis, which related to: the participants' pursuit of new knowledge; educational delivery modes in DEWE; learning gains due to DEWE; and adaptations recommended for future programs. Each theme comprised subthemes, as shown in Figure 9.

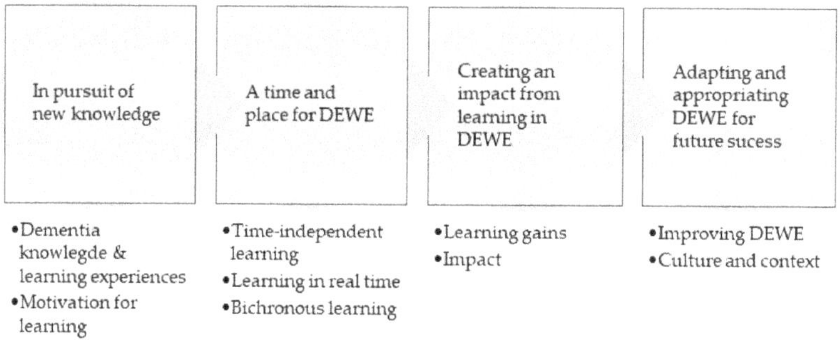

Figure 9. Themes and subthemes.

4.3. Theme 1: In Pursuit of New Knowledge

4.3.1. Dementia Knowledge and Learning Experiences

Participants from India often reported superficial knowledge about dementia [P3-02-01; P4-01-01; P5-01-01; P8-02-01] and limited prior experience of dementia education [P2-01-01; P3-02-01; P6-01-01]. Despite this, there was awareness of the increasing dementia prevalence in India and limitations in national dementia surveillance systems and health programs.

> "*Dementia is also a very important disorder that is on the rise, you know, like, more and more elderly patients are having this disorder and because of that I think, yeah, we should be really into understanding more about dementia, learning more about dementia and all that*". [P4-01-01]

Participants were critical of dementia education in India which was limited in undergraduate nursing curricula with basic content considered inadequate to support future practice.

> "*It is just a very small, small, minute part of the curriculum which, by the time the student becomes the staff, they would have forgotten, they wouldn't even sometimes remember I feel*". [P4-01-01]

Dissatisfaction with professional and vocational development in dementia care resulted from training using in-person and didactic delivery methods.

> "*We are used to like monotonous resource person going on and on and sometimes very few programs have some participation, but there is no variety in the program, you know, live program*". [P5-01-01]

Among participants from the UK, dementia was described to be an unattractive career option which intensified the need for comprehensive undergraduate dementia education despite competing demands within existing curricula.

> "*I don't know how familiar you are with nursing curricula but they're always very challenging to get everything into a relatively short period of time, three years is never long enough*". [P7-01-02]

In-house and online dementia education were common modes for professional development in the UK. Online training was often mandated and risked disengagement due to asynchronous delivery.

> *"The system that we use for our staff . . .you log in by yourself, you watch twenty plus videos and after each video clip you have a multiple-choice question. . .its quite basic".* [P9-02-02]

4.3.2. Motivation for Learning

DEWE provided participants with opportunities to develop new dementia knowledge which participants valued for their own professional development but also to pass on to others.

> *"I've been a caregiver for last 20 years now to my in-laws and three years ago my mother-in-law suffered a stroke and then she had an onset of dementia. . .and also at [workplace] we focus a lot on senior citizens care, that is one of our main areas of work, so, I thought both professionally and personally this is going to give me a lot of insights".* [P8-02-01]

> *"As an educator, always keen to try to enrich any students learning and, so, ...it was really good to sort of develop my own learning and understand things that are really helpful in others, in helping others to learn as well, you know, around dementia".* [P7-01-02]

The expert facilitation in DEWE provided a sense of credibility, which motivated learner engagement. Motivation for learning was also enhanced as the course was delivered free of charge with certification of completion particularly valued by participants from India [P5-01-01; P6-01-01].

4.4. Theme 2: A Time and a Place for DEWE

4.4.1. Time-Independent Learning

The online workbooks allowed for time-independent learning with opportunities for participants to assimilate and reflect on new concepts. The resources provided participants with ongoing access to information which could be revisited and stored with the aim of supporting learning.

> *"I just found them really helpful and the fact that you can then revisit things because, you know, because my memories good at some points but others it isn't. . . being able to revisit it and you could download some of the pages from that. . .which again was just helpful".* [P7-01-02]

The use of active learning strategies including quizzes and games supported information retention. Real-life and emotive videos provided a proxy for experiential learning and resulted in emotional engagement which supported information retention and development of compassionate care and empathy for people with dementia.

> *"Seeing videos like that, you're seeing it from the other person's point of view. . .I understand now that they can't help it, you know, it's confusing for them".* [P9-02-02]

A potential barrier to self-directed learning was self-motivation for engagement. Additional barriers included isolation during learning, which was perceived problematic in the context of dementia education.

> *"I don't think you learn in the same way when something is strictly online. . .a topic like dementia is about people, and you almost want to test out, sort of, you know, your own learning with others".* [P7-01-02]

4.4.2. Learning in Real Time

Synchronous sessions made learning more interesting through group interactions with peers, facilitators, and guest speakers, allowing participants to gain knowledge from diverse experiences and perspectives. Learning was enriched from the cultural and professional diversity within the learning groups and opportunities to learn from a variety of professional and personal experiences.

> *"Like it says like 'none of us is smarter than all of us', so, it's like the years of wisdom comes in a room and all that, all those years of experience and learning, so that was very rich".* [P1-01-01]

Sessions involving people with lived experience of dementia resulted in depth of emotional engagement and an appreciation of the realities of informal dementia care.

> *"Lived experiences of people was more encouraging and practical and to learn from their life experiences, so that was very good and that was really touching our hearts".* [P5-01-01]

Participants were motivated and inspired by the facilitator/s who contributed to live sessions.

> *"I just thought she was amazing, so much passion, and you could tell that she loved making the lives better for the people that they had living with dementia, and it was just, yeah, it was heart-warming".* [P09-02-02]

The weekly sessions provided consistent facilitation and opportunities to build on prior learning. The synchronous platform enabled active group learning whilst simultaneously encouraging introspection and personal reflection.

> *"We had lots of opportunities to understand our perspectives as well as other perspectives, like it was a platform for us to introspect whether our understanding or our perspectives about dementia is right or what else I can look for when it comes to the care of patients".* [P6-01-01]

Barriers to synchronous sessions included poor online etiquette and time limitations, which would require skillful moderation and opportunities for all participants to be heard.

> *"I think that is just a fact of, you know, learning this way. . .obviously we encounter it all the time. . .there's usually somebody who's quite vocal, somebody else is trying to talk, but because you can't see them you aren't really aware of that, so that to me was probably a drawback".* [P7-01-02]

Participants from India were less accustomed to the WebEx platform and occasionally experienced connectivity issues and difficulty joining synchronous sessions.

> *"We did have challenges using Webex because many times our people were not able to join, we are so accustomed to Zoom, that was the first time I think many of us were using Webex".* [P5-01-01]

4.4.3. Bichronous Learning

Participants considered the bichronous delivery to be a novel approach using multiple methods to meet the needs of a diverse audience and learning styles.

> *"It was actually perfect blending or perfect package of all three components, like all three domains of teaching, affective, cognitive, and psychomotor. . .so, it's a perfect blending of all three domains of teaching".* [P6-01-01]

The asynchronous resources enriched participation in synchronous sessions from prior preparation. Correspondingly, synchronous sessions elaborated on asynchronous content. This reciprocity seemed to influence enhanced learning.

> *"I was able to take away much from the class because I was able to read and then come to the class, otherwise I don't think it would have been so much of beneficial to me".* [P8-02-01]

Benefits of the bichronous approach also included the potential to revisit/reuse asynchronous resources and recordings of synchronous sessions as often and for as long as required to support learning.

"We can go over and over whenever we have a doubt, we can go back and learn from them, so the freedom to access that has been given to us...that is a positive thing". [P5-01-01]

DEWE had become more relevant since the COVID-19 pandemic and was considered to be an enjoyable and motivating learning experience.

"Because this sort of fell during the pandemic, you know, we were adapting to online, you know, very quickly anyway...we were getting so familiar with the way that we were teaching anyway". [P7-01-02]

4.5. Theme 3: Impact from Learning in DEWE

4.5.1. Learning Gains

Aspects of new knowledge gained by participants in DEWE are shown in Table 3.

Table 3. Aspects of knowledge gained.

Knowledge Aspect	Quote
Types of dementia	*"We learned that there is like 200 different types of dementia...I had no idea, and I've got twenty plus years' experience, like, in health and social care".* [P9-02-02]
Neurophysiology	*"The role of hippocampus...so what is the difference between normal ageing and dementia, especially when we talk about memory changes...that is what is more important to know".* [P6-01-01]
Stress & Distress	*"I really learned from this course...like analyzing a situation using the ABC chart...when something happens".* [P5-01-01]
Delirium	*"Particularly in my clinical role, you know, in acute trauma, being able to identify things like delirium is so helpful, so those tools were really good".* [P7-01-02]
Person-centered care	*"I have learned tools on how to handle different situations and how to understand why the person is behaving in a certain way and therefore how you kind of adapt your care to suit that person's needs".* [P8-02-01]
Relationship-centered care	*"I really liked the six senses approach, I thought that was really, really useful".* [P7-01-02]
Care for caregivers	*"I understood that not only people living with dementia that needs attention, but we have to pay special attention even to the carers of people living with dementia".* [P4-01-01]
Dignity & Respect	*"Taking your time with people, never getting cross, and the fact that you might have to answer the same thing...you're answering the same questions but doing so every time with patience rather than frustration can make a huge difference".* [P7-01-02]
Care environment	*"I remember some of the classes where they said how does the environment impact a person living with dementia, so, I think even the environment also is very, very important, the type of environment that we create around these people".* [P4-01-01]
Care empathy	*"It can be very frustrating to have dementia and to place ourselves in their shoes, like some of those case studies we looked at, and listening to the various talks, that really helped me".* [P1-01-01]

DEWE had broadened participants' understanding about dementia and also resulted in the development of positive dementia care attitudes.

"I have learned on how to be...an empathetic caregiver... an informed caregiver". [P8-02-01]

4.5.2. Impact

Participants reported having a greater awareness of the signs and symptoms of dementia following DEWE including the behaviors of older adults in their care and communities.

"Earlier, it was not in my thinking, or it was not in part of my internal function, to think of something like this... to wonder if a person could have dementia". [P1-01-01]

One participant who worked in clinical areas shared an anecdote of using the knowledge gained with greater confidence to support people living with dementia in practice:

"On the last shift I did, I actually was in a bay, you know, with six ladies and one of whom, you know, did have dementia, so, you know, constantly I was just going back, you know,

reiterating what I'd said, holding her hand and everything else and it was only when I was going back to another lady and they went 'oh we're going to have a quiet day today' and I said 'oh, have things been, you know, disturbing you?' and she said, 'yes' she said 'that's the most attention she's had since we've been here'". [P7-01-02]

The course provided participants with the confidence to provide informal health education and support for friends and relatives. Learning from DEWE created a positive ripple effect as participants confidently shared knowledge with others.

"There was something I learned, it was so profound, I put it on my social page. . .it was nice that some of the people within my friends circle who saw that, they replied back, and they told that, thank you so much it was a very good information and because they have somebody in their family who are living with dementia". [P4-01-01]

Participants identified potential to incorporate concepts from DEWE into nursing curricula and educational resources for practitioners and dissemination on a wider scale both in India and the UK.

"It was a particularly big blessing for me because I've written like some modules on elderly care, so I could apply this into that, and see, these modules and curriculum that we've designed is being used to train primary health level workers, nurses across India". [P1-01-01]

"I think it should be rolled out everywhere, I think it should be like teamed up with the NHS, I think it should be done with all new staff starting, even old staff. . .. I think it would be a fantastic program to roll out". [P9-02-02]

Several participants were motivated to engage with further learning about dementia in other online courses [P3-02-01], masters [P9-02-02], and PhD programs [P2-01-01].

The impact from DEWE also motivated participants from India to develop programs of research including timely inquiries into dementia prevalence in local communities.

"I started to read articles on dementia related to India and South Asian countries, I found that there were very few nursing related articles, so, a colleague and I decided to conduct a small study and we're in the process of doing that". [P3-02-01]

4.6. Theme 4: Adapting and Appropriating DEWE for Future Success

4.6.1. Improving DEWE

Several participants suggested that future modifications to DEWE were not necessary [P1-01-01; P3-02-01; P5-01-01; P7-01-02]. Despite benefits of the bichronous online delivery, some participants noted a preference for in-person [P1-01-01] and practice-based learning [P4-01-01].

Discussion in DEWE had focused on participants' experience, perceptions, and perspectives of dementia care. Recommendations to improve synchronous sessions were to include case presentations based on actual experiences using a systematic approach incorporating patient assessment, evaluation, and care planning [P6-01-01]. Assessment and evaluation of learning were recommended using multiple choice questions and concept mapping techniques [P2-01-01]. Other suggestions to improve DEWE included even greater focus on neurophysiology [P2-01-01] and the dementia care environment [P6-01-01].

Participants recommended that DEWE is updated regularly to reflect evidence-based changes in dementia care.

"We want this to be given again and again with some other changes or a kind of recap, recapitulation, or kind of refresher course, we want this to be at least once a year or twice a year . . . I feel that it has to be refreshed". [P6-01-01]

4.6.2. Culture and Context

DEWE was thought to benefit from greater contextualization. Cultural adaptations were thought necessary to convey the unique challenges of dementia care in India. Greater emphasis on familial systems of support was considered the most relevant adaptation to the Indian context.

> *"The context was good, but I think some of the tools which are available for people in probably UK settings are not available for people here, for example, like, xxxx shared about having a community of people with dementia and community helping each other so, we don't have that kind of a network here".* [P8-02-01]

Contextualization of DEWE to the Indian context would also require content adapted to address unique cultural perspectives and challenges including regional language variations.

> *"For Northern India must have to think about the Hindi language and their perspectives, and South India might have to think a little different. . .like that, we might have to add a few videos or something. . . so that it feels that, yes, it is our own problems here and it is what our people are going through".* [P5-01-01]

5. Results: Mixed Methods

Integration of quantitative and quantitative findings highlighted several motivating factors for engagement in DEWE including support with continuing professional development, access to expert facilitation, certification for learning, and education at no cost. The integrated findings also resulted in the identification of strengths and areas for improvements in DEWE (Table 4).

Table 4. Summary of DEWE strengths and areas for improvement. The arrow up symbol denotes "increasing levels".

	Strengths	Areas for Development
Satisfaction		
Asynchronous	High quality resources Easy to use Time for learning Learning on demand Active learning Real-life videos Preparation for synchronous sessions	Consider cultural adaptations Provide more assessments Improve placement of videos Improve quality of resources in print form Update content regularly Consider strategies for learner motivation
Synchronous	Interactive Active learning and reflection Diversity of participants Includes dementia experts Includes people with lived experience Provides expert facilitation Consolidates asynchronous learning	Include interactive icebreakers session *Discuss/mitigate technical issues* *Discuss/mitigate poor online etiquette* Optimize session duration Optimize delivery platform Include more discussions on actual cases Provide follow-up sessions
Bichronous	Highly rated Mutual learning between resources Ongoing access to resources Relevance post-COVID-19	-
Learning	New knowledge New skills Positive attitudes	-
Behaviors	Positive behavior change	-
Results	↑ Dementia awareness ↑ Knowledge transfer ↑ Development of educational resources ↑ Engagement with dementia education ↑ Engagement with dementia research Dissemination of DEWE (wider audience)	-

6. Discussion

Dementia training that is dependent on learner-initiated asynchronous instruction involving episodic or standardized elements of care often fails to accurately depict the trajectory of the illness and risks assumptions that such criteria are ubiquitous to the dementia syndrome [29]. One might also presume that such training has the potential to inadvertently introduce unconscious negative bias and reinforce stigma when certain training packages, e.g., Management of Stress & Distress, are recommended as mandatory dementia training. Such an approach unfortunately does not seem to help practitioners understand dementia as a neurodegenerative disorder and the complexities associated with the progression of the disease. Acknowledging the inherent uniqueness of the dementia trajectory for each person ensured that DEWE prioritized and enabled learning for participants to see the person behind the illness rather than the condition itself or focus on managing isolated behaviors associated with the condition [30]. DEWE, as both a unique and comprehensive dementia training program, used a "journey-based approach" to help participants to appreciate the essentials, priorities, and enablers for high-quality person and relationship-centered dementia care.

The COVID-19 pandemic prompted a shift in educational delivery and a transition to online programs which was particularly notable in India where e-learning has only started to gain popularity [31]. DEWE was developed during the pandemic to provide dementia education through a balance of flexibility (asynchronous workbooks) and immediacy (synchronous sessions). Previous research has demonstrated that the combination of asynchronous and synchronous (bichronous) online learning has several advantages including improved learning outcomes [17].

Asynchronous workbooks provided participants with access to dementia education at any time and place. Convenience and flexibility are benefits of technology-enabled dementia education [32–34]; however, asynchronous learning may result in feelings of isolation [35]. DEWE implemented various active learning strategies to compensate the effects of learner isolation. Adherence to principles of adult learning [36] combined with established motivating factors for participation, e.g., certification for learning [37], optimized learner interest and enthusiasm. Feedback is an integral element of teaching and learning across educational delivery modes [38,39]. Formal assessment of learning in DEWE may indicate whether specified learning outcomes were achieved and enhance learner motivation by fostering engagement with course content [40].

It is recommended that effective dementia education be relevant to the roles, experiences, and practices of learners, rather than adopting a one-size-fits-all approach [41]. However, diverse and multidisciplinary learning cohorts are also known to be beneficial [42]. DEWE replicated in-person teaching in synchronous sessions involving various practitioners and educators in real-time group discussions. This rich diversity of participants shared a passion for dementia and actively sought improvements in dementia care which led to a vibrant community of engagement and expertise [43].

Online programs should be designed to focus on pedagogical issues which emphasize collaborative and case-based learning (CBL) [31]. CBL aimed to connect theory and practice in both asynchronous and synchronous resources through emotional engagement with authentic clinical cases [44]. CBL using actual learner experience is aligned with the experiential learning model [45]. Greater emphasis on participants' direct experience may develop higher order thinking whilst encouraging group reflection and collaborative problem solving [46]. Experience-based CBL during synchronous sessions could be enhanced using frameworks rooted in nursing processes to guide discussions and the effective articulation of cases [47].

DEWE was deemed highly relevant to the participants' current practice; however, it fell short in addressing cultural differences between the UK and India. Both countries share many common goals, such as providing quality healthcare and addressing the needs of the growing elderly population [48]. Culturally appropriate education is crucial in India to address the rising burden of dementia and effectively address the unique socio-economic, cultural, linguistic, geographical, and lifestyle characteristics of this population [49]. Learner motivation can be enhanced where educational content includes references to national dementia prevalence, incidence, and related factors, along with information on local professional and community services [50]. Incorporating relevant material is crucial as participants anticipate applying new knowledge locally in practice.

DEWE was enriched through the involvement of individuals with lived experience of dementia and their family carers. Involvement in dementia education may foster a sense of worth and altruism among people with dementia and can provide carers with opportunities to share experiences and address caregiving challenges. The involvement of lived experience in DEWE fostered emotional connections with participants for deeper engagement [51]. Engagement was further enhanced from expert facilitation and input from credible and relatable dementia care experts who served as positive dementia care role models [52].

Surr [41] suggested that the total duration of dementia education programs should be more than eight hours with individual sessions being at least 90 min. Limited evidence exists on the optimal duration for online synchronous sessions; however, during or after these sessions, learners often report feelings of fatigue [53]. The average duration of synchronous sessions in DEWE was 82 min with most exceeding the 90 min recommendation and were regularly interspaced with breakout opportunities. Nonetheless, the duration of synchronous sessions in future iterations of DEWE might be minimized to mitigate cognitive overload and learner fatigue.

Delivery via WebEx posed challenges to participants from India due to an unfamiliarity with the platform. Engagement may have been further compromised as several participants used mobile phones to access DEWE. Mobile devices including smartphones are promising as learning devices due to their portability and ability to facilitate rapid information retrieval, collaborative interaction, and situated learning [54]; however, mobile devices may not be ideal for online learning due to software compatibility issues and small screen sizes [55].

Technical challenges and poor online etiquette can risk misunderstanding and miscommunication [56]. Setting rules for online etiquette in synchronous sessions may encourage a sense of community and active participation amongst learners [57]. In future courses, it will be important to provide 'netiquette' guidance in the first synchronous session, with contingency plans to resolve potential technical issues. These enhancements will ensure that DEWE provides a seamless and efficient online learning experience.

Limitations

The survey did not include demographic information to establish the impact of the training based on country of origin. Social care practitioners who completed the survey consisted of care home and home care professionals; however, specific counts for the subgroups were not reported.

Most (78%) interview participants were from India which limits the transferability of the findings to the UK. This disparity also highlights the need for culturally sensitive learning content should DEWE be provided for learners based exclusively in the UK or India. Interviews were conducted up to 18 months post-training which allowed participants time to observe and comment on practice-based behavioral changes; however, this timeframe may also have introduced recall bias. The research team frequently discussed qualitative analytical procedures; however, the absence of respondent validation for interview transcripts may have compromised the methodological rigor of the inductive analytical process. The final sample size (n = 9) represented over a quarter of all DEWE participants that completed the online survey. Whilst practical, this approach did not adhere to robust principles of data saturation and potentially limited the emergence of additional insights and assurances of analytical rigor.

7. Conclusions

DEWE is an innovative resource and response to dementia education and training during the COVID-19 pandemic, integrating asynchronous and synchronous instruction. The person- and relationship-centered approach across the trajectory of the illness has relevance to diverse participants and educational settings which fosters an inclusive and supportive learning environment. Communities of engagement and expertise play a crucial role in enriching the overall learning experience. By bringing together participants with individuals with lived experiences and specialist knowledge, these communities can flourish to enhance learning and foster personal and professional growth. DEWE offers a notable advantage in its ability to overcome geographical boundaries; however, international dissemination will require cultural adaptations to ensure that the program aligns with cultural contexts for maximum impact. Future research will be useful to assess the effectiveness of DEWE using pre- and post-test methodologies or in comparative studies involving alternative modes of dementia education, including face-to-face or asynchronous instruction alone.

Supplementary Materials: The following supporting information can be downloaded at: https://www.mdpi.com/article/10.3390/healthcare12050590/s1, Interview Schedule.

Author Contributions: Conceptualization, L.M.; data curation, K.M.; formal analysis, K.M.; funding acquisition, L.M.; investigation, K.M.; methodology, L.M. and K.M.; supervision, L.M.; writing—original draft, K.M.; writing—review and editing, L.M. All authors have read and agreed to the published version of the manuscript.

Funding: This project was funded by the COVID-19 Action Fund of The Churchill Fellowship, UK.

Institutional Review Board Statement: Ethics approval to conduct the study was secured from the Research Ethics Committee of the University of the Highlands and Islands (UHI) [ETH2122-0481], approved on 31 March 2022.

Informed Consent Statement: Informed consent was obtained from all subjects involved in the study. Written informed consent has been obtained from the participants to publish this paper.

Data Availability Statement: The data that support the findings of this study are not openly available since participant consent was not gained for this purpose.

Acknowledgments: Chat GDP software version 3.5 was used to improve readability and clarity of language in some sections of the manuscript draft with full author (K.M.) oversight and control.

Conflicts of Interest: L.M. conceptualized DEWE and facilitated synchronous online sessions. L.M. disseminated project information to DEWE participants but did not participate in recruitment, data collection, or analysis to avoid any conflict of interest with interpretation of results. The funders had no role in the design of the study; in the collection, analyses, or interpretation of data; in the writing of the manuscript; or in the decision to publish the results.

References

1. World Health Organization. Dementia A Public Health Priority. 2012. Available online: https://www.who.int/publications/i/item/dementia-a-public-health-priority (accessed on 3 April 2023).
2. Alzheimer's Society. Facts for the Media about Dementia. 2023. Available online: https://www.alzheimers.org.uk/about-us/news-and-media/facts-media (accessed on 3 April 2023).
3. World Health Organization. Dementia: Key Facts. 2023. Available online: https://www.who.int/news-room/fact-sheets/detail/dementia (accessed on 3 April 2023).
4. Scutti, S. New Estimate of Dementia Prevalence Indicates Magnitude of India's Challenge. 2023. Available online: https://www.fic.nih.gov/News/GlobalHealthMatters/march-april-2023/Pages/new-estimate-dementia-prevalence-magnitude-india-challenge.aspx (accessed on 10 April 2023).
5. Lee, J.; Meijer, E.; Langa, K.M.; Ganguli, M.; Varghese, M.; Banerjee, J.; Khobragade, P.; Angrisani, M.; Kurup, R.; Chakrabarti, S.S.; et al. Prevalence of dementia in India: National and state estimates from a nationwide study. *Alzheimer's Dement. J. Alzheimer's Assoc.* **2023**, *19*, 2898–2912. [CrossRef] [PubMed]
6. Dias, A.; Patel, V. Closing the treatment gap for dementia in India. *Indian J. Psychiatry* **2009**, *51* (Suppl. S1), S93–S97.

7. Alzheimer's and Related Disorders Society of India. *The Dementia India Report: Prevalence, Impact, Costs and Services for Dementia;* Executive Summary; Alzheimer's and Related Disorders Society of India: New Delhi, India, 2010.
8. Department of Health. Prime Minister's Challenge on Dementia. Delivering Major Improvements in Dementia Care and Research by 2015. 2012. Available online: https://assets.publishing.service.gov.uk/government/uploads/system/uploads/attachment_data/file/215101/dh_133176.pdf (accessed on 10 April 2023).
9. Department of Health and Social Care. Prime Ministers Challenge on Dementia 2020. 2015. Available online: https://www.gov.uk/government/publications/prime-ministers-challenge-on-dementia-2020/prime-ministers-challenge-on-dementia-2020#why-dementia-remains-a-priority (accessed on 10 April 2023).
10. Scottish Government. *Scotland's National Dementia Strategy 2010*; The Scottish Government: Edinburgh, UK, 2010.
11. Scottish Government. Standard of Care for Dementia in Scotland. 2011. Available online: https://www.gov.scot/publications/standards-care-dementia-scotland-action-support-change-programme-scotlands-national-dementia-strategy/ (accessed on 10 April 2023).
12. Scottish Government. Scotland's National Dementia Strategy 2013–2016. 2013. Available online: https://webarchive.nrscotland.gov.uk/3000/https://www.gov.scot/Resource/0042/00423472.pdf (accessed on 10 April 2023).
13. Scottish Government. National Dementia Strategy: 2017–2020. 2017. Available online: https://www.gov.scot/publications/scotlands-national-dementia-strategy-2017-2020/pages/3/ (accessed on 10 April 2023).
14. Scottish Government. Promoting Excellence 2021: A framework for All Health and Social Services Staff Working with People with Dementia, Their Families and Carers. 2021. Available online: https://www.gov.scot/publications/promoting-excellence-2021-framework-health-social-services-staff-working-people-dementia-families-carers/ (accessed on 10 April 2023).
15. Muirhead, K.; Macaden, L.; Smyth, K.; Chandler, C.; Clarke, C.; Polson, R.; O'malley, C. Establishing the effectiveness of technology-enabled dementia education for health and social care practitioners: A systematic review. *Syst. Rev.* **2021**, *10*, 252. [CrossRef] [PubMed]
16. Muirhead, K.; Macaden, L.; Smyth, K.; Chandler, C.; Clarke, C.; Polson, R.; O'malley, C. The characteristics of effective technology-enabled dementia education: A systematic review and mixed research synthesis. *Syst. Rev.* **2022**, *11*, 34. [CrossRef] [PubMed]
17. Martin, F.; Kumar, S.; Ritzhaupt, A.D.; Polly, D. Bichronous online learning: Award-winning online instructor practices of blending asynchronous and synchronous online modalities. *Internet High. Educ.* **2023**, *56*, 100879. [CrossRef]
18. Macaden, L. Being Dementia Smart (BDS): A Dementia Nurse Education Journey in Scotland. *Int. J. Nurs. Educ. Scholarsh.* **2016**, *13*, 45–53. [CrossRef]
19. Baillie, L.; Sills, E.; Thomas, N. Educating a health service workforce about dementia: A qualitative study. *Qual. Ageing Older Adults* **2016**, *17*, 119–130. [CrossRef]
20. Bute, J. Glorious Opportunity. Available online: https://www.gloriousopportunity.org/ (accessed on 17 April 2023).
21. Gallagher, R. The lived experience of people with dementia. *Br. Columbia Med. J.* **2019**, *61*, 39–40.
22. Nolan, M.R.; Davies, S.; Brown, J.; Keady, J.; Nolan, J. Beyond 'person-centred' care: A new vision for gerontological nursing. *J. Clin. Nurs.* **2004**, *13*, 45–53. [CrossRef] [PubMed]
23. UK Government. Adults with Incapacity (Scotland) Act 2000. Available online: https://www.legislation.gov.uk/asp/2000/4/contents/enacted (accessed on 17 April 2023).
24. NHS Education for Scotland. Staff Wellbeing Resources. 2021. Available online: https://www.nes.scot.nhs.uk/news/staff-wellbeing-resources/ (accessed on 17 April 2023).
25. Kirkpatrick, D. Great Ideas Revisited. Techniques for evaluating training programs. Revisiting Kirkpatrick's Four-Level Model. *Train. Dev.* **1996**, *50*, 54–59.
26. Online Surveys. 2023. Available online: https://www.onlinesurveys.ac.uk/ (accessed on 24 April 2023).
27. Braun, V.; Clarke, V. *Thematic Analysis: A Practical Guide*, 1st ed.; Sage: London, UK, 2021.
28. Lincoln, Y.; Guba, E. *Naturalistic Inquiry*; Sage: Newbury Park, CA, USA, 1985.
29. Fazio, S.; Pace, D.; Flinner, J.; Kallmyer, B. The Fundamentals of Person-Centered Care for Individuals with Dementia. *Gerontologist* **2018**, *58* (Suppl. S1), S10–S19. [CrossRef]
30. Kitwood, T. *Dementia Reconsidered: The Person Comes First*; Open University Press: Maidenhead, UK, 1997.
31. Dhawan, S. Online Learning: A Panacea in the Time of COVID-19 Crisis. *J. Educ. Technol. Syst.* **2020**, *49*, 5–22. [CrossRef]
32. Almutairi, H.; Stafford, A.; Etherton-Beer, C.; Flicker, L.; Saunders, R. Aged care staff perceptions of an online training program for responsive behaviours of residents with dementia. *Australas. J. Ageing* **2022**, *41*, e112–e121. [CrossRef]
33. Gallant, N.; Hadjistavropoulos, T.; Winters, E.M.; Feere, E.K.; Wickson-Griffiths, A. Development, evaluation, and implementation of an online pain assessment training program for staff in rural long-term care facilities: A case series approach. *BMC Geriatr.* **2022**, *22*, 336. [CrossRef]
34. Jones, C.; Moyle, W. Sexuality & dementia: An eLearning resource to improve knowledge and attitudes of aged-care staff. *Educ. Gerontol.* **2016**, *42*, 563–571. [CrossRef]
35. Cleveland-Innes, M.; Wilton, D.; Guide to Blended Learning. Chapter 7: Synchronous and Asynchronous Activities. 2018. Available online: https://openbooks.col.org/blendedlearning/chapter/chapter-7-synchronous-and-asynchronous-activities/ (accessed on 24 April 2023).
36. Knowles, M. Adult learning. In *The ASTD Training and Development Handbook*, 4th ed.; Craig, R., Ed.; McGraw-Hill: New York, NY, USA, 1996.

37. Surr, C.A.; Parveen, S.; Smith, S.J.; Drury, M.; Sass, C.; Burden, S.; Oyebode, J. The barriers and facilitators to implementing dementia education and training in health and social care services: A mixed-methods study. *BMC Health Serv. Res.* **2020**, *20*, 512. [CrossRef]
38. Enders, N.; Gaschler, R.; Kubik, V. Online Quizzes with Closed Questions in Formal Assessment: How elaborate feedback can promote learning. *Psychol. Learn. Teach.* **2021**, *20*, 91–106. [CrossRef]
39. Mate, K.; Weidenhofer, J. Considerations and strategies for effective online assessment with a focus on the biomedical sciences. *FASEB BioAdv.* **2021**, *4*, 9–21. [CrossRef]
40. Perera-Diltz, D.; Moe, J. Formative and summative assessment in online education. *J. Res. Innov. Teach.* **2014**, *7*, 130–142.
41. Surr, C.A.; Gates, C.; Irving, D.; Oyebode, J.; Smith, S.J.; Parveen, S.; Drury, M.; Dennison, A. Effective Dementia Education and Training for the Health and Social Care Workforce: A systematic review of the literature. *Rev. Educ. Res.* **2017**, *87*, 966–1002. [CrossRef]
42. Toubøl, A.; Moestrup, L.; Thomsen, K.; Ryg, J.; Hansen, D.L.; Foldager, M.; Jakobsen, S.; Nielsen, D.S. The impact of an education intervention on the approach of hospital staff to patients with dementia in a Danish general hospital setting: An explanatory sequential mixed-methods study. *Nord. J. Nurs. Res.* **2022**, *42*, 28–41. [CrossRef]
43. Wenger-Trayner, E.; Wenger-Trayner, B. Introduction to Communities of Practice: A Brief Overview of the Concept and Its Uses. 2015. Available online: https://www.wenger-trayner.com/introduction-to-communities-of-practice/ (accessed on 8 May 2023).
44. McLean, S.F. Case-Based Learning and Its Application in Medical and Health-Care Fields: A Review of Worldwide Literature. *J. Med. Educ. Curric. Dev.* **2016**, *3*, JMECD.S20377. [CrossRef]
45. Kolb, D. *Experiential Learning: Experience as the Source of Learning and Development*; Prentice-Hall: Englewood Cliffs, NJ, USA, 1984.
46. Seshan, V.; Matua, G.A.; Raghavan, D.; Arulappan, J.; Al Hashmi, I.; Roach, E.J.; Sunderraj, S.E.; Prince, E.J. Case Study Analysis as an Effective Teaching Strategy: Perceptions of Undergraduate Nursing Students from a Middle Eastern Country. *SAGE Open Nurs.* **2021**, *7*, 23779608211059265. [CrossRef]
47. Toney-Butler, T.J.; Thayer, J.M. Nursing Process. In *StatPearls*; StatPearls Publishing: Treasure Island, FL, USA, 2023.
48. HealthcareUK. India and the UK: Partners in Healthcare. 2014. Available online: https://assets.publishing.service.gov.uk/government/uploads/system/uploads/attachment_data/file/311349/Healthcare_UK_India_and_the_UK_LOW.pdf (accessed on 8 May 2023).
49. Ravindranath, V.; Sundarakumar, J.S. Changing demography and the challenge of dementia in India. *Nat. Rev. Neurol.* **2021**, *17*, 747–758. [CrossRef]
50. Kember, D.; Ho, A.; Hong, C. The importance of establishing relevance in motivating student learning. *Act. Learn. High. Educ.* **2008**, *9*, 249–263. [CrossRef]
51. Cashin, Z.; Daley, S.; Hebditch, M.; Hughes, L.; Banerjee, S. Involving people with dementia and their carers in dementia education for undergraduate healthcare professionals: A qualitative study of motivation to participate and experience. *Int. Psychogeriatr.* **2019**, *31*, 869–876. [CrossRef]
52. Birden, H.; Glass, N.; Wilson, I.; Harrison, M.; Usherwood, T.; Nass, D. Teaching professionalism in medical education: A Best Evidence Medical Education (BEME) systematic review. BEME Guide No. 25. *Med. Teach.* **2013**, *35*, e1252–e1266. [CrossRef]
53. Lepp, M.; Luik, P.; Tark, T.M. How Can Web Lessons Be Taught to Reduce Screen Fatigue, Motivational, and Concentration Problems in Different Disciplines? *Front. Sociol.* **2022**, *7*, 871770. [CrossRef]
54. Sophonhiranrak, S. Features, barriers, and influencing factors of mobile learning in higher education: A systematic review. *Heliyon* **2021**, *7*, e06696. [CrossRef]
55. Nikpeyma, N.; Zolfaghari, M.; Mohammadi, A. Barriers and facilitators of using mobile devices as an educational tool by nursing students: A qualitative research. *BMC Nurs.* **2021**, *20*, 226. [CrossRef]
56. Oza, P. Digital Etiquette in Online Teaching Learning. 2022. Available online: https://ssrn.com/abstract=4217177 (accessed on 15 May 2023).
57. Iqbal, S.; Hanif, R.; Ali, F.; Tahir, M.; Minhas, R.; Yasmeen, R.; Khokhar, A.; Laique, T. Teachers' Perceptions of Netiquette Practices by undergraduate Dental Students During Online Classes in COVID-19 Pandemic. *Pak. J. Med. Health Sci.* **2021**, *15*, 3498–3500. [CrossRef]

healthcare MDPI

Systematic Review

Emerging Therapeutic Strategies for Diffuse Intrinsic Pontine Glioma: A Systematic Review

Shahrukh Farrukh [1], Shagufta Habib [2], Amna Rafaqat [3], Zouina Sarfraz [3], Azza Sarfraz [4,*], Muzna Sarfraz [5], Karla Robles-Velasco [6], Miguel Felix [7] and Ivan Cherrez-Ojeda [6,*]

[1] Department of Research, Khawaja Muhammad Safdar Medical College, Sialkot 51310, Pakistan
[2] Department of Research, University Medical and Dental College Faisalabad, Faisalabad 38800, Pakistan
[3] Department of Research and Publications, Fatima Jinnah Medical University, Lahore 54000, Pakistan
[4] Department of Pediatrics and Child Health, The Aga Khan University, Karachi 74000, Pakistan
[5] Independent Researcher, Lahore 54000, Pakistan
[6] Department of Allergy, Immunology and Pulmonary Medicine, Universidad Espíritu Santo, Samborondón 092301, Ecuador
[7] Department of Internal Medicine, New York City Health + Hospitals, Lincoln, The Bronx, NY 10451, USA
* Correspondence: azza.sarfraz@aku.edu (A.S.); ivancherrez@gmail.com (I.C.-O.)

Abstract: Background: Of all central nervous systems tumors, 10–20% are located in the brainstem; diffuse intrinsic pontine glioma (DIPG) is diagnosed in 80% of them. With over five decades of clinical trial testing, there are no established therapeutic options for DIPG. This research article aims to collate recent clinical trial data and provide a landscape for the most promising therapies that have emerged in the past five years. Methods: PubMed/MEDLINE, Web of Science, Scopus, and Cochrane were systematically searched using the following keywords: Diffuse intrinsic pontine glioma, Pontine, Glioma, Treatment, Therapy, Therapeutics, curative, and/or Management. Both adult and pediatric patients with newly diagnosed or progressive DIPG were considered in the clinical trial setting. The risk of bias was assessed using the ROBINS-I tool. Results: A total of 22 trials were included reporting the efficacy and safety outcomes among patients. First, five trials reported outcomes of blood–brain barrier bypass via single or repeated-dose intra-arterial therapy or convection-enhanced delivery. Second, external beam radiation regimens were assessed for safety and efficacy in three trials. Third, four trials administered intravenous treatment without using chemotherapeutic regimens. Fourth, eight trials reported the combinations of one or more chemotherapeutic agents. Fifth, immunotherapy was reported in two trials in an adjuvant monotherapy in the post-radiotherapy setting. Conclusion: This research article captures a clinical picture of the last five years of the direction toward which DIPG research is heading. The article finds that re-irradiation may prolong survival in patients with progressive DIPG; it also instills that insofar palliative radiotherapy has been a key prognostic choice.

Keywords: diffuse intrinsic pontine glioma; CNS; tumor; therapies; palliative; quality of life; advances

1. Introduction

Central nervous system (CNS) tumors have a higher mortality rate among all cancers in US children aged 1–19 years [1–3]. Of all CNS tumors, 10–20% are located in the brainstem, with diffuse intrinsic pontine glioma (DIPG) diagnosed in 80% of them [4]. The prognosis is dismal with DIPG with the overall survival rate being lower than 10% at 2 years [5]. The median survival rates are less than 12 months and the 5-year survival rates are below 2% [6,7]. Radiation therapy is the current standard of treatment, yet it remains a palliative option as radiotherapy only temporarily relieves symptoms [8]. DIPG has been classified histopathologically as high-grade astrocytoma (HGA) with most cases being consistent with histological grade III or IV (anaplastic astrocytoma or glioblastoma, respectively) but certain less aggressive cases are histologically classified as grade II (diffuse astrocytoma) [9]. More recently, the World Health Organization (WHO) classified DIPG as diffuse midline gliomas with histone H3K27M mutation [9]. With over five decades of clinical trials exploring different chemotherapy and radiotherapy regimens, there are no promising therapeutic options in DIPG [10]. Several clinical trials of systematic therapies have been tested or are ongoing [11].

Certain therapies have recently gained traction for their potential efficacy in DIPG [12]. Thereby, this research article aims to collate data from recent clinical trials and provide a landscape for the most promising therapeutic options that have emerged in the last five years.

2. Materials and Methods

2.1. Search Strategy

A comprehensive systematic search was conducted using the following databases, adhering to Preferred Reporting Items for Systematic Reviews and Meta-Analyses (PRISMA) Statement 2020 guidelines: PubMed/MEDLINE, Web of Science, Scopus, and Cochrane. The search was conducted from 1 January 2017, until 16 October 2022, without any language limitations (non-English studies were translated to English using Google Translate). Applying the Boolean (and/or) logic, the following keywords were applied: Diffuse intrinsic pontine glioma, Pontine, Glioma, Treatment, Therapy, Therapeutics, curative, and/or Management. The titles and abstracts of shortlisted studies from the given databases were screened independently by two mid-career authors (Z.S., A.S.). In the screening phase, the reference lists were also reviewed, in line with the umbrella methodology to ensure no data were omitted. In the case of any disagreements, a third author (I.C.-O.) was present to resolve them and to reach a consensus. Cohen's coefficient of the inter-reviewer agreement was computed using Statistical Package for Social Sciences (SPSS, v.25, IBM).

2.2. Inclusion and Exclusion Criteria

The inclusion criteria comprised clinical trials enrolling both adult and pediatric patients of any gender with newly diagnosed or progressive DIPG. The treatment could consist of any of the following: (i) blood–brain barrier bypass (intra-arterial therapy or convection enhanced delivery), (ii) external beam radiation, (iii) intravenous treatment regimens without administering chemotherapeutic agents, (iv) combination regimens with the use of one or more chemotherapeutic agents.

Studies intervening with only surgical procedures were not included. Further, cohorts (retrospective/prospective), case series, case reports, systematic reviews and meta-analyses, brief reports, and letters to editors were excluded.

2.3. Data Extraction (Selection and Coding)

Two mid-career authors (Z.S., A.S.) independently extracted the data from the included trials into a spreadsheet. The third author (I.C.-O.) was present for any disagreements. The pair identified the trials and treatments of the screened studies. Once the independent review of the studies was conducted, the third author (I.C.-O.) assessed the extracted domains from the spreadsheet and conducted the final review against the inclusion criteria.

The data were extracted as follows: Author, Year, Title, Journal, Country, Study design, Inclusion criteria, Intervention given, Method of administration; Number of patients with DIPG, Age at diagnosis (in years), Sex (percentage of males), Previous treatment, Outcome measures; Median OS (in months), Median EFS/PFS (in months), Radiological response (percentage), Clinical improvement (proportion), Tolerance and safety, and Steroid use discontinuation.

Individual study data were prepared in a presentable format during the inclusion phase and the concluding remarks were also added. EndNote X9 (Clarivate, London, UK) was the software used to omit duplicates during the study selection process. In addition, Mendeley (Elsevier, Amsterdam, The Netherlands) was used for bibliographic management.

2.4. Risk of Bias (Quality Assessment)

The Risk of Bias in Non-randomized Studies of Interventions (ROBINS-I) tool was used to assess the risk of bias in the included trials. This tool comprised seven domains. (1) Bias due to confounding; (2) bias due to selection of participants; (3) bias in classification of interventions; (4) bias due to deviations from intended interventions; (5) bias due to missing data; (6) bias in the measurement of outcomes; (7) bias in the selection of the reported result.

Domain-level judgments about the risk of bias were classified as the following: (1) low risk; (2) moderate risk; and (3) serious risk. The traffic light plot of bias assessment and the weighted summary plot of the overall type of bias encountered is illustrated in Section 3.6.

3. Results

During the phase I, the identification phase, a total of 1249 studies were identified. Of these, 234 duplicates were removed. In phase II, the screening phase, 1015 study titles and abstracts were screened, of which 897 were omitted as they did not warrant inclusion against the inclusion criteria. Subsequently, 118 full-text studies were reviewed and assessed for eligibility. Of these, 96 studies were excluded as 28 were non-human studies, 43 of them were model/experimental papers, and 25 were not clinical trials. In phase III, the inclusion phase, a total of 22 trials were included (Figure 1). Kappa's score was calculated to be 0.91.

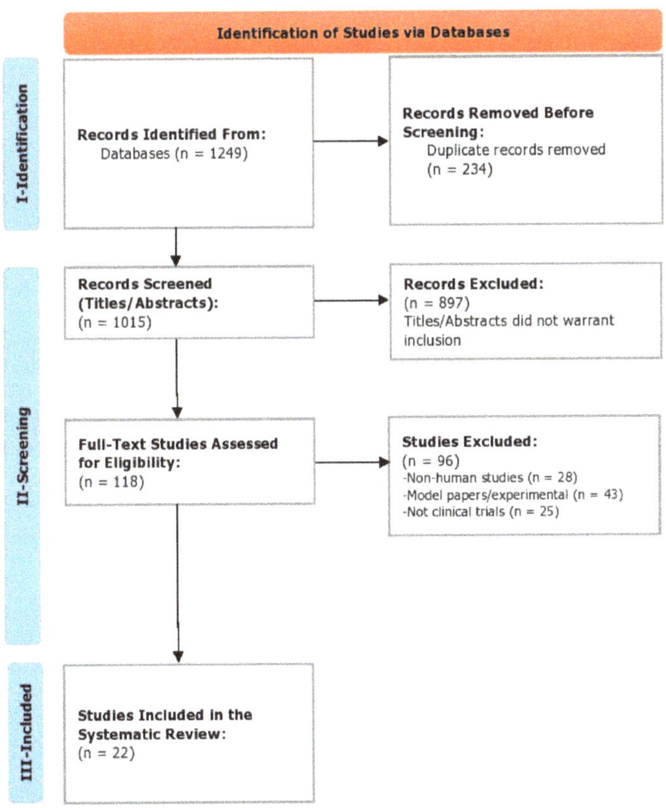

Figure 1. PRISMA flowchart depicting the study selection process.

A total of 22 trials were found that reported efficacy and safety outcomes among patients with newly diagnosed or progressive DIPG (Tables 1–3). First, trials that reported bypassing of the blood–brain barrier (BBB) are reported. In five phase I trials, authors evaluated outcomes of blood–brain barrier (BBB) bypass via single or repeated-dose intra-arterial therapy [13] or convection-enhanced delivery (CED) [14–17].

Second, trials that explored different external beam radiation regimens are elaborated. In two randomized controlled trials [18,19], the authors explored the efficacy and safety of different radiotherapy regimens including conventionally fractionated and hypofractionated radiotherapy in newly diagnosed DIPG. Re-irradiation at three dose levels among patients who had received initial radiotherapy $\geq$10 months ago was compared with patients with progressive DIPG in a phase I/II trial [20].

Third, trials are listed that administered intravenous treatment regimens without administering chemotherapeutic agents. In a phase III trial, authors evaluated the outcomes of epidermal growth factor receptor (EGFR) inhibitors, nimoztuzumab with radiotherapy in newly diagnosed DIPG patients [21]. In a phase I/II trial, the authors evaluated the outcomes of vorinostat given concomitantly and as adjuvant to radiotherapy in newly diagnosed DIPG [22]. Adavosertib, a Wee 1 kinase inhibitor, was given with cranial radiation therapy (CRT) in newly diagnosed DIPG in a phase I trial [23]. A phase II trial administered EBT and valproic acid (VPA), an anti-convulsant, followed by bevacizumab, an anti-vascular endothelial growth factor, and VPA in newly diagnosed DIPG patients [24].

Fourth, trials that evaluated combination regimens with the use of one or more chemotherapeutic agents are listed. One phase II trial with newly diagnosed DIPG combined radiotherapy and cefuximab, an epidermal growth factor receptor (EGFR) inhibitor, followed by cefuximab and irinotecan, a topoisomerase I inhibitor [25]. Another phase I/II trial combined erlotinib, an EGFR inhibitor, with bevacizumab, a vascular endothelial growth factor (VEGF) inhibitor, and irinocetan among patients with progressive DIPG [26]. Two trials explored outcomes of ribociclib (kinase inhibitor) concomitantly with radiotherapy and everolimus (kinase inhibitor) (phase I trial [27]) and as adjuvant monotherapy (in phase II [28]) in newly diagnosed patients with DIPG. One phase I/II trial administered concomitant EBT and veliparib, a PARP inhibitor, followed by veliparib and temozolomide, an alkylating agent [29]. Capecitabine, an alkylating agent, was given in combination with EBT and as adjuvant monotherapy in newly diagnosed DIPG patients in a phase II trial [30]. Gemcitabine, a nucleoside metabolic inhibitor, was combined with initial EBT among newly diagnosed DIPG patients in a phase I/II trial [31]. One trial explored the maximum tolerated dose (MTD) and efficacy of cabazitaxel, a microtubule inhibitor, as adjuvant monotherapy in progressive DIPG patients in a phase I/II dose-escalating trial [32].

Fifth, trials that administered immunotherapeutic agents as adjuvant monotherapy after radiotherapy are reported. One phase II trial administered pomalidomide, an immunomodulatory drug, among patients with progressive DIPG. One phase I trial administered pelareorep, an immunomodulatory oncolytic virus, combined with sargramostin, a recombinant human granulocyte-macrophage colony-stimulating factor, in patients with progressive DIPG.

Table 1. Baseline characteristics of the trial and dosing regimens.

Author	Year	Title	Journal	Country	Study Design	Inclusion Criteria	Intervention Given	Method of Administration
				Blood-brain Barrier Bypass				
McCrea	2021 [13]	Intraarterial delivery of bevacizumab and cetuximab utilizing blood-brain barrier disruption in children with high-grade glioma and diffuse intrinsic pontine glioma: results of a phase I trial	*Journal of Neurosurgery*	USA	Phase I trial (NCT01884740)	Patients aged <22 years with a histological diagnosis of relapsed or refractory HCG or radiological diagnosis of DIPG	Single intraarterial dose of 15 mg/kg bevacizumab and 200 mg/m^2 cetuximab after BBBD with mannitol	Superselective intraarterial cerebral infusion
Heiss	2018 [14]	Phase I trial of convection-enhanced delivery of IL13-Pseudomonas toxin in children with diffuse intrinsic pontine glioma	*Journal of NeuroSurgery: Pediatrics*	USA	Phase I dose-escalation trial (NCT00088061)	Patients aged <18 years with clinical and radiological evidence of progressive DIPG, >2 weeks after their last chemotherapy dose or neurosurgical procedure, and >4 weeks from the last dose of radiation	IL13-PE38QQR and surrogate marker of IL13-PE38QQR distribution, Gd-DTPA co-infused, initial concentration of 0.125 μg/mL followed by 0.25 μg/mL IL13-PE38QQR	Intratumoral CED
Pérez-Larraya	2022 [15]	Oncolytic DNX-2401 Virus for Pediatric Diffuse Intrinsic Pontine Glioma	*The New England Journal of Medicine*	Spain	Phase 1 trial (NCT03178032)	Patients who were diagnosed with treatment-naive DIPG and aged 3–18 years	Single infusion of oncolytic adenovirus DNX-2401 (1 × 1010 or 5 × 1010 viral particles) followed by radiotherapy	CED, virus infused through a catheter placed in the cerebellar peduncle
Bander	2020 [16]	Repeat convection-enhanced delivery for diffuse intrinsic pontine glioma	*Journal of Neurosurgery*	USA	Phase I trial (NCT01502917)	Patients who were radiographically diagnosed with DIPG and previously treated with external-beam radiation therapy; showed no dose-limiting toxicity or disease progression in the 30-day observation window after first round of CED	≥2 infusions of I-8H9 monoclonal antibody (124I-omburtamab, Y-mAbs Therapeutics) via CED	CED through supratentorial trajectory with intraprocedural MRI-guided stereotactic placement
Majzner	2022 [17]	GD2-CAR T cell therapy for H3K27M-mutated diffuse midline gliomas	*Nature*	USA	Phase I dose-escalation trial (NCT04196413)	Patients who had H3K27M-mutated DIPG at any stage and aged 5–25 years	GD2-CAR T cells at dose level 1 (1 × 106 GD2-CAR T cells per kg administered intravenously) and subsequent GD2-CAR T-cell infusions administered intracerebroventricularly if there was a clinical benefit with first dose	Intravenously followed by intracerebroventricularly
Author	**Year**	**Title**	**Journal**	**Country**	**Study Design**	**Inclusion Criteria**	**Intervention Given**	**Method of Administration**
				Different Radiotherapy Regimens				
Zaghloul	2022 [18]	Hypofractionated Radiation Therapy For Diffuse Intrinsic Pontine Glioma: A Noninferiority Randomized Study Including 253 Children	*International Journal of Radiation Oncology*	Egypt	Randomized clinical trial	Patients with diagnosed DIPG	HF radiotherapy regimens: HF1, receiving 39 Gy in 13 fractions; HF2, receiving 45 Gy in 15 fractions; and CF, receiving 54 Gy in 30 fractions	External beam radiotherapy

Table 1. *Cont.*

Author	Year	Title	Journal	Country	Study Design	Inclusion Criteria	Intervention Given	Method of Administration
				Different Radiotherapy Regimens				
Izzuddeen	2019 [19]	Hypofractionated radiotherapy with temozolomide in diffuse intrinsic pontine gliomas: a randomized controlled trial	*Journal of Neuro-Oncology*	India	Phase II randomized trial	Patients aged 3 to 40 years with newly diagnosed patients with DIPG, confirmed radiologically on MRI with involvement of more than half of pons and basilar artery	Arm A received conventional fractionated RT of 60 Gy in 30 fractions over 6 weeks while patients in arm B received hypo-fractionated radiotherapy of 39 Gy in 13 fractions over 2.6 weeks along with concurrent TMZ 75 mg/m^2 from day 1 to day 17 followed by adjuvant TMZ for six cycles.	Orally and external beam radiotherapy
Amsbaugh	2019 [20]	A Phase 1/2 Trial of Reirradiation for Diffuse Intrinsic Pontine Glioma	*International Journal of Radiation Oncology*	India	Phase I/II trial	Patients with radiologically confirmed DIPG by MRI who received radiation therapy at least 10 months previously with progressive disease confirmed clinically and radiologically	Re-irradiation at three doses, dose level 1: 24 Gy in 12 fractions, dose level 2: 26.4 Gy in 12 fractions, dose level 3: 30.8 Gy in 14 fractions	External beam radiotherapy
Author	**Year**	**Title**	**Journal**	**Country**	**Study Design**	**Inclusion Criteria**	**Intervention Given**	**Method of Administration**
				Non-Chemotherapeutic Agent Regimens				
Fleischhack	2019 [21]	Nimotuzumab and radiotherapy for treatment of newly diagnosed diffuse intrinsic pontine glioma (DIPG): a phase III clinical study	*Journal of Neuro-Oncology*	Germany, Italy, Russia	Phase III trial	Patients between 3 and 20 years with clinically and radiologically confirmed DIPG, diagnosed in the last 3 months	Nimotuzumab was given intravenously at 150 mg/m^2 weekly for 12 weeks and radiotherapy at a total dose of 54 Gy between week 3 and week 9	Intravenously and external beam radiotherapy
Su	2022 [22]	Phase I/II trial of vorinostat and radiation and maintenance vorinostat in children with diffuse intrinsic pontine glioma: A Children's Oncology Group report	*Neuro-Oncology*	USA	Phase I/II trial	Children aged 3 to 21 years with newly diagnosed DIPG, radiographically defined as tumors with a pontine epicenter and diffuse involvement of at least two-thirds of the pons; if aforementioned criteria were not met then tumors were biopsied, children who had anaplastic astrocytoma, glioblastoma, gliosarcoma, or anaplastic mixed glioma were included	Vorinostat once daily from Monday till Friday, during radiation therapy (54 Gy in 30 fractions), then 230 mg/m^2 daily for a maximum of twelve 28-day cycles	Orally and external beam radiotherapy
Mueller	2022 [23]	Wee1 kinase inhibitor adavosertib with radiation in newly diagnosed diffuse intrinsic pontine glioma: A Children's Oncology Group phase I consortium study	*Neuro-Oncology Advances*	USA	Phase I trial (NCT01922076)	Patients aged 3–21 years with newly diagnosed DIPG	On days of cranial radiation therapy, 7 adavosertib DLs (50 mg/m^2 alternating weeks, 50 mg/m^2 alternating with weeks of every other day, 50 mg/m^2, then 95, 130, 160, 200 mg/m^2)	Orally

Table 1. *Cont.*

Author	Year	Title	Journal	Country	Study Design	Inclusion Criteria	Intervention Given	Method of Administration
				Non-Chemotherapeutic Agent Regimens				
Su	2020 [24]	A phase 2 study of valproic acid and radiation, followed by maintenance valproic acid and bevacizumab in children with newly diagnosed diffuse intrinsic pontine glioma or high-grade glioma	*Pediatric Blood & Cancer*	USA	Phase II trial (NCT00879437)	Patients between 3 and 21 years with newly diagnosed radiologically confirmed DIPG	Radiation therapy and VPA (15 mg/kg/day and dose adjustment to maintain a trough range of 85 to 115 µg/mL), VPA continued post-radiation, bevacizumab (10 mg/kg) intravenously biweekly, four weeks after completing radiation therapy	Intravenously and external beam radiotherapy
Author	**Year**	**Title**	**Journal**	**Country**	**Study Design**	**Inclusion Criteria**	**Intervention Given**	**Method of Administration**
				Chemotherapeutic Agent Regimens				
Macy	2017 [25]	A pediatric trial of radiation/cetuximab followed by irinotecan/cetuximab in newly diagnosed diffuse pontine gliomas and high-grade astrocytomas: A Pediatric Oncology Experimental Therapeutics Investigators' Consortium study	*Pediatric Blood & Cancer*	USA	Phase II trial	Patients 3 to 21 years of age with newly diagnosed DIPG confirmed clinically and radiologically (MRI)	EBT (5940 cGy in 33 fractions (180 cGy)) with concomitant cetuximab (250 mg/m^2 IV weekly for six doses) with a recovery period of 26–52 days and followed by irinotecan (16 mg/m^2/day over one hour for five days, given two consecutive weeks) and cetuximab once weekly (250 mg/m^2/dose IV in 21-day cycles)	Intravenously and external beam radiotherapy
El-Khouly	2021 [26]	A phase I/II study of bevacizumab, irinotecan, and erlotinib in children with progressive diffuse intrinsic pontine glioma	*Journal of Neuro-Oncology*	The Nether-lands	Phase I/II trial (EudraCT 2009-016080-11, Dutch Trial Register NTR2391)	Patients aged 3–18 years with progressive DIPG (clinical or radiological) after initial radiotherapy	Biweekly bevacizumab (10 mg/kg) and irinotecan (125 mg/m^2) combined with daily erlotinib, dose increased for erlotinib for 2 cohorts (65 and 85 mg/m^2) following a 3 + 3 dose-escalation schedule, until disease progression for a maximum of one year	Through central venous catheter and intravenously
DeWire	2022 [27]	Phase I study of ribociclib and everolimus in children with newly diagnosed DIPG and high-grade glioma: A CONNECT pediatric neuro-oncology consortium report	*Neuro-Oncology Advances*	USA	Phase I trial (NCT02607124)	Patients with newly diagnosed DIPG or HIG who initiated radiotherapy within 30 days of radiographic diagnosis or definitive surgery (whichever was later)	Ribociclib 170 mg/m^2 daily for 21 days and everolimus 1.5 mg/m^2 daily for 28 days	Orally, via g-tube, or nasogastric tube
DeWire	2020 [28]	A phase I/II study of ribociclib following radiation therapy in children with newly diagnosed diffuse intrinsic pontine glioma (DIPG)	*Journal of Neuro-Oncology*	USA	Phase I/II trial (NCT02607124)	Patients aged 1–30 years with newly-diagnosed DIPG confirmed radiologically or histologically, within 30 days of radiographic diagnosis or definitive surgery	350 mg/m^2 ribociclib daily for 21 days/7 days of every 28 days for up to 12 courses, 2–4 weeks after radiotherapy	Orally or via nasogastric/gastric tube

Table 1. *Cont.*

Author	Year	Title	Journal	Country	Study Design	Inclusion Criteria	Intervention Given	Method of Administration
				Chemotherapeutic Agent Regimens				
Baxter	2020 [29]	A phase I/II study of veliparib (ABT-888) with radiation and temozolomide in newly diagnosed diffuse pontine glioma: a Pediatric Brain Tumor Consortium study	*Neuro-Oncology*	USA	Phase I/II trial (NCT01514201)	Children aged 21 years or younger with newly diagnosed DIPG, defined as tumors with a pontine epicenter and diffuse intrinsic involvement of the pons	Veliparib was given Monday through Friday (50 mg/m^2/dose twice daily with 2 planned dose escalations, 65 and 85 mg/m^2/dose twice daily and 1 planned de-escalation (35 mg/m^2/dose twice daily) during radiation (5400 cGy in 30 fractions over 6 weeks) and a 4-week gap, followed by veliparib at 25 mg/m^2 b.i.d. and TMZ 135 mg/m^2 daily for 5 days every 28 days	Orally
Kilburn	2018 [30]	A pediatric brain tumor consortium phase II trial of capecitabine rapidly disintegrating tablets with concomitant radiation therapy in children with newly diagnosed diffuse intrinsic pontine gliomas	*Pediatric Blood & Cancer*	USA	Phase II trial	Children aged 3 to 17 years with newly diagnosed DIPG	Capecitabine, 650 mg/m^2/dose BID (MTD in children with concurrent radiation) was administered for 9 weeks starting the first day of RT. Following a 2-week break, 3 courses of capecitabine, 1250 mg/m^2/dose BID for 14 days followed by a 7-day rest, were administered	Orally and external beam radiation
Zanten	2017 [31]	A phase I/II study of gemcitabine during radiotherapy in children with newly diagnosed diffuse intrinsic pontine glioma	*Journal of Neuro-Oncology*	The Nether-lands	Phase I/II trial	Patients with newly-diagnosed DIPG	Gemcitabine (weekly dose for 6 weeks, increasing doses of 140, 175, and 200 mg/m^2 gemcitabine, respectively, following a 3 + 3 dose-escalation schedule) concomitant to 6 weeks of hyper fractionated radiotherapy	Intravenously and external beam radiation
Manley	2018 [32]	A phase 1/2 dose-finding, safety, and activity study of cabazitaxel in pediatric patients with refractory solid tumors including tumors of the central nervous system	*Pediatric Blood & Cancer*	USA	Phase I/II dose-escalating trial (NCT01751308)	Patients aged 2–18 years old with progressive DIPG and recovered from any acute toxic effects of all prior therapy to grade ≤1 before enrollment	Cabazitaxel infused over 1 h (20 mg/m^2 initially and if tolerated, escalated to 25, 30, 35, and 40 mg/m^2) on day 1 of every 21-day cycle	Intravenously

Table 1. *Cont.*

Author	Year	Title	Journal	Country	Study Design	Inclusion Criteria	Intervention Given	Method of Administration
					Immunotherapy			
Fangusaro	2021 [33]	Phase 2 Study of Pomalidomide (CC-4047) Monotherapy for Children and Young Adults With Recurrent or Progressive Primary Brain Tumors	*Frontiers in Oncology*	USA, France, Italy, Spain, UK	Phase II trial (NCT03257631)	Patients aged 1 to <21 years with a diagnosis of recurrent or progressive DIPG, must have received ≥1 prior standard therapy	Pomalidomide (2.6 mg/m^2/day once daily) on days 1–21 of each 28-day treatment cycle, followed by a 7-day rest period for up to 24 cycles	Orally
Schuelke	2022 [34]	Phase I trial of sargramostim/pelareorep therapy in pediatric patients with recurrent or refractory high-grade brain tumors	*Neuro-Oncology Advances*	USA	Phase I trial (NCT02444546)	Patients aged 10 to 21 years with progressive high-grade DPIG and life expectancy >3 months	Sargramostim (subcutaneously at 250 mcg/m^2) for 2 days followed by 3 days of pelareorep (IV over 60 min)	Intravenously and subcutaneously

Abbreviations: BBBD: blood–brain barrier disruption; BID: two times a day; CED: convection-enhanced delivery; CF: conventional fractionation; DLs: dose levels; Gd-DTPA: gadolinium-diethylenetriamine-pentaacetic acid; Gy: gray; HCG: high-grade glioma; HF: hypofractioned; MRI: magnetic resonance imaging; MTD: maximum tolerated dose; TMZ: temozolomide; VPA: valproic acid.

Table 2. Patient characteristics and outcome measures.

Author	Number of Patients with DIPG	Age at Diagnosis (Years)	Sex (% Male)	Previous Treatment	Outcome Measures
			Blood–Brain Barrier Bypass		
McCrea	10 patients	5.5 years (5–7)	5 patients (50%)	All patients had received standard radiotherapy, 6 patients (60%) had received immunotherapy, convection-enhanced delivery, MK-1775/Wee1 inhibitor, and oral panobinostat	Clinical response, safety, objective response (T1-weighted pre- and postcontrast sequences and T2-weighted FLAIR sequences)
Heiss	5 patients	Mean: 13 years (SD: 5)	3 patients (60%)	Standard radiotherapy	Clinical response, radiological response, corticosteroid dose, QoL
Pérez-Larraya	12 patients	NR	NR	None	Safety, overall survival, quality of life, objective response, tumor biopsy and peripheral-blood samples for correlative studies of the molecular features of DIPG and antitumor immune responses
Bander	7 patients	Mean: 5.4 years	4 patients (57.14%)	All patients received external-beam RT	Postinfusion deficits, distribution volume, targeting accuracy
Majzner	3 patients	Mean: 13.3 years	1 patient (33.3%)	All patients received standard radiotherapy ≥ 6 months before enrollment	Safety, clinical improvement, radiological improvement

Table 2. *Cont.*

Author	Number of Patients with DIPG	Age at Diagnosis (Years)	Sex (% Male)	Previous Treatment	Outcome Measures
Different Radiotherapy Regimens					
Zaghloul	253 patients	NR	NR	NR	OS, PFS
Izzuddeen	33 patients (conventional treatment arm: $n = 16$, experimental arm: $n = 17$)	<7 years: conventional arm: 9 patients (52%), experimental arm: 9 patients (50%); 8–18 years: conventional arm: 5 patients (29%), experimental arm: 5 patients (27%); >18 years: conventional arm: 3 patients (17%), experimental arm: 4 patients (22%)	Conventional arm: 8 patients (47%), treatment arm: 7 patients (38%)	None	Toxicities, PFS, OS
Amsbaugh	12 patients (group 1: $n = 6$, group 2: $n = 4$, group 3: $n = 2$)	Group 1: 5.5 years (4–20), group 2: 10 years (5–26) group 3: 6 years (5–7)	7 patients (58.3%)	Radiotherapy (at least 10 months before)	Toxicities, OS, PFS, clinical improvement, radiological response, QoL
Author	**Number of Patients with DIPG**	**Age at Diagnosis (Years)**	**Sex (% Male)**	**Previous Treatment**	**Outcome Measures**
Non-Chemotherapeutic Agent Regimens					
Su	61 patients	7.1 years (3.3–19.4)	32 patients (45.7%)	None	Toxicities, EFS, OS
Fleischhack	42 patients	Median: 7.4 years (3–15)	16 patients (38.1%)	None	PFS, clinical response, radiological response (RECIST criteria), adverse events
Mueller	46 patients	Median: 6 years (3–21)	22 patients (48%)	None (except surgery)	Tolerability, pharmacokinetics, OS, radiological response, peripheral blood γH2AX levels
Su	20 patients	Median: 7.69 years (5.2–9.9)	10 patients (50%)	May have received surgery and/or corticosteroids	Safety, radiological response (WHO bidimensional criteria), EFS, OS
Author	**Number of Patients with DIPG**	**Age at Diagnosis (Years)**	**Sex (% Male)**	**Previous Treatment**	**Outcome Measures**
Chemotherapeutic Agent Regimens					
Macy	25 patients	Median: 8 years (3–19)	21 patients (47%)	None (except surgery)	Tolerability, OS, PFS, TTP
El-Khouly	9 patients	Mean: 9.39 years	5 patients (55.5%)	Radiotherapy (all 9 patients, 100%) combined with gemcitabine (4 patients, 44.4%) in the previous phase I of the trial, re-irradiation during the current trial (4 patients, 44.4%)	Safety (DLTs), sPFS, OS, radiological response (MRI images scored with the modified RANO-criteria), QoL
DeWire	15 patients	Median: 6.5 years (2–15)	5 patients (26%)	Patients were eligible if they received 10% of standard dose of radiotherapy (54 Gy across 1.8 Gy daily fractions over 6 weeks to the planning target volume)	Toxicities, OS, radiological response (MRI based on RANO criteria)
DeWire	9 patients	7.3 years (5–14.7)	4 patients (40%)	Patients were eligible if they received 10% of standard dose of radiotherapy (54 Gy across 1.8 Gy daily fractions over 6 weeks to the planning target volume)	Safety, OS, feasibility
Baxter	65 patients	6.6 years (2.2–15.8)	40 (61.5%)	None	OS, radiological response, DLT

Table 2. *Cont.*

Author	Number of Patients with DIPG	Age at Diagnosis (Years)	Sex (% Male)	Previous Treatment	Outcome Measures
			Chemotherapeutic Agent Regimens		
Kilburn	44 patients	7.2 (3.4–16.2)	22 (50%)	None (except surgery and corticosteroid therapy)	PFS, safety
Zanten	9 patients	10.8 years (7.5–17.3)	5 patients (55.5%)	None	DLTs, radiological response (based on modified RANO criteria), PFS, OS, QoL
Manley	12 patients	Phase 1: 9.0 years (4–18), phase 2: 9.5 years (3–16)	Phase 1: 15 patients (65%), phase 2: 8 patients (50%)	Systemic anticancer therapy within ≤3 weeks, investigational agents, or small field radiotherapy ≤4 weeks, craniospinal radiation therapy ≤6 months	Radiological response (as per the modified RANO criteria), PFS, DLTs
Author	**Number of Patients with DIPG**	**Age at Diagnosis (Years)**	**Sex (% Male)**	**Previous Treatment**	**Outcome Measures**
			Immunotherapy		
Fangusaro	9 patients	7.0 (4–12)	7 (63.6%)	Radiation (11 patients, 100%), surgery (5 patients, 55.55%), systemic therapy (7 patients, 63.6%)	OR, LTSD, OS, PFS, safety
Schuelke	2 patients	10 and 17 years	0	Radiation (2 patients, 100%), chemotherapy (2 patients, 100%)	DLTs, radiological response, OS

Abbreviations: DLTs: dose limiting toxicities; EFS: event free survival; LTSD: long-term stable disease; MRI: magnetic resonance imaging; NR: not reported; OS: overall survival; PFS: progression-free survival; QoL: quality of life; RT: radiotherapy; sPFS: secondary progression-free survival; TTP: time to progression; WHO: World Health Organization.

Table 3. Efficacy and safety outcomes of the trials.

Author	Median OS (Months)	Median EFS/PFS (Months)	Radiological Response (%)	Clinical Improvement (n, %)	Tolerance and Safety	Steroid Use Discontinuation	Concluding Remarks
				Blood–Brain Barrier Bypass			
McCrea	17.3 months (221–761 days)	NR	T1-weighted postcontrast sequence: progressive disease (4 patients, 40%), stable disease (2 patients, 20%), partial response (2 patients, 20%), complete response (1 patient, 10%); T2-weighted FLAIR imaging: progressive disease (5 patients, 50%), stable disease (5 patients, 50%)	6 patients (60%)	Well-tolerated; 4 (40%) patients had minor adverse events (grade I epistaxis in 2 patients and grade I rash in 2 patients)	2 patients (20%)	Intraarterial therapy of bevacizumab and cetuximab is well-tolerated in children with DIPG and warrants further investigation
Heiss	NR	NR	Disease progression: 3 patients (60%)	1 patient (20%)	Elevated serum creatine kinase (2 patients, 40%), renal calculi (1 patient, 20%), somnolence (1 patient, 20%), suspected aspiration prompting hospitalization (1 patient, 20%)	4 patients (80%)	Direct brainstem infusion of IL13-PE using CED temporarily arrested disease progression in 2 out of 5 patients and adverse events were due to infusion-related brainstem edema with no signs of toxicity noted

Table 3. *Cont.*

Author	Median OS (Months)	Median EFS/PFS (Months)	Radiological Response (%)	Clinical Improvement (*n*, %)	Tolerance and Safety	Steroid Use Discontinuation	Concluding Remarks
				Blood–Brain Barrier Bypass			
Pérez-Larraya	17.8 months (5.9–33.5)	NR	MRI: complete response (9 patients, 75%) partial response (3 patients, 25%), stable disease (8 patients, 66.7%)	NR	Grade 1 and 2 events: headache, nausea, vomiting, fatigue, hemiparesis (1 patient, 8.3%), tetraparesis (1 patient, 8.3%)	NR	Intratumoral infusion of oncolytic virus DNX-2401 followed by radiotherapy in pediatric patients with DIPG has molecular changes including T-cell activity and a reduction in or stabilization of tumor size but there may be adverse events
Bander	NR	NR	NR	NR	Grade 1 and 2 events: contralateral hemiparesis (5 patients, 71.4%), nystagmus (2 patients, 28.6%), dysmetria (1 patient, 14.3%), cranial nerve VI and/or VII palsy (4 patients, 51.1%)	NR	Repeated CED in the brainstem for children with DIPG is safe
Majzner	Patient 1: 13 months, Patient 2: 20 months, Patient 3: 26 months	NR	MRI: 20% enlargement (1 patient, 33.3%), improved T2/FLAIR signal (2 patients, 66.7%), 17% smaller tumor volume (1 patient, 33.3%)	2 patients (66.7%)	CAR T cell-mediated inflammation at the local tumor site, termed TIAN in all 3 patients (100%)	3 patients (100%)	Toxicity management algorithm for TIAN offers potentially safe delivery of targeted CAR T-cell therapy locally
Author	**Median OS (Months)**	**Median EFS/PFS (Months)**	**Radiological Response (%)**	**Clinical Improvement (*n*, %)**	**Tolerance and safety**	**Steroid Use Discontinuation**	**Concluding Remarks**
				Different Radiotherapy Regimens			
Zaghloul	HF1: 9.6 months, HF2: 8.2 months, CF: 8.7 months	NR	NR	NR	Well-tolerated	NR	Hypofractioned radiation therapy is non-inferior to conventional fractionation with younger age (2–5 years) showing superiority with HF1 (low hypofractionated therapy dose of 39 Gy in 13 fractions)
Izzuddeen	Conventional arm: 11 months (95% CI: 7.5–14.5), experimental arm: 12 months (95% CI: 10.5–13.5)	PFS: conventional arm—7 months (95% CI: 3.6–10.3), experimental arm—8 months (95% CI: 6.7–9.3)	NR	NR	5 patients (28%) in the experimental arm developed $\geq$ grade 3 hematological toxicity; 1 patient (7%) developed $\geq$ grade 3 toxicity	NR	Hypofractionated radiotherapy with concurrent and adjuvant temozolomide did not improve survival rates and has higher hematological toxicity
Amsbaugh	19.5 months (95% CI: 15.6–21.1)	PFS: 4.5 months	Improvement: 8 patients (66.7%)	11 (91.7%)	Dose level 3: $\geq$Grade 3 events: hypoxia and dysphagia (1 patient, 50%)	NR	Re-irradiation was safe and had improved survival outcomes among patients with progressive DIPG

Table 3. *Cont.*

Author	Median OS (Months)	Median EFS/PFS (Months)	Radiological Response (%)	Clinical Improvement (n, %)	Tolerance and safety	Steroid Use Discontinuation	Concluding Remarks
Non-Chemotherapeutic Agent Regimens							
Su	1-year OS: 39.2% (95% CI: 27.8–50.5%).	1-year EFS: 5.85% (95% CI 1.89–13.1%)	NR	NR	42 patients (60%) had at least 1 DLT	NR	Vorinostat given together with radiation and afterward was well-tolerated but did not improve survival outcomes
Fleischhack	9.4 months	PFS: 5.8 months	ORR: 4.2%, Partial response (2 patients, 4.8%), stable disease (27 patients, 64.3%), progressive disease (10 patients, 23.8%)	NR	Alopecia (6 patients, 14.3%), vomiting (3 patients, 7.1%), headache (3 patients, 7.1%) radiation skin injury (3 patients, 7.1%), intra-tumoral bleeding (1 patient, 2.4%), acute respiratory failure (1 patient, 2.4%)	NR	Nimotuzumab combined with RT is well-tolerated and has comparable efficacy with RT and intensive chemotherapy without requiring prolonged hospitalization among children with newly diagnosed DIPG
Mueller	11.8 months (9–13.9)	NR	Stable disease: 33 patients (80.5%), progressive disease: 8 patients (19.5%)	NR	≥Grade 3 events: ALT elevation (1 patient, 6.7%), neutropenia (1 patient, 6.7%)	NR	Adavosertib in combination with CRT is well tolerated in children with newly diagnosed DIPG, however, compared to historical controls, did not improve OS. These results can inform future trial designs in children with high-risk cancer.
Su	10.3 (7.4–13.4) months	EFS: 7.8 (95% CI 5.6–8.2)	Partial response (8 patients, 40%), minor response (9 patients, 45%), stable disease (1 patient, 5%), not available (2 patients, 10%)	NR	≥Grade 3 events with VPA and RT: thrombocytopenia (3 patients), somnolence (1 patient), fatigue (3 patients), weight gain (2 patients); ≥grade 3 events with VPA and bevacizumab maintenance: thrombocytopenia (3 patients), intracranial/intratumoral hemorrhage (1 patient), hypertension (4 patients), subacute bone infarction (1 patient), fatigue (3 patients), weight gain (2 patients)	NR	VPA and bevacizumab given in combination with radiation is well-tolerated but there is no improvement in EFS or OS among children with newly diagnosed DIPG
Author	**Median OS (Months)**	**Median EFS/PFS (Months)**	**Radiological Response (%)**	**Clinical Improvement (n, %)**	**Tolerance and safety**	**Steroid Use Discontinuation**	**Concluding Remarks**
Chemotherapeutic Agent Regimens							
Macy	12.1 months (95% CI: 9.93, 18)	PFS: 7.12 months (95% CI: 6.89, 12.5)	Stable disease: 6 patients (24%)	NR	≥Grade 3 events: lymphopenia (26 patients, 57.7%), hypokalemia (18 patients, 40%), neutropenia (6 patients, 13.3%), anorexia (9 patients, 20%)	NR	Combination of EGFR inhibitor to radiation and irinotecan is a treatment regimen that may improve progression-free survival and is well-tolerated but did not improve survival rates

Table 3. *Cont.*

Author	Median OS (Months)	Median EFS/PFS (Months)	Radiological Response (%)	Clinical Improvement (n, %)	Tolerance and safety	Steroid Use Discontinuation	Concluding Remarks
Chemotherapeutic Agent Regimens							
El-Khouly	Overall: 13.8 months (9.3–33.0), patients who were re-irradiated: 16.2 months (12.8–20.0)	PFS: 7.3 months (3.5–10.0), sPFS: 3.2 months (1.0–10.9)	3 months: Partial response (3 patients, 33.3%), stable disease (1 patient, 11.1%), progressive disease (5 patients, 55.5%); 6 months: progressive disease (2 patients, 50%). stable disease (2 patients, 50%)	4 patients (44.4%)	Grade III acute diarrhea (1 patient, 11/1%), grade II acute secretory diarrhea (1 patient, 11.1%). grade I/II late-onset diarrhea (5 patients, 55.5%), grade I/II nausea and vomiting (4 patients, 44.4%), grade I acneiform rash (5 patients, 55.5%), grade I/II mucositis (1 patient, 11.1%), grade I/II constipation (1 patient, 11.1%), grade II keratitis (1 patient, 11.1%), grade II urinary tract infection (2 patients, 22.2%), and grade II adrenal insufficiency as a result of chronic dexamethasone use (2 patients, 22.2%)	NR	Daily erlotinib (up to 85 mg/m^2) with biweekly bevacizumab and irinotecan is safe and improves median OS in children with progressive DIPG
DeWire	13.9 months	NR	Pseudoprogression: 4 patients (8.3%), progression: 2 patients (4.2%)	NR	≥Grade 3 events: neutropenia (6 patients, 33%), leucopenia (3 patients, 17%), lymphopenia (2 patients, 11%), pulmonary infection (1 patient, 6%), elevated ALT and hypokalemia (1 patient, 6%), cardiac toxicity (1 patient, 6%)	NR	Ribociclib and everolimus following radiotherapy in children with newly diagnosed DIPG is well-tolerated and requires further exploration for efficacy potential
DeWire	16.1 months (10–30)	NR	Disease progression: 9 patients (90%)	NR	≥grade 3 events: neutropenia (9 patients, 90%), lymphopenia (5 patients, 50%), and leukopenia (7 patients, 70%)	NR	Ribociclib administered following radiotherapy has survival benefits but increased tumor necrosis may be a treatment effect represent a treatment effect
Baxter	One-year OS: 37.2% (SE 7%)	NR	PR: 7 patients (14%)	NR	DLTs: 4 patients (33.3%)during radiation in phase I (Grade 2 intratumoral hemorrhage (n = 1), grade 3 maculopapular rash (n = 2), and grade 3 nervous system disorder (generalized neurologic deterioration) (n = 1)), 4 patients (50%) during intrapatient dose escalation	NR	Veliparib used in combination with radiation followed by TMZ and veliparib was well-tolerated and did not improve survival rates in patients with newly diagnosed DIPG
Kilburn	NR	6-month PFS: 33.7% (SE = 7.1%), 1-year PFS: 7.2% (SE = 3.5%)	Progressive disease (8 patients, 18.2%)	Deterioration (3 patients, 6.8%)	DLTs: 5 patients (grade 4 neutropenia (n = 1), grade 2 CNS necrosis (n = 2), grade 4 neutropenia that did not resolve within 7 days (n = 1), and persistent toe infection (n = 1)	NR	Concomitant and adjuvant Capecitabine with radiotherapy was well-tolerated but did not improve survival outcomes for children with newly-diagnosed DIPG

Table 3. *Cont.*

Author	Median OS (Months)	Median EFS/PFS (Months)	Radiological Response (%)	Clinical Improvement (*n*, %)	Tolerance and safety	Steroid Use Discontinuation	Concluding Remarks
				Chemotherapeutic Agent Regimens			
Zanten	Intermediate risk: 12.4 months, high risk: 8.1 months	PFS for intermediate risk: 6.4 months, PFS for high risk: 4.5 months	Stable disease: 2 patients, progressive disease: 3 patients, pseudoprogression: 4 patients	9 patients (100%)	Grade 3 hepatotoxicity (2 patients, 22.2%), grade 3 neutropenia (1 patient, 11.1%)	3 patients (75%)	Gemcitabine in combination with radiotherapy is well-tolerated but does not improve survival outcomes in patients with newly-diagnosed DIPG
Manley	2.7 months (95% CI: 1.7–4.5)	Median PFS: 1.3 months (95% CI: 0.6–2.1)	Progressive disease 25 patients (75.8%), stable disease: 6 patients (18.2%), partial response: 1 patient (3%), complete response: 1 patient (3%)	NR	≥grade 3 events: 12 patients (52%)	Steroid treatment used as part of protocol	Cabazitaxel in pediatric patients with progressive DIPG does not improve survival outcomes but is well-tolerated and safe at the established MTD
Author	**Median OS (Months)**	**Median EFS/PFS (Months)**	**Radiological Response (%)**	**Clinical Improvement (*n*, %)**	**Tolerance and safety**	**Steroid Use Discontinuation**	**Concluding Remarks**
				Immunotherapy			
Fangusaro	3.78 months	Median PFS: 2.6 months	Disease progression: 6 (66.7%)	NR	≥grade 3 events: neutropenia (3 patients, 27.3%), lymphopenia (1 patient, 9.1%), leucopenia (1 patient, 9.1%), vertigo (1 patient, 9.1%)	NR	Pomalidomide monotherapy in progressive DIPG did not improve survival rates
Schuelke	1.1 months	NR	Disease progression: 2 patients (100%)	Death: 82 and 60 days	No DLTs	NR	Sargramostim/pelareorep was well-tolerated but did not improve survival rates

Abbreviations: ALT: alanine transaminase; CAR: chimeric antigen receptor; CED: convection-enhanced delivery; CI: confidence interval; EFS: event-free survival; EGFR: epidermal growth factor receptor; MTD: maximum tolerated dose; NR = not reported; PFS: progression free survival; RT: radiotherapy; SE: standard error; TIAN: tumor inflammation-associated neurotoxicity; VPA: valproic acid.

3.1. Bypassing the Blood–Brain Barrier

3.1.1. Intra-Arterial Therapy

McCrea et al. explored the tolerability and efficacy of super selective intraarterial cerebral infusion (SIACI) among 10 patients with DIPG who had all previously received radiotherapy, as well as other systemic therapies [13]. Mannitol (12.5 mL of 20%) was administered to disrupt the blood–brain barrier (BBB), followed by bevacizumab (15 mg/kg), a vascular endothelial growth factor A (VEGF-A) inhibitor, and cetuximab (200 mg/m^2), an epidermal growth factor receptor (EGFR) inhibitor, respectively [13]. The treatment and technique were well-tolerated with no dose-limiting toxicities. In terms of efficacy, the median OS was 17.3 months, which is higher than that for historical controls despite DIPG patients being heavily treated [13]. This method of delivery warrants further investigation to establish efficacy in DIPG patients [13].

3.1.2. Convection-Enhanced Delivery

Heiss et al. evaluated the outcomes including the safety and tolerability of single-dose IL13-PE38QQR, a recombinant cytotoxic chimera of human interleukin 13 (IL-13), and the enzymatic portion of pseudomonas exotoxin A, infused via single-catheter CED (0.125 μg/mL) into 5 patients with progressive DIPG [14]. The intervention was safe and well-tolerated which occurred due to infusion-related brainstem edema [14]. There was a temporary improvement in clinical and radiological status in 2 patients (40%) and their dose was escalated to 0.25 μg/mL. CED-supported delivery of IL13-PE did not reach optimal volumes in the tumor and only temporary anti-tumoral effects were observed in 2 patients [14].

Pérez-Larraya et al. determined the safety and efficacy outcomes of single-dose CED infusion of DNX-2401, an oncolytic adenovirus that only replicates in tumor cells, through the cerebellar peduncle, followed by radiotherapy in 12 newly diagnosed DIPG patients [15]. The median OS was favorable at 17.8 months; 11 of the 12 patients had a reduction or stabilization of tumor size but certain adverse events (hemiparesis in 1 patient and tetraparesis in 1 patient) were reported [15].

Bander et al. evaluated the efficacy and safety of $\geq$2 doses of CED, via the supratentorial trajectory with intraprocedural stereotactic placement using MRI guidance, infusing I-8H9 monoclonal antibody among 7 DIPG patients who previously received radiotherapy [16]. Sequential CED infusions were well-tolerated and the second infusion significantly reduced radial error and absolute tip error compared to the first infusion [16]. This was a phase I trial whereby Bander et al. lay support for repeated CED in DIPG patients for further evaluation of improved survival rates [16].

Majzner et al. similarly delivered two doses of disialoganglioside GD2-directed chimeric antigen receptor (CAR) T cell; the first dose administered intravenously and the second dose delivered intracerebroventricularly to 3 patients with K27M mutation in genes encoding histone H3 (H3K27M) at any stage. All patients had received radiotherapy $\geq$ 6 months before enrollment. Of the three patients, two had improvement radiologically and one had tumor progression [17]. All patients had infusion-related toxicity which was reversible with intensive support [17]. With the necessary management algorithm for tumor inflammation-associated neurotoxicity (TIAN), delivery of CAR T-cell therapy via CED is a promising treatment option that may be explored further in trial settings [17].

3.2. Different Radiotherapy Regimens

3.2.1. Hypofractionated Radiation Therapy

Zagloul et al. confirmed the noninferiority of hypofractionated (HF) radiation therapy with three arms, arm 1 received HF therapy of 39 Gy in 13 fractions, arm 2 received HF therapy of 45 Gy in 15 fractions, and arm 3 received conventional fractionation (CF) of 54 Gy in 30 fractions [18]. The median OS was the highest in low-dose HF across arm 1 (9.6 months) followed by CF in arm 3 (8.7 months) and high-dose HF in arm 2 (8.2 months).

Younger age (2–5 years) had a higher prognosis with lower HF dose given in arm 1 which was not found in arm 2 recipients [18].

Izzuddeen et al. compared the efficacy and tolerability of CF radiotherapy and low-dose HF radiotherapy (39 Gy in 13 fractions) with concurrent and adjuvant temozolomide, an alkylating agent [19]. The group that received HF radiotherapy and temozolomide did not show any improved survival rates (12 months vs. 11 months) and there was an increase in grade 3/4 hematological toxicity (n = 5, 28%) [19].

3.2.2. Re-Irradiation

Amsbaugh et al. found clinical improvement and improved quality of life with conventionally fractionated re-irradiation among patients who had ≥10 months from the end of initial radiotherapy [20]. The lowest dose arm of 24 Gy in 12 fractions had the highest utility and is considered safe and effective for re-irradiation in DIPG patients [20].

3.3. *Non-Chemotherapeutic Agent Regimens*

Fleischhack et al. assessed the safety and efficacy of intravenous nimotuzumab, an anti-EGFR humanized monoclonal antibody, combined with external beam radiotherapy (EBT) among treatment-naïve patients with DIPG diagnosed in the last 3 months. The intervention was well-tolerated and no adverse events were observed, such as those produced by other EGFR-targeting agents e.g., severe acneiform rash, hypokalemia, or hypomagnesemia [21]. Nimotuzumab administered concomitantly and continued after EBT had comparable efficacy to intensive chemotherapy and EBT among newly diagnosed DIPG e.g., median OS of 9.4 months while offering the benefit of being administered in outpatient settings and associated with reduced hospitalization stays [21].

Su et al. reported the efficacy and tolerability of Vorinostat, an oral histone deacetylase inhibitor, given with initial radiotherapy and as monotherapy afterward [22]. While it was well tolerated, there were no survival benefits in patients with newly diagnosed DIPG [22].

Mueller et al. determined the tolerability of Adavosertib, an orally administered blood–brain barrier penetrant, Wee 1 kinase inhibitor when combined with cranial radiation therapy (CRT) among patients with newly diagnosed DIPG [23]. While the treatment was well-tolerated, there was no survival benefit with a median OS of 11.1 months [23].

Su et al. explored the tolerability and efficacy of valproic acid (VPA), an anti-convulsant, and radiation, followed by VPA and bevacizumab, an anti-VEGF humanized monoclonal antibody, among patients with newly diagnosed DIPG in a phase II trial [24]. While the concomitant use of VPA and bevacizumab was well-tolerated, there was no improvement in survival outcomes with a median OS of 10.3 months [24].

3.4. *Chemotherapeutic Agent Regimens*

Macy et al. evaluated the efficacy and safety of cetuximab, anti-EGFR humanized with concurrent radiation therapy followed by cetuximab and irinotecan, a topoisomerase I inhibitor, among patients with newly diagnosed DIPG [25]. While there was some improvement in PFS, the median OS was 12.1 months and the therapy regimen does not warrant further investigation [25].

El-Khouly et al. conducted a phase I/II trial to determine the safety, tolerability, and efficacy of bevacizumab, a VEGF inhibitor, irinotecan, a topoisomerase I inhibitor, and Erlotinib, an EGFR inhibitor, among 9 patients with progressive DIPG. The median OS was 13.8 months which was higher than that of historical controls for this subset of patients and the regimen was well-tolerated [26].

DeWire et al. conducted a phase I trial to determine the tolerability and efficacy of Ribociclib (CDK4/6-inhibitor) and Everolimus (kinase inhibitor) for patients newly diagnosed with DIPG within 30 days of receiving a 10% standard dose of radiotherapy [27]. The treatment was well-tolerated and apparently improved median OS to 13.9 months; however, when two patients who were less than 3 years at diagnosis e.g., associated with better prognosis were removed, the median OS decreased to 10.8 months which suggests no additional efficacy of treatment [27].

DeWire et al. also conducted a phase I/II trial to identify the safety, feasibility, and early efficacy of ribociclib (CDK4/6-inhibitor) in 9 newly diagnosed DIPG patients [28]. Ribociclib adjuvant monotherapy post-radiotherapy had improved median OS (16.1 months) [28]. Yet, its safety is not clear as there was increased tumor necrosis volume in 4 patients (40%) warranting further volumetric analyses of necrosed tumors [28].

Baxter et al. conducted a phase I/II trial of 65 patients with newly diagnosed DIPG who received concomitant veliparib (PARP inhibitor) and radiation therapy followed by veliparib and temozolomide (alkylating agent) [29]. While the treatment was generally well-tolerated with limited DLTs, there were no survival benefits categorized as 1-year and 2-year survival rates of 37.2% and 5.3%, respectively [29].

Kilburn et al. conducted a phase II trial with capecitabine (alkylating agent) given concomitantly with radiotherapy followed by adjuvant capecitabine among 44 patients with newly diagnosed DIPG [30]. There was no survival benefit (OS and PFS were comparable to historical controls) with the treatment regimen but it was well-tolerated [30].

Zanten et al. conducted a phase I/II trial to determine the efficacy, safety, and tolerability of gemcitabine, a nucleoside metabolic inhibitor, during radiotherapy among 9 children with newly diagnosed DIPG [31]. The treatment was well-tolerated and a dose of up to 200 mg/m^2/once weekly with radiotherapy was safe [31]. There were, however, no survival benefits with a median OS of 12.4 months and 8.7 months in intermediate- and high-risk patients [31].

Manley et al. explored the maximum tolerated dose (MTD), safety, and efficacy of Cabazitaxel, a chemotherapeutic agent, in patients with progressive treatment-refractory DIPG in a phase I/II dose-escalating trial [32]. The maximum tolerated dose (MTD) was found to be 30 mg/m^2 and was well-tolerated. There was no anti-tumor activity with the MTD and there was no improvement in survival outcomes [32].

3.5. Immunotherapy

Fangusaro et al. conducted a phase II trial and determined the efficacy and safety of Pomalidomide, an immunomodulatory drug, among 9 patients with progressive DIPG [33]. There were no favorable survival outcomes of pomalidomide monotherapy with no objective response (OR) or long-term stable disease (LTSD) found in the patients and a median OS of 3.78 months [33].

Schuelke et al. determined the safety of sargramostin, a recombinant human granulocyte-macrophage colony-stimulating factor, and pelareorep, an immunomodulatory oncolytic virus, among 2 patients with progressive DIPG in a phase I trial [34]. While the treatment was well-tolerated, the sample size was too small to evaluate survival rates; the treatment warrants further investigation for efficacy [34].

3.6. Risk of Bias Synthesis

Overall, 19 studies (86.4%) had a low risk of bias, 2 (9.1%) had moderate risks and 1 (4.5%) had a serious risk of bias (Figure 2). On noting bias due to confounding, 17 studies (77.3%) had a low risk of bias, 4 (18.2%) had moderate risk, whereas 1 (4.5%) had a serious risk of bias. When assessing bias due to the selection of participants, a total of 14 studies (63.6%) had a low risk of bias, whereas 7 (31.8%) had a moderate risk of bias and 1 (4.5%) had a serious risk of bias. Noting the bias in the classification of interventions, 20 studies (90.9%) had low risks of bias while 2 studies (9.1%) had a moderate risk of bias. Bias due to deviations from intended interventions had low risk in 21 studies (95.5%) and moderate risk in 1 study (4.5%). On noting bias due to missing outcome data, 18 studies (81.8%) had a low risk of bias, and 2 studies each (9.1%) had moderate and serious risks of bias. Assessment of bias in the measurement of outcomes yielded 18 studies (81.8%) with a low risk of bias and 4 studies (18.2%) with a moderate risk of bias. The risk of bias in the selection of the reported result was low in 12 studies (54.4%), moderate in 9 studies (40.9%), and serious in 1 study (4.5%) (Figure 2).

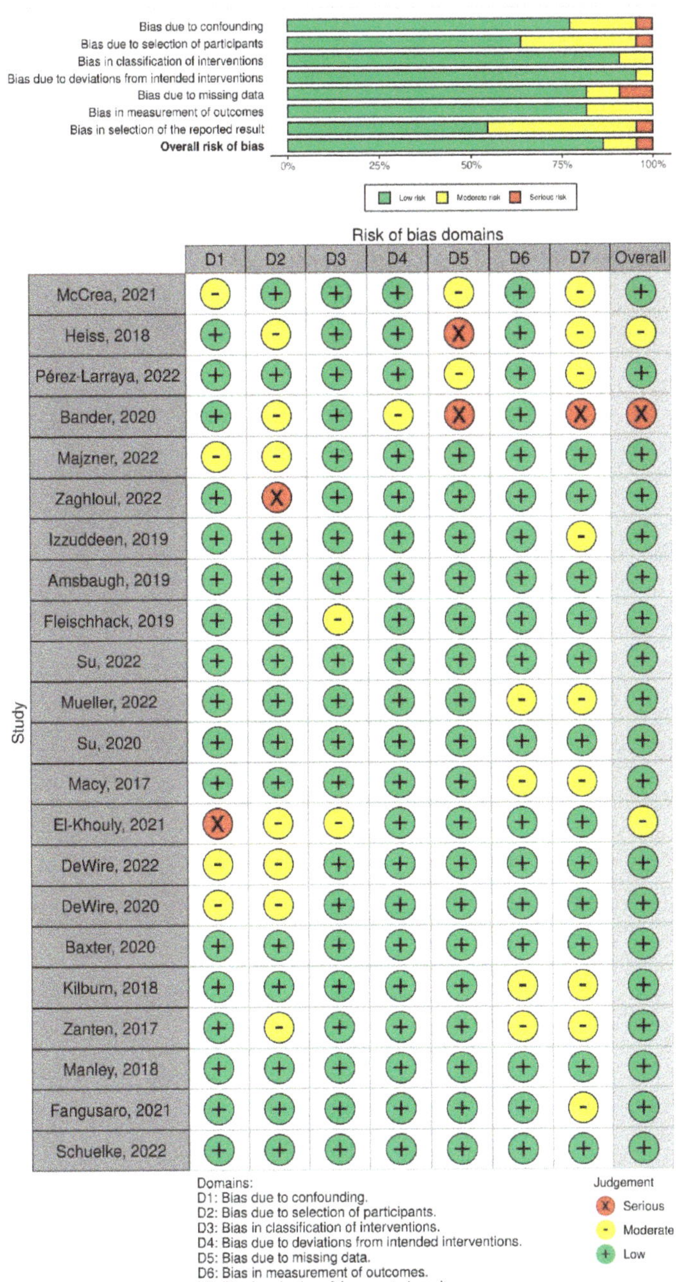

Figure 2. Summary plot and traffic light plot depicting risk of bias among the included studies [13–34].

4. Discussion

This research article aimed to collate evidence from all trials conducted in the last five years to evaluate the efficacy and safety of different treatments for DIPG. We assessed 22 trials and five key therapeutic regimen themes emerged including blood–brain barrier (BBB) bypass (intra-arterial delivery or convection-enhanced delivery (CED)), radiotherapy regimens, non-chemotherapeutic agent regimens, chemotherapeutic agent regimens, and immunotherapy. The 22 trials included in this study are likely to constitute all available clinical trial evidence, due to the robust search strategy and rigorous screening process.

Of the 5 trials reporting BBB bypass techniques, 3 reported overall survival (OS), 4 reported radiological responses, 3 reported clinical improvement, all 5 reported tolerance and safety, and 3 reported steroid discontinuation. All 3 trials that explored radiotherapy regimens and doses did report OS, 2 trials reported progression-free survival (PFS), 1 reported radiological response, 1 reported clinical improvement, and all 3 reported tolerance and safety outcomes. Four trials that explored non-chemotherapeutic agents and OS were reported across all 4 trials, PFS in 1 trial, event-free survival (EFS) in 2 trials, radiological response in 3 trials, and safety/tolerance in all 4 trials. A total of 8 trials administered chemotherapeutic agents in combination with other therapeutics and all 8 trials reported OS, 5 trials reported PFS, all 8 trials reported radiological response, 3 trials reported clinical improvement, and all 8 reported tolerability/safety. Lastly, of the 2 trials that administered immunotherapy agents, both reported OS, 1 reported PFS, 2 reported radiological response, 1 reported clinical improvement, and both identified safety/tolerance. There were differences among studies, even within the same theme, with regard to outcome measures, specifically radiological response.

All therapeutic agents were initiated at different time points in the natural clinical course of DIPG. The most commonly observed subset of patients was newly diagnosed across 12 trials, followed by progressive DIPG in 8 trials. One trial enrolled patients at any stage and 1 trial did not specify the stage of DIPG. Patient demographics were similar across the 22 trials. Age at diagnosis was primarily mid-childhood. The gender ratio was somewhat well-balanced, ranging from 35–65% across the studies.

4.1. Intra-Arterial Delivery

Superselective intraarterial cerebral infusion (SIACI) improved survival rates (median OS: 17.3 months) when offered to patients with progressive DIPG. SIACI offers an advantage over intravenous drug delivery through selective blood–brain barrier (BBB) opening. Our synthesis supports the intraarterial delivery of cetuximab and bevacizumab with the initial administration of mannitol to increase the absorption of the drugs. As we found support for safe and well-tolerated repeated CED infusions, further trials can consider expanding the number of patients and determining the efficacy of SIACI. A phase I trial (NCT05271240) is underway that is planning enrollment of 432 patients with glioblastoma multiforme (GBM) and comparing repeated mannitol-infusion followed by SIACI of bevacizumab with temozolomide and standard radiation to temozolomide and standard radiation only. As data are still emerging regarding the safety and tolerability of intra-arterial delivery, further trials can consider using a labeling agent to assess drug delivery distribution. Another consideration is to identify molecular targets with a biopsy to optimize the agent of choice. With evidence of safe bypassing of the BBB, it is of note to consider targeting tumor cells based on the biology e.g., EGFR and/or VEGF positive.

4.2. Convection-Enhanced Delivery

CED is an emerging therapy for DIPG due to its ability to bypass the BBB and deliver pertinent doses of treatment in relevant brain volumes. The agents tested in clinical trials via CED were ^{124}I-8H9 [16], IL13-Pseudomonas toxin [14], DNX-2401 (an oncolytic virus) [15], and GD2-CAR T cells [17]. Of the 4 trials evaluating the role of convection-enhanced delivery (CED) in the treatment of DIPG, there were somewhat favorable outcomes based on different techniques, agents used, and stages of DIPG. Intra-tumoral infusion with an oncolytic virus had the most favorable outcomes with a median OS of 17.8 months in newly diagnosed DIPG but there was an increased risk of adverse events related to infusion-related brainstem edema. Augmentation of CED-infused pharmacological agents gained support from observational studies such as Tsvankin et al. who found improvement in median OS with CED of dasatinib, a tyrosine kinase inhibitor, in a transgenic H3.3K27M mutant murine model [35]. It remains unclear which pharmacological agent offers the highest survival rates and it is reasonable to consider CED to have a plateau effect given its ability to target localized disease.

Repeated CED infusions were well-tolerated but neurological signs and symptoms are present. Hollingworth et al. [36] measured infusion-related side effects of CED in DIPG with the Pontine Neurological Observation Score (PONScore), a standardized tool with a 57-point scale, to determine their frequency and recovery during infusion. As CED is gaining preliminary support from the literature for its efficacy in DIPG, there is a gap in standardized documentation of its side effects for which a scale such as PONScore [36] can highlight the nature and timing of neurological injury during infusion. Further clinical trials must consider it imperative to consider meticulously documenting infusion-related side effects to address patient outcomes. As of now, CED is being tested in early phase clinical trials for treatment with DIPG which has the potential to control the regional disease. However, CED as a standalone may not be able to control spread to distant areas e.g., outside the brainstem [37] or leptomeningeal involvement [38], by nature of its delivery and it may be advantageous to consider combination approaches e.g., craniospinal radiation or intrathecal delivery [39], to meaningfully improve survival rates in DIPG patients who already have a dismal prognosis.

4.3. Radiotherapy

The mainstay of treatment for DIPG is conventionally fractionated radiation therapy (RT), delivered across a 6-week period. However, such RT only transiently improves symptoms without prominent survival benefits. Hypofractionated RT regimens did not demonstrate survival benefits across two trials in our study but may provide temporary relief. In a trial, re-irradiation did improve survival outcomes and quality of life among DIPG patients who had received initial radiotherapy $\geq$ 10 months ago (strongest support for low-dose conventional RT at 24 Gy in 12 fractions). Gallitto et al. [8] corroborate the findings of the trial and suggests re-irradiation at first progression as an effective palliative therapy with a mean increase of ~3 months to OS compared to controls. Combination immunotherapy agents (PD-1 inhibitor, nivolumab) [40] with re-irradiation have also shown improved life spans in progressive DIPG patients. Overall, certain patients can tolerate re-irradiation, have reduced symptoms, and improve survival rates by a few months. Current trials have compared different radiation doses and fractionation for re-irradiation; support for conventional fractionation and low-dose radiation is found in clinical trials. Further clinical trials can address the frequency of re-irradiation, the gap between radiotherapy, and optimal radiation dose and fractionation for children with progressive DIPG [41].

4.4. Other Regimens

Other trials explored the efficacy of radiotherapy with neoadjuvant non-chemotherapeutic interventions (nimotuzumab, bevacizumab, adavosertib, and vorinostat) with or without adjuvant therapy afterward in newly diagnosed DIPG patients and found no additional survival benefit compared to historical controls. Similarly, there was no significant improvement in survival outcomes with a neoadjuvant chemotherapeutic alkylating agent (temozolomide) or anti-metabolites (capecitabine, gemcitabine, cabazitaxel) in combination with radiotherapy, and other agents (cetuximab, an EGFR inhibitor, and veliparib, a PARP inhibitor). Moreover, immunotherapy regimens did not improve median OS with pomalidomide and pelareorep combined with sargramostim. There were, however, two trials by DeWire et al. [27,28] that found some improvement in median OS with combination regimens in newly diagnosed DIPG patients: median OS of 13.9 months with ribociclib and everolimus, both kinase inhibitors, within 30 days of receiving 10% standard radiation doses, and median OS of 16.1 months with ribociclib together with radiotherapy and adjuvant monotherapy. There is emerging support for ribociclib, a CDK4/6 inhibitor, together with targeted radiotherapy among treatment-naïve DIPG patients. However, in both these trials, there was a prominent frequency of ≥grade 3 events which may be due to the treatment. Another trial [26] administered bevaziumab, a VEGF inhibitor, erlotinib, an EGFR inhibitor, and irinotecan, a topoisomerase I inhibitor among progressive DIPG patients. Of note, this trial indicated that anti-EGFR agents and anti-VEGF antibodies when combined with chemotherapy have some additive antitumor activity (median OS of 13.8 months) and are well-tolerated. These findings provide support for the collaboration of anti-VEGF and anti-EGFR for inhibiting tumor growth and angiogenesis in aggressive DIPG, combined with chemotherapy.

4.5. Potential Molecular Targets

The lack of targeted therapies for DIPG is in part due to the lack of routine biopsies conducted in these tumors. Neurosurgeons have been reluctant to perform biopsies due to more risks than direct benefits to the patients. As molecular genetic techniques are expanding in oncology, many centers have begun conducting stereotactic biopsy to support ongoing research which requires molecular characterization and potentially druggable targets toward more individualized treatments [42,43]. About 80% of all DIPG cases have a specific point mutation that results in the substitution of lysine 27 on the amino-terminal tail with methionine (H3K27M) in histone isoforms H3.1 or H3.3, encoded by genes *HIST1H3B* and *H3F3A* respectively [44–46]. There are subtle differences in prognosis and outcomes with both; H3.1 histone mutations have a better prognosis and this has been recognized by the World Health Organization of CNS tumors [9,47]. Along with these histone modifications, molecular profiling has enumerated numerous targets for therapeutic interventions. These include ACVR1 mutations (~30% of DIPG tumors) and co-occur with H3.1 and TP53 mutations (~22–40% of DIPG tumors) which co-occur with PDFR amplification [48–50]. PDFR amplification (PDFRA) is common and present in nearly 1/3rd of high-grade gliomas; when co-segregated with H3.3 mutations (H3.3K27M), these tumors are clinically aggressive [51]. PDFRA combined with PIK3R1 and PIK3CA are drivers of the PI3K pathway which contributes to aggressive DIPG [48,52].

4.6. Strengths and Future Directions

The 22 studies in this study constitute the latest clinical trends for DIPG therapeutics with an inclusive search strategy and rigorous screening process. Two independent reviewers screened the full text and there was 91.6% agreement. As part of the search strategy, an umbrella review methodology was also applied which revealed four potential papers, though none were included. Another strength was the double-checking of data entry by the second reviewer. The conclusions made from this study are based on all the latest available evidence from clinical trials in the past 5 years. Therefore, the data included in this study are not observational, which means that the quality of included studies is not compromised. Lastly, the study was flexible in terms of eligibility criteria in relation to the nature of treatment which allowed for a comprehensive synthesis.

The risk of bias among the included trials was largely low with 86.4% depicting low concerns. However, two studies had moderate risks (El-Khouly, 2021; Heiss, 2018) and one had a serious risk of bias (Bander, 2020). Based on the biases we reported in this study, future trials in this discipline of research ought to ensure datasets reporting of patient outcomes including follow-up. Furthermore, in an effort to improve outcomes for patients with DIPG, confounding variables including multi-disciplinary therapies must be assessed in a manner that may quantify various approaches both singularly or combined for survival (OS, EFS, PFS) and associated outcomes.

4.7. Limitations

There are certain limitations of this study. This study included early phase clinical trials that had a small sample size. We omitted case series and case reports to ensure only high-tier evidence was included, which may have led to omission of specific cases in literature. As such, the findings must be explored in further clinical trials to prove the safety, characterization of adverse events, and clinical outcomes if given in a larger sample size. While certain trials have demonstrated efficacy with prolonged survival rates, the results cannot be generalized and must be corroborated in further multi-center, blinded, randomized controlled trials to prove its benefits.

5. Conclusions

DIPG is a pediatric brain tumor that has a dismal prognosis with a median survival rate of nine months. There is currently no effective treatment beyond palliative radiotherapy. Our analysis of all clinical trials in the last five years captures 22 studies that point toward the direction in which the ongoing research is headed. Importantly, we show that a promising therapeutic strategy is a blood–brain barrier (BBB) bypass. We also find support for chemotherapeutic agents combined with VEGF- and EGFR inhibitors. Finally, our synthesis suggests re-irradiation as another strategy that can prolong survival in progressive DIPG patients. We collate current evidence to guide future research and therapeutic candidates in DIPG.

Author Contributions: Conceptualization, S.F., S.H. and A.R.; methodology, Z.S., A.S., M.S. and K.R.-V.; software, Z.S., A.S. and M.S.; formal analysis, S.F., S.H. and A.R.; investigation, S.F., S.H., A.R., Z.S., A.S., M.S., K.R.-V., M.F. and I.C.-O.; resources, S.F., S.H., A.R., Z.S. and A.S.; data curation, S.F., S.H., A.R., Z.S. and A.S.; writing—original draft preparation, S.F., S.H., A.R., Z.S., A.S., M.S., K.R.-V., M.F. and I.C.-O.; writing—review and editing, S.F., S.H., A.R., Z.S., A.S., M.S., K.R.-V., M.F. and I.C.-O.; visualization, S.F., S.H., A.R. and A.S.; supervision, M.F. and I.C.-O.; project administration, M.F., A.S. and I.C.-O. are co-guarantors of this study. All authors have read and agreed to the published version of the manuscript.

Funding: This research received no external funding.

Institutional Review Board Statement: Not applicable.

Informed Consent Statement: Not applicable.

Data Availability Statement: All data utilized for the purpose of this study are available publicly and online. Additional data may be requested by the corresponding author (A.S.) on reasonable request.

Conflicts of Interest: The authors declare no conflict of interest.

References

1. Linabery, A.M.; Ross, J.A. Trends in childhood cancer incidence in the US (1992–2004). *Cancer Interdiscip. Int. J. Am. Cancer Soc.* **2008**, *112*, 416–432.
2. Ostrom, Q.T.; Cioffi, G.; Waite, K.; Kruchko, C.; Barnholtz-Sloan, J.S. CBTRUS statistical report: Primary brain and other central nervous system tumors diagnosed in the United States in 2014–2018. *Neuro Oncol.* **2021**, *23*, iii1–iii105. [CrossRef] [PubMed]
3. Ostrom, Q.T.; de Blank, P.M.; Kruchko, C.; Petersen, C.M.; Liao, P.; Finlay, J.L.; Stearns, D.S.; Wolff, J.E.; Wolinsky, Y.; Letterio, J.J. Alex's Lemonade Stand Foundation infant and childhood primary brain and central nervous system tumors diagnosed in the United States in 2007–2011. *Neuro Oncol.* **2015**, *16*, x1–x36. [CrossRef]
4. Li, G.; Mitra, S.S.; Monje, M.; Henrich, K.N.; Bangs, C.D.; Nitta, R.T.; Wong, A.J. Expression of epidermal growth factor variant III (EGFRvIII) in pediatric diffuse intrinsic pontine gliomas. *J. Neurooncol.* **2012**, *108*, 395–402. [CrossRef]
5. Rashed, W.M.; Maher, E.; Adel, M.; Saber, O.; Zaghloul, M.S. Pediatric diffuse intrinsic pontine glioma: Where do we stand? *Cancer Metastasis Rev.* **2019**, *38*, 759–770. [CrossRef] [PubMed]
6. Janssens, G.O.; Gandola, L.; Bolle, S.; Mandeville, H.; Ramos-Albiac, M.; van Beek, K.; Benghiat, H.; Hoeben, B.; La Madrid, A.M.; Kortmann, R.-D. Survival benefit for patients with diffuse intrinsic pontine glioma (DIPG) undergoing re-irradiation at first progression: A matched-cohort analysis on behalf of the SIOP-E-HGG/DIPG working group. *Eur. J. Cancer* **2017**, *73*, 38–47. [CrossRef]

7. Wiese, M.; Hamdan, F.H.; Kubiak, K.; Diederichs, C.; Gielen, G.H.; Nussbaumer, G.; Carcaboso, A.M.; Hulleman, E.; Johnsen, S.A.; Kramm, C.M. Combined treatment with CBP and BET inhibitors reverses inadvertent activation of detrimental super enhancer programs in DIPG cells. *Cell Death Dis.* **2020**, *11*, 673. [CrossRef] [PubMed]
8. Gallitto, M.; Lazarev, S.; Wasserman, I.; Stafford, J.M.; Wolden, S.L.; Terezakis, S.A.; Bindra, R.S.; Bakst, R.L. Role of radiation therapy in the management of diffuse intrinsic pontine glioma: A systematic review. *Adv. Radiat. Oncol.* **2019**, *4*, 520–531. [CrossRef] [PubMed]
9. Louis, D.N.; Perry, A.; Reifenberger, G.; Von Deimling, A.; Figarella-Branger, D.; Cavenee, W.K.; Ohgaki, H.; Wiestler, O.D.; Kleihues, P.; Ellison, D.W. The 2016 World Health Organization classification of tumors of the central nervous system: A summary. *Acta Neuropathol.* **2016**, *131*, 803–820. [CrossRef]
10. El-Khouly, F.E.; Veldhuijzen van Zanten, S.E.M.; Santa-Maria Lopez, V.; Hendrikse, N.H.; Kaspers, G.J.L.; Loizos, G.; Sumerauer, D.; Nysom, K.; Pruunsild, K.; Pentikainen, V. Diagnostics and treatment of diffuse intrinsic pontine glioma: Where do we stand? *J. Neurooncol.* **2019**, *145*, 177–184. [CrossRef]
11. Long, W.; Yi, Y.; Chen, S.; Cao, Q.; Zhao, W.; Liu, Q. Potential new therapies for pediatric diffuse intrinsic pontine glioma. *Front. Pharmacol.* **2017**, *8*, 495. [CrossRef]
12. Srikanthan, D.; Taccone, M.S.; Van Ommeren, R.; Ishida, J.; Krumholtz, S.L.; Rutka, J.T. Diffuse intrinsic pontine glioma: Current insights and future directions. *Chin. Neurosurg. J.* **2021**, *7*, 6. [CrossRef]
13. McCrea, H.J.; Ivanidze, J.; O'Connor, A.; Hersh, E.H.; Boockvar, J.A.; Gobin, Y.P.; Knopman, J.; Greenfield, J.P. Intraarterial delivery of bevacizumab and cetuximab utilizing blood-brain barrier disruption in children with high-grade glioma and diffuse intrinsic pontine glioma: Results of a phase I trial. *J. Neurosurg. Pediatr.* **2021**, *28*, 371–379. [CrossRef]
14. Heiss, J.D.; Jamshidi, A.; Shah, S.; Martin, S.; Wolters, P.L.; Argersinger, D.P.; Warren, K.E.; Lonser, R.R. Phase I trial of convection-enhanced delivery of IL13-Pseudomonas toxin in children with diffuse intrinsic pontine glioma. *J. Neurosurg. Pediatr.* **2018**, *23*, 333–342. [CrossRef]
15. Gállego Pérez-Larraya, J.; Garcia-Moure, M.; Labiano, S.; Patiño-García, A.; Dobbs, J.; Gonzalez-Huarriz, M.; Zalacain, M.; Marrodan, L.; Martinez-Velez, N.; Puigdelloses, M. Oncolytic DNX-2401 virus for pediatric diffuse intrinsic pontine glioma. *N. Engl. J. Med.* **2022**, *386*, 2471–2481. [CrossRef]
16. Bander, E.D.; Ramos, A.D.; Wembacher-Schroeder, E.; Ivasyk, I.; Thomson, R.; Morgenstern, P.F.; Souweidane, M.M. Repeat convection-enhanced delivery for diffuse intrinsic pontine glioma. *J. Neurosurg. Pediatr.* **2020**, *26*, 661–666. [CrossRef]
17. Majzner, R.G.; Ramakrishna, S.; Yeom, K.W.; Patel, S.; Chinnasamy, H.; Schultz, L.M.; Richards, R.M.; Jiang, L.; Barsan, V.; Mancusi, R. GD2-CAR T cell therapy for H3K27M-mutated diffuse midline gliomas. *Nature* **2022**, *603*, 934–941. [CrossRef]
18. Zaghloul, M.S.; Nasr, A.; Tolba, M.; Refaat, A.; Youssef, A.; Mosaab, A.; Enayet, A.; Arafa, O.; Maher, E.; Eldebawy, E. Hypofractionated Radiation Therapy For Diffuse Intrinsic Pontine Glioma: A Noninferiority Randomized Study Including 253 Children. *Int. J. Radiat. Oncol. Biol. Phys.* **2022**, *113*, 360–368. [CrossRef]
19. Izzuddeen, Y.; Gupta, S.; Haresh, K.P.; Sharma, D.; Giridhar, P.; Rath, G.K. Hypofractionated radiotherapy with temozolomide in diffuse intrinsic pontine gliomas: A randomized controlled trial. *J. Neurooncol.* **2020**, *146*, 91–95. [CrossRef]
20. Amsbaugh, M.J.; Mahajan, A.; Thall, P.F.; McAleer, M.F.; Paulino, A.C.; Grosshans, D.; Khatua, S.; Ketonen, L.; Fontanilla, H.; McGovern, S.L. A phase 1/2 trial of reirradiation for diffuse intrinsic pontine glioma. *Int. J. Radiat. Oncol. Biol. Phys.* **2019**, *104*, 144–148. [CrossRef]
21. Fleischhack, G.; Massimino, M.; Warmuth-Metz, M.; Khuhlaeva, E.; Janssen, G.; Graf, N.; Rutkowski, S.; Beilken, A.; Schmid, I.; Biassoni, V. Nimotuzumab and radiotherapy for treatment of newly diagnosed diffuse intrinsic pontine glioma (DIPG): A phase III clinical study. *J. Neurooncol.* **2019**, *143*, 107–113. [CrossRef] [PubMed]
22. Su, J.M.; Kilburn, L.B.; Mansur, D.B.; Krailo, M.; Buxton, A.; Adekunle, A.; Gajjar, A.; Adamson, P.C.; Weigel, B.; Fox, E. Phase I/II trial of vorinostat and radiation and maintenance vorinostat in children with diffuse intrinsic pontine glioma: A Children's Oncology Group report. *Neuro Oncol.* **2022**, *24*, 655–664. [CrossRef]
23. Mueller, S.; Cooney, T.; Yang, X.; Pal, S.; Ermoian, R.; Gajjar, A.; Liu, X.; Prem, K.; Minard, C.G.; Reid, J.M. Wee1 kinase inhibitor Adavosertib with radiation in newly diagnosed diffuse intrinsic pontine glioma: A Children's Oncology Group phase 1 consortium study. *Neuro-Oncol. Adv.* **2022**, *4*, vdac073. [CrossRef] [PubMed]
24. Su, J.M.; Murray, J.C.; McNall-Knapp, R.Y.; Bowers, D.C.; Shah, S.; Adesina, A.M.; Paulino, A.C.; Jo, E.; Mo, Q.; Baxter, P.A. A phase 2 study of valproic acid and radiation, followed by maintenance valproic acid and bevacizumab in children with newly diagnosed diffuse intrinsic pontine glioma or high-grade glioma. *Pediatr. Blood Cancer* **2020**, *67*, e28283. [CrossRef]
25. Macy, M.E.; Kieran, M.W.; Chi, S.N.; Cohen, K.J.; MacDonald, T.J.; Smith, A.A.; Etzl, M.M.; Kuei, M.C.; Donson, A.M.; Gore, L. A pediatric trial of radiation/cetuximab followed by irinotecan/cetuximab in newly diagnosed diffuse pontine gliomas and high-grade astrocytomas: A Pediatric Oncology Experimental Therapeutics Investigators' Consortium study. *Pediatr. Blood Cancer* **2017**, *64*, e26621. [CrossRef] [PubMed]
26. El-Khouly, F.E.; Veldhuijzen van Zanten, S.E.M.; Jansen, M.H.A.; Bakker, D.P.; Sanchez Aliaga, E.; Hendrikse, N.H.; Vandertop, W.P.; van Vuurden, D.G.; Kaspers, G.J.L. A phase I/II study of bevacizumab, irinotecan and erlotinib in children with progressive diffuse intrinsic pontine glioma. *J. Neurooncol.* **2021**, *153*, 263–271. [CrossRef]
27. DeWire, M.; Lazow, M.; Campagne, O.; Leach, J.; Fuller, C.; Senthil Kumar, S.; Stanek, J.; de Blank, P.; Hummel, T.R.; Pillay-Smiley, N. Phase I study of ribociclib and everolimus in children with newly diagnosed DIPG and high-grade glioma: A CONNECT pediatric neuro-oncology consortium report. *Neuro-Oncol. Adv.* **2022**, *4*, vdac055. [CrossRef] [PubMed]

28. DeWire, M.; Fuller, C.; Hummel, T.R.; Chow, L.M.L.; Salloum, R.; de Blank, P.; Pater, L.; Lawson, S.; Zhu, X.; Dexheimer, P. A phase I/II study of ribociclib following radiation therapy in children with newly diagnosed diffuse intrinsic pontine glioma (DIPG). *J. Neurooncol.* **2020**, *149*, 511–522. [CrossRef]
29. Baxter, P.A.; Su, J.M.; Onar-Thomas, A.; Billups, C.A.; Li, X.-N.; Poussaint, T.Y.; Smith, E.R.; Thompson, P.; Adesina, A.; Ansell, P. A phase I/II study of veliparib (ABT-888) with radiation and temozolomide in newly diagnosed diffuse pontine glioma: A Pediatric Brain Tumor Consortium study. *Neuro Oncol.* **2020**, *22*, 875–885. [CrossRef] [PubMed]
30. Kilburn, L.B.; Kocak, M.; Baxter, P.; Poussaint, T.Y.; Paulino, A.C.; McIntyre, C.; Lemenuel-Diot, A.; Lopez-Diaz, C.; Kun, L.; Chintagumpala, M. A pediatric brain tumor consortium phase II trial of capecitabine rapidly disintegrating tablets with concomitant radiation therapy in children with newly diagnosed diffuse intrinsic pontine gliomas. *Pediatr. Blood Cancer* **2018**, *65*, e26832. [CrossRef] [PubMed]
31. Veldhuijzen van Zanten, S.E.M.; El-Khouly, F.E.; Jansen, M.H.A.; Bakker, D.P.; Sanchez Aliaga, E.; Haasbeek, C.J.A.; Wolf, N.I.; Zwaan, C.M.; Vandertop, W.P.; van Vuurden, D.G. A phase I/II study of gemcitabine during radiotherapy in children with newly diagnosed diffuse intrinsic pontine glioma. *J. Neurooncol.* **2017**, *135*, 307–315. [CrossRef] [PubMed]
32. Manley, P.E.; Trippett, T.; Smith, A.A.; Macy, M.E.; Leary, S.E.S.; Boklan, J.; Cohen, K.J.; Goldman, S.; Kilburn, L.B.; Dhall, G. A phase 1/2 dose-finding, safety, and activity study of cabazitaxel in pediatric patients with refractory solid tumors including tumors of the central nervous system. *Pediatr. Blood Cancer* **2018**, *65*, e27217. [CrossRef]
33. Fangusaro, J.; Cefalo, M.G.; Garré, M.L.; Marshall, L.V.; Massimino, M.; Benettaib, B.; Biserna, N.; Poon, J.; Quan, J.; Conlin, E. Phase 2 Study of Pomalidomide (CC-4047) Monotherapy for Children and Young Adults With Recurrent or Progressive Primary Brain Tumors. *Front. Oncol.* **2021**, *11*, 660892. [CrossRef] [PubMed]
34. Schuelke, M.R.; Gundelach, J.H.; Coffey, M.; West, E.; Scott, K.; Johnson, D.R.; Samson, A.; Melcher, A.; Vile, R.G.; Bram, R.J. Phase I trial of sargramostim/pelareorep therapy in pediatric patients with recurrent or refractory high-grade brain tumors. *Neuro-Oncol. Adv.* **2022**, *4*, vdac085. [CrossRef] [PubMed]
35. Tsvankin, V.; Hashizume, R.; Katagi, H.; Herndon, J.E.; Lascola, C.; Venkatraman, T.N.; Picard, D.; Burrus, B.; Becher, O.J.; Thompson, E.M. ABC transporter inhibition plus dexamethasone enhances the efficacy of convection enhanced delivery in H3. 3K27M mutant diffuse intrinsic pontine glioma. *Neurosurgery* **2020**, *86*, 742–751. [CrossRef] [PubMed]
36. Hollingworth, M.; Zacharoulis, S. Infusion-related side-effects during convection enhanced delivery for brainstem-diffuse midline glioma/diffuse intrinsic pontine glioma. *J. Neurooncol.* **2022**, *159*, 417–424. [CrossRef] [PubMed]
37. Buczkowicz, P.; Hawkins, C. Pathology, molecular genetics, and epigenetics of diffuse intrinsic pontine glioma. *Front. Oncol.* **2015**, *5*, 147. [CrossRef]
38. Sethi, R.; Allen, J.; Donahue, B.; Karajannis, M.; Gardner, S.; Wisoff, J.; Kunnakkat, S.; Mathew, J.; Zagzag, D.; Newman, K. Prospective neuraxis MRI surveillance reveals a high risk of leptomeningeal dissemination in diffuse intrinsic pontine glioma. *J. Neurooncol.* **2011**, *102*, 121–127. [CrossRef]
39. Fowler, M.J.; Cotter, J.D.; Knight, B.E.; Sevick-Muraca, E.M.; Sandberg, D.I.; Sirianni, R.W. Intrathecal drug delivery in the era of nanomedicine. *Adv. Drug Deliv. Rev.* **2020**, *165*, 77–95. [CrossRef]
40. Kline, C.; Liu, S.J.; Duriseti, S.; Banerjee, A.; Nicolaides, T.; Raber, S.; Gupta, N.; Haas-Kogan, D.; Braunstein, S.; Mueller, S. Reirradiation and PD-1 inhibition with nivolumab for the treatment of recurrent diffuse intrinsic pontine glioma: A single-institution experience. *J. Neurooncol.* **2018**, *140*, 629–638. [CrossRef]
41. Cacciotti, C.; Liu, K.X.; Haas-Kogan, D.A.; Warren, K.E. Reirradiation practices for children with diffuse intrinsic pontine glioma. *Neuro-Oncol. Pract.* **2021**, *8*, 68–74. [CrossRef] [PubMed]
42. Puget, S.; Beccaria, K.; Blauwblomme, T.; Roujeau, T.; James, S.; Grill, J.; Zerah, M.; Varlet, P.; Sainte-Rose, C. Biopsy in a series of 130 pediatric diffuse intrinsic Pontine gliomas. *Child's Nerv. Syst.* **2015**, *31*, 1773–1780. [CrossRef] [PubMed]
43. Hamisch, C.; Kickingereder, P.; Fischer, M.; Simon, T.; Ruge, M.I. Update on the diagnostic value and safety of stereotactic biopsy for pediatric brainstem tumors: A systematic review and meta-analysis of 735 cases. *J. Neurosurg. Pediatr.* **2017**, *20*, 261–268. [CrossRef] [PubMed]
44. Somatic histone H3 alterations in pediatric diffuse intrinsic pontine gliomas and non-brainstem glioblastomas. *Nat. Genet.* **2012**, *44*, 251–253. [CrossRef]
45. Mackay, A.; Burford, A.; Carvalho, D.; Izquierdo, E.; Fazal-Salom, J.; Taylor, K.R.; Bjerke, L.; Clarke, M.; Vinci, M.; Nandhabalan, M. Integrated molecular meta-analysis of 1000 pediatric high-grade and diffuse intrinsic pontine glioma. *Cancer Cell* **2017**, *32*, 520–537. [CrossRef] [PubMed]
46. Schwartzentruber, J.; Korshunov, A.; Liu, X.-Y.; Jones, D.T.W.; Pfaff, E.; Jacob, K.; Sturm, D.; Fontebasso, A.M.; Quang, D.-A.K.; Tönjes, M. Driver mutations in histone H3.3 and chromatin remodelling genes in paediatric glioblastoma. *Nature* **2012**, *482*, 226–231. [CrossRef]
47. Jones, C.; Baker, S.J. Unique genetic and epigenetic mechanisms driving paediatric diffuse high-grade glioma. *Nat. Rev. Cancer* **2014**, *14*, 651–661. [CrossRef]
48. Grill, J.; Puget, S.; Andreiuolo, F.; Philippe, C.; MacConaill, L.; Kieran, M.W. Critical oncogenic mutations in newly diagnosed pediatric diffuse intrinsic pontine glioma. *Pediatr. Blood Cancer* **2012**, *58*, 489–491. [CrossRef]
49. Puget, S.; Philippe, C.; Bax, D.A.; Job, B.; Varlet, P.; Junier, M.-P.; Andreiuolo, F.; Carvalho, D.; Reis, R.; Guerrini-Rousseau, L. Mesenchymal transition and PDGFRA amplification/mutation are key distinct oncogenic events in pediatric diffuse intrinsic pontine gliomas. *PLoS ONE* **2012**, *7*, e30313. [CrossRef]

50. Buczkowicz, P.; Hoeman, C.; Rakopoulos, P.; Pajovic, S.; Letourneau, L.; Dzamba, M.; Morrison, A.; Lewis, P.; Bouffet, E.; Bartels, U. Genomic analysis of diffuse intrinsic pontine gliomas identifies three molecular subgroups and recurrent activating ACVR1 mutations. *Nat. Genet.* **2014**, *46*, 451–456. [CrossRef]
51. Paugh, B.S.; Zhu, X.; Qu, C.; Endersby, R.; Diaz, A.K.; Zhang, J.; Bax, D.A.; Carvalho, D.; Reis, R.M.; Onar-Thomas, A. Novel Oncogenic PDGFRA Mutations in Pediatric High-Grade GliomasPDGFRA Mutations in Gliomagenesis. *Cancer Res.* **2013**, *73*, 6219–6229. [CrossRef] [PubMed]
52. Hoffman, L.M.; DeWire, M.; Ryall, S.; Buczkowicz, P.; Leach, J.; Miles, L.; Ramani, A.; Brudno, M.; Kumar, S.S.; Drissi, R. Spatial genomic heterogeneity in diffuse intrinsic pontine and midline high-grade glioma: Implications for diagnostic biopsy and targeted therapeutics. *Acta Neuropathol. Commun.* **2016**, *4*, 1–8. [CrossRef] [PubMed]

healthcare

MDPI

Article

Palliative Care Survey: Awareness, Knowledge and Views of the Styrian Population in Austria

Ulrike Spary-Kainz [1], Nicole Posch [1,*], Muna Paier-Abuzahra [1], Melanie Lieb [1], Alexander Avian [2], Erika Zelko [3] and Andrea Siebenhofer [1,4]

1 Institute of General Practice and Evidence-Based Health Services Research, Medical University of Graz, Neue Stiftingtalstraße 6, 8010 Graz, Austria; ulrike.spary-kainz@medunigraz.at (U.S.-K.); muna.paier-abuzahra@medunigraz.at (M.P.-A.); melaniesoper26@gmail.com (M.L.); andrea.siebenhofer@medunigraz.at (A.S.)

2 Institute of Medical Informatics, Statistics and Documentation, Medical University of Graz, Auenbruggerplatz 2, 8036 Graz, Austria; alexander.avian@medunigraz.at

3 Institute of General Practice, Johannes Kepler University Linz, The Life Science Park, 4040 Linz, Austria; erika.zelko@jku.at

4 Institute for General Practice, Goethe University Frankfurt am Main, Theodor-Stern-Kai 7, D-60590 Frankfurt, Germany

* Correspondence: nicole.posch@medunigraz.at; Tel.: +43-316-3857-3560

Abstract: Background: No population-based data on awareness and knowledge of palliative care currently exist in Austria. We therefore conducted a survey to determine the general awareness and knowledge of palliative care in Styria, a federal state in Austria. We also asked participants to imagine what services they would need as a patient or family member, where they themselves would like to receive such services, and what fears they imagined patients with a terminal illness would have. Methods: A descriptive cross-sectional survey consisting of 18 questions that address several aspects of palliative care was carried out in the adult population of Styria, Austria, from October 2019 to March 2020. Results: A total of 419 questionnaires were analyzed, whereby 70.3% of respondents had at least heard of palliative care. Of these, significantly more were female, had a university degree and were aged 50 to 64. The main goal of palliative care was chosen correctly by 67.1% of participants, with the proportion of correct answers increasing in line with education and reaching 82.0% among university graduates. Overall, 73.2% believed that the greatest need of terminally ill persons was a reduction in physical suffering, whereas the greatest perceived need of relatives was the availability of specialist care around the clock. About one-third believed that the greatest fear of palliative patients was that of death, which was chosen significantly more often by men than women. If terminally ill, some 39% of respondents would wish to be looked after at home by professional carers, and women and people that had completed high school chose this answer significantly more often. The most desired service that should be provided to patients and relatives was home pain management at 69.9%, followed by time off for family caregivers at 58.0%. This item was chosen significantly more often by women. Conclusions: To facilitate the care of severely ill patients at home, it would make sense to develop targeted information campaigns. These should also attempt to deliver targeted information to less informed groups of people, such as young, poorly educated men, in order to raise their awareness of the difficulties and challenges of providing care to terminally ill patients and thus increase the acceptance of support options.

Keywords: palliative care; awareness of palliative care; information campaign; health literacy

1. Introduction

Palliative care and palliative medicine have a positive influence on the lives of severely ill patients. The World Health Organization (WHO) defines palliative care as an approach that improves the quality of life of patients and their families who are facing the problems associated with life-threatening illness. It achieves this through the prevention and relief of suffering by means of early identification and the correct assessment and treatment of pain and other problems, whether physical, psychosocial or spiritual [1].

Palliative care improves symptom burden and the health-related quality of life of those affected and increases the likelihood that patients can die at home if they prefer [2]. Although not the primary goal, life can even be prolonged in some cases [3]. In addition to clinical advantages, it also makes financial sense to expand the palliative care network, especially in populations whose life expectancy is increasing [2–4].

However, expanding the palliative care network requires raising community awareness, eliminating prejudice and teaching people about it. Awareness and knowledge of palliative care vary considerably between countries but also between different groups of people, depending on their age, education and gender. For example, over 80% of respondents to a survey in Northern Ireland said they had heard the term "palliative care", but most (75%) of them knew little or nothing about it [5], whereas only 32% of respondents to a Turkish survey were aware of it at all [6]. A survey of 3194 persons in the U.S. carried out by Huo et al. showed that fewer than 30% of respondents had any knowledge of palliative care [7]. A Slovenian survey conducted in 2020 showed that women, people of older age and those that had completed higher education were more aware of palliative care [8]. Furthermore, the term "palliative" may be mistakenly associated with hospice care or even euthanasia. A study published in 2013 showed that the term "palliative care" was less familiar to the general population than the term "supportive care", although they essentially mean the same thing [9]. The term palliative care also carries the stigma of being associated with the very last weeks of life, although early access would be beneficial in terms of quality of life and clinical outcomes [10]. In Styria, a federal state in Austria, institutions specializing in the care of patients with life-limiting illnesses have existed since 1998 [11]. As no population-based awareness data are currently available, we conducted a survey to determine the general awareness and knowledge of palliative care in the general population of Styria, a federal state in Austria. We also asked participants to imagine what services they would need as a patient or family member, where they themselves would like to receive such services, and what fears they would have as a patient.

2. Materials and Methods

2.1. Study Design

The study is based on a descriptive cross-sectional survey addressing several aspects of palliative care. We therefore surveyed people and asked them to imagine that they were terminally ill patients or family members of such patients. The data were collected as part of an international study performed in Slovenia, Hungary and Croatia. Ethics approval was granted by the Medical University of Graz (EK Nr: 1382/2019 Version 1).

2.2. Participants

Participants included a community-based sample of adults ($\geq$18 years) residing in Styria, a federal state in Austria. Participants were required to understand German, the official language in Austria, and provide their written consent by signing a consent form.

2.3. Recruitment and Data Collection

Two medical practices consecutively recruited the participants, who were subsequently asked to answer an anonymous questionnaire (paper-and-pencil). Names, insurance numbers and other data that could be used to identify any of the respondents were not collected. Data were collected from 9 October 2019 to 25 March 2020. Participants completed the study in one sitting lasting approximately 15 min.

2.4. Outcome Measures

We used an existing Slovenian questionnaire [8] that had been used in 1015 Slovenian adults. This survey consists of 18 questions, some multiple choice and some single choice. It was translated from Slovenian into German by a professional translator. To ensure the accuracy of the translated questionnaire, it was proofread by a native Slovenian who is fluent in both German and Slovene and works in the medical field. The questionnaire was linguistically adapted to take into account the differences between the Austrian and Slovenian healthcare and education systems. We were therefore in regular contact with the Slovenian research team during the translation process to ensure that the survey was not only valid and suitable for international comparisons but also appropriate for use in Austria. The German questionnaire was tested using the Cognitive Debriefing method [12]. This is a process by which an instrument is actively tested among representatives of the target population and target language group to determine whether respondents understand the questionnaire properly.

The questionnaire asked about awareness and knowledge of palliative care, and it further asked participants to put themselves in the position of terminally ill patients and their relatives and to provide their views on the services they thought such patients or the family members of such patients should have, where they themselves would like to receive such services (at home, in a hospice, etc.) and what fears they would have if they were a patient. The full questionnaire can be found in the Appendix A.

2.5. Statistical Analyses

SPSS 28 (IBM Corp., Armonk, NY, USA) was used for data analysis; $p < 0.05$ was considered as significant. Missing data were not imputed. Data are presented as absolute or relative frequencies. Differences between groups (gender, age groups, educational levels) were analyzed using the Chi-square test or Fisher's exact test, as appropriate. For this analysis, age was grouped into 18–34 years, 35–49 years, 50–64 years, ≥65 years, and educational level was grouped into EL1: compulsory school, EL2: apprenticeship, EL3: trade school, EL4: high school, EL5: university.

3. Results

3.1. Description of the Sample

A total of 419 questionnaires were analyzed. A further 37 questionnaires were not taken into consideration because they were incomplete.

The age of the respondents ranged from 18 to 93 years. Overall, 58% were female, 8.3% had completed compulsory schooling (EL1), 28.2% had completed an apprenticeship (EL2), 16.7% had been trained at a technical college or trade school (EL3), 18.1% had finished high school (EL4) and 28.6% had graduated from a university or university of applied sciences (EL5). Overall, 303 lived in a rural area (72.3%) and 116 in an urban area (27.7%).

3.2. Awareness and Knowledge of Palliative Medicine

Of the 419 respondents, 70.3% (n = 295) had at least heard of palliative medicine in Styria. Of these, 11.2% reported knowing a fair amount about it and 3.3% reported having extensive knowledge. More of the participants that had heard of palliative medicine were female (78.3%, $p < 0.001$), had a university degree (74.2%, $p = 0.033$) and were aged 50 to 64 (79.6% $p = 0.003$). Only the 295 (70.3%) that had at least heard of palliative care were asked what its main aim was. The right answer, which was to "improve quality of life", was chosen by 67.1% of them (wrong answers: 25.4%; did not know: 7.5%). While the responses did not differ according to sex ($p = 0.503$) and age group ($p = 0.227$), the proportion of correct answers increased in line with education, reaching 82.0% in graduates from universities of applied sciences or universities ($p = 0.003$).

3.3. Survey Participants' Views on the Greatest Needs of Palliative Care Patients and Their Relatives

Overall, 73.2% believed that the greatest need of terminally ill persons at the end of their lives was a *reduction in physical suffering*, while 9.5% said it was *home nursing care*, 6.4% *medical specialist care*, 4.4% *psychological care*, 3.4% *caregiver support* and 1.4% *spiritual support*. Views on the greatest needs of terminally ill persons depended on the respondent's age. Younger respondents more often believed that *psychological care* was the greatest need of terminally ill persons (age < 35 years: 10.1%, 35–49 years: 4.0%, 50–64 years: 3.7%, ≥65 years: 0.0%; $p = 0.031$). No other significant correlations existed between the provided responses and the variables of age, education and gender. For more details, see Figure 1 and Table A1 in Appendix C.

Around–the–clock availability of specialist care was the most common response to the question on the greatest needs of relatives (35.3%), followed by *home nursing* care (26.1%) and *psychological care* (16.3%). A perceived need for home nursing care was stronger in males than females (f: 22.0%, m: 33.7%; $p = 0.029$), while age influenced a perceived need for *around–the–clock availability of specialist care* (<35 years: 22.9%, 35–49 years: 33.3%, 50–64 years: 36.6%, ≥65 years: 48.5%; $p = 0.017$) and *psychological care* (<35 years: 27.1%, 35–49 years: 20.0%, 50–64 years: 14.6%, ≥65 years: 2.9%; $p = 0.001$). The level of education influenced the ratings for *around-the-clock availability of specialist care* (EL2: 47.1%, EL 3: 38.9%, EL1: 38.1%, EL4: 34.1%, EL5: 21.3%; $p = 0.010$), as well as for *hospice care* (EL5: 12.4%, EL2: 10.3%, EL3: 11.1%, EL4: 0.0%, EL1: 0.0%; $p = 0.048$), *psychological care* (EL4: 27.3%, EL5: 21.3%, EL3: 16.7%, EL2: 9.2%, EL1: 0.0%; $p = 0.010$) and *grief counseling* (EL1: 19.0%, EL4: 9.1%, EL3: 5.6%, EL2: 1.1%, EL5: 1.1%; $p = 0.002$). See Figure 2.

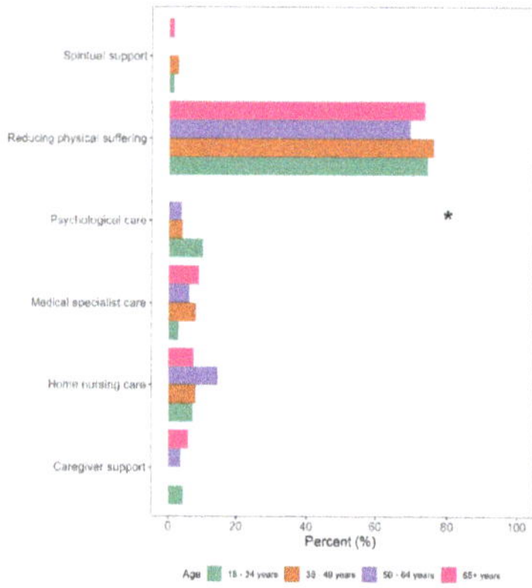

(a)

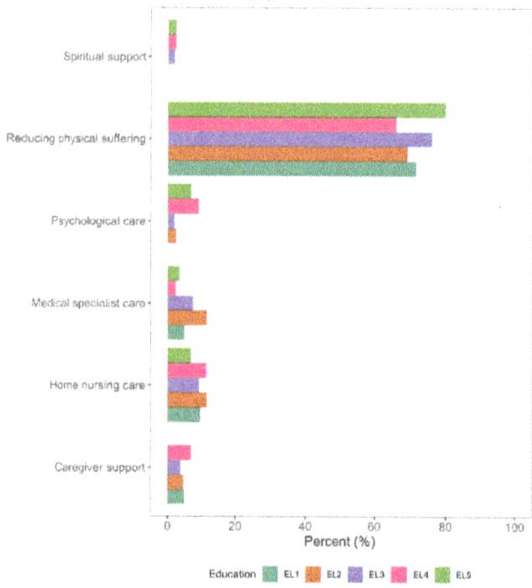

(b)

Figure 1. *Cont.*

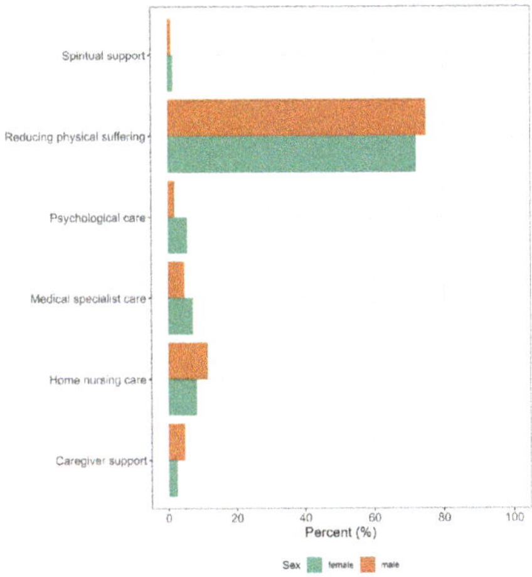

(c)

Figure 1. Differences in survey participants' views on the greatest needs of palliative care patients according to the participating's age, educational level (EL1: compulsory school, EL2: apprenticeship, EL3: trade school, EL4: high school, EL5: university) and sex. * Significant; (**a**) age; (**b**) education; (**c**) sex; n = 295.

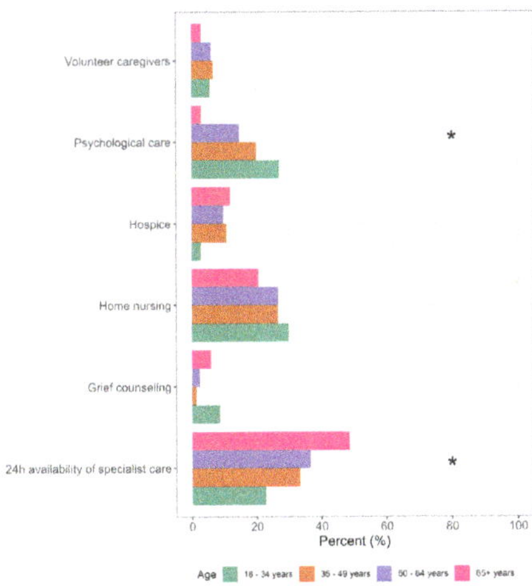

(a)

Figure 2. *Cont.*

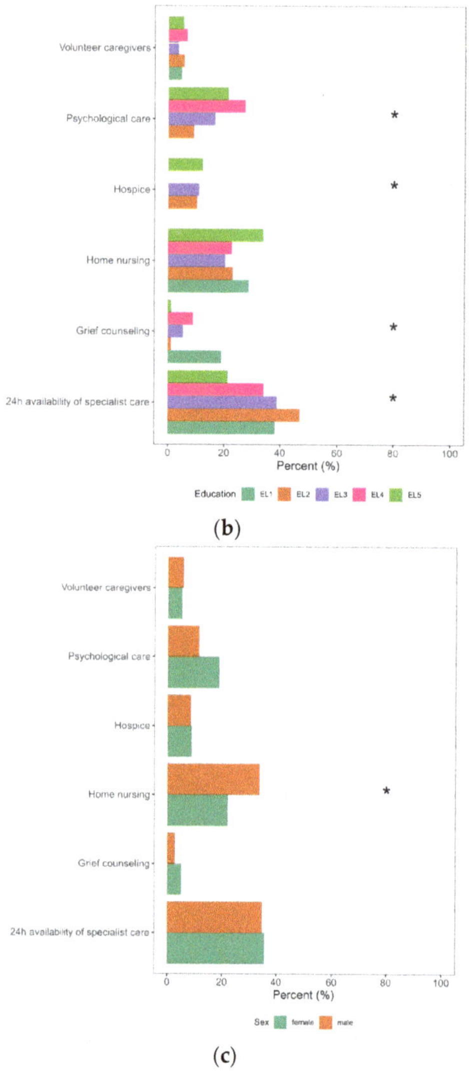

Figure 2. Differences in survey participants' views on the greatest needs of their relatives according to the participant's age, educational level (EL1: compulsory school, EL2: apprenticeship, EL3: trade school, EL4: high school, EL5: university) and sex. * Significant; (**a**) age; (**b**) education; (**c**) sex; n = 295.

3.4. Survey Participants' Views on the Fears of Palliative Care Patients

About one–third of participants (32.9%) said they believed the greatest fear of terminally ill people was that of *death*, followed by *pain* (24.1%), *losing independence* (16.9%), *being a burden to someone* (9.3%), *losing mental abilities* (7.6%), *becoming disabled* (6.0%), *loneliness* (1.0%) and *financial burdens* (0.5%). Age influenced expectations that fear of *death* was the greatest concern and was higher in participants in the group aged 35–49 years (47.5%) and lowest in the 65+ age group (11.3%; $p < 0.000$). Fear of *death* was chosen significantly more often by men than women (41.7% vs. 26.6%; $p = 0.001$).

A quarter of respondents (24.1%) believed the greatest fear was *pain*, but the results also depended considerably on age, with the youngest respondents (≤34 years) having the least fear of *pain* (15.8%) and respondents in the group aged 50–64 years having the greatest (32.0%) ($p = 0.030$). See Figure 3 and Table A3 in Appendix C for more details.

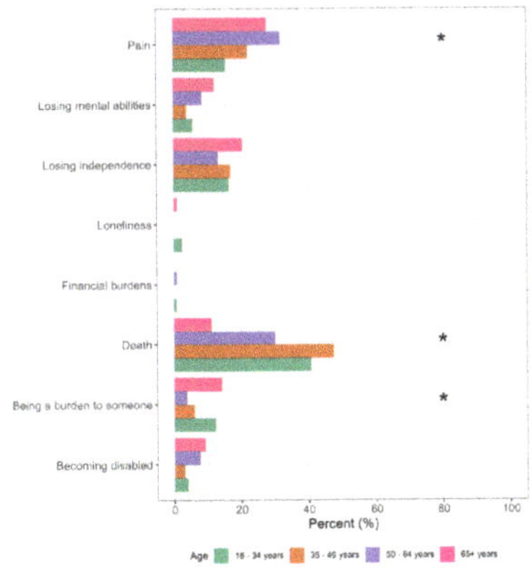

(**a**)

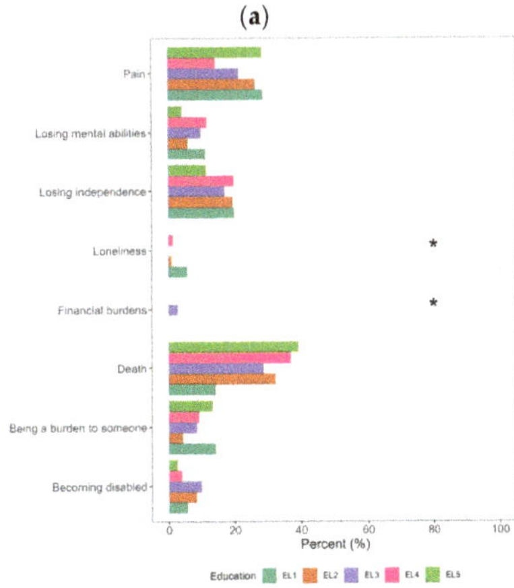

(**b**)

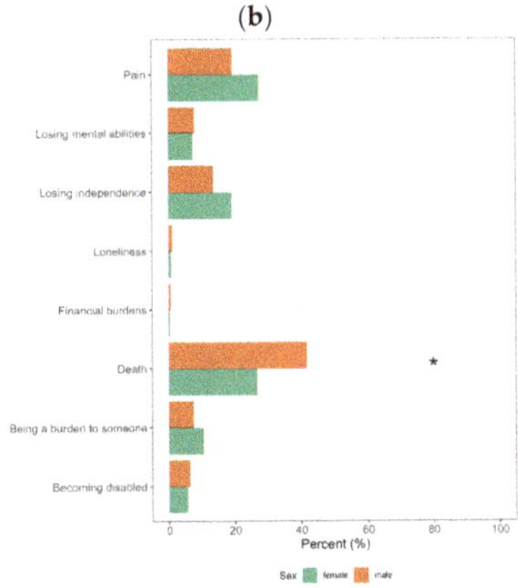

(**c**)

Figure 3. Differences in survey participants' views on the fears of palliative care patients according to the participant's age, educational level (EL1: compulsory school, EL2: apprenticeship, EL3: trade school, EL4: high school, EL5: university) and sex. * Significant; (**a**) age; (**b**) education; (**c**) sex; n = 419.

3.5. Survey Participants' Views on the Best Place for Palliative Care Patients to Receive Care

When terminally ill, 39.0% of respondents believed it is best to be cared for *at home by professional caregivers*, followed by cared for *at home by relatives* (21.7%), *hospices* (21.4%) and *hospitals* (11.9%). Results depended strongly on sex, with females more often choosing to be cared for *at home by professional caregivers* (f: 40.3%, m: 36.5%) and *hospices* (f: 25.7%, m: 13.5%) and less often cared for *at home by relatives* (f: 20.4%, m: 24.0%) and *hospitals* (f: 7.3%, m: 20.2%; $p = 0.005$). Respondents with EL2 (44.8%), EL4 (47.7%) and EL 5 (37.1%) considered it best to be cared for *at home by professional caregivers*, while respondents that had EL 1 thought it best to be cared for *at home by relatives* (52.4%) and those that had EL 3 were in favor of *hospices* (31.5%) ($p = 0.003$). No differences were found between the various age groups ($p = 0.533$).

3.6. Survey Participants' Views on the Services That Should Be Provided to Palliative Care Patients and Their Relatives

The service that was mentioned most often was home pain management 69.9% (n = 293), followed by time off for family caregivers (58%), daycare (49.4%), nightcare (42.0%), home assistance (40.1%), information on financial support (35.1%), availability of social workers (27.4%), complementary and alternative medicine (22.4%) and pastoral care (20.5%). Sex differences in preferred services were only found in time off for family caregivers, which were significantly more popular among females (64.3%) than males (49.1%) ($p = 0.002$). Age groups significantly influenced preferences for complementary and alternative medicine ($p = 0.001$), pastoral care ($p < 0.001$), availability of social workers ($p = 0.009$) and information on financial support ($p < 0.001$). Educational level also had a significant influence on the preference for pastoral care ($p < 0.001$), availability of social workers ($p = 0.004$) and information on financial support ($p = 0.012$). See Figure 4 and Table A4 in Appendix C.

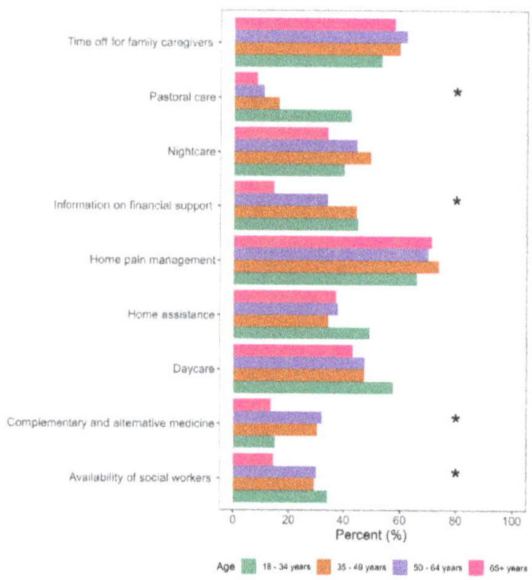

(a)

Figure 4. *Cont.*

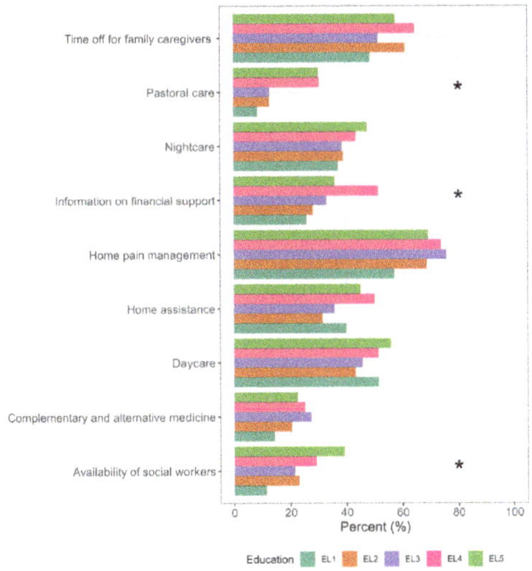

(**b**)

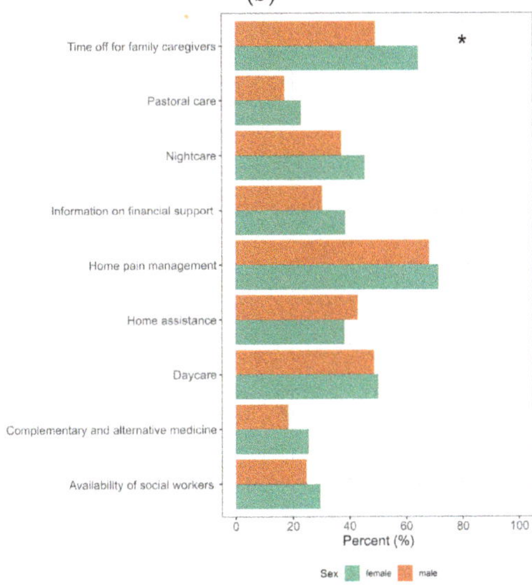

(**c**)

Figure 4. Differences in survey participants' views on the services that should be provided to palliative care patients and their relatives according to the participating's age, educational level (EL1: compulsory school, EL2: apprenticeship, EL3: trade school, EL4: high school, EL5: university) and sex. * Significant; (**a**) age; (**b**) education; (**c**) sex; n = 419.

4. Discussion

With over 400 participants, this cross-sectional survey showed that in our sample, more people had heard of palliative care in Styria, Austria, than in many other countries [6]. In similar countries to Austria, a relatively large number of people (70%) had heard of palliative care but had no precise idea of what it really was [5,13]. Our survey also indicated that as few as 13.5% of respondents knew a fair amount or had extensive knowledge of it. It is interesting to note that there were major differences in terms of gender, with 40.6% of men saying they knew nothing about palliative care, as compared to only 21.7% of women.

The difference may reflect gender roles, as informal caregiving is generally provided by women [14,15], which would explain why they knew more about it. At the same time, female caregivers report greater burden, stress, anxiety, depression, and adverse health outcomes than male caregivers [16]. A Canadian study found that the majority of spousal caregivers were female and that these female caregivers reported a significantly greater level of caregiving strain than their male counterparts [17]. In our survey, this was reflected in the question of what the respondents thought families and their relatives should be provided in terms of support. Here, significantly more women (64.3%) than men (49.1%) said that additional support should be offered to caregivers at home, so that caregiving relatives could have more time for themselves. It is evident that caring for relatives is still largely the responsibility of women [18] and that awareness of caregiver burden is therefore stronger in women. It has further been shown that care recipients with a female caregiver are less likely to receive informal support from family and friends in carrying out tasks associated with personal care than male caregivers, to whom others are more likely to offer such support [17].

Another field in which gender differences were observed was in response to the question where it is best to be provided palliative care when terminally ill. Women more often chose to be cared for at home by professional caregivers (f: 40.3%, m: 36.5%) or cared for in hospices (f: 25.7%, m: 13.5%) and less often to be cared for at home by relatives (f: 20.4%, m: 24.0%). This difference may also reflect the traditional distribution of roles, with women more frequently wanting to avoid burdening their families with their need for care. Another interesting aspect is that significantly more men (41.7%) than women (26.6%) said they thought the greatest fear of a terminally ill person was likely to be the fear of death. A survey conducted in Germany found that significantly more women than men found the thought of their own death less painful than that of a loved one [19].

However, differences were not only related to gender but also to age. Younger respondents tended to know less about palliative care, as has also been found in previous studies [20]. In the group aged 18–35 years, 10.1% of respondents believed that psychological support was the greatest need of terminally ill patients, whereas no respondents in the group aged 65 years and older thought so. For older people, around-the-clock availability of specialist care for relatives appeared to be more important than for younger people, while psychological support was more important to younger people than to older people. There were significant differences in opinions on the greatest fears of terminally ill patients. In the middle-aged group, 47.5% thought it was the fear of death, while only 11.3% believed this in the 65+ group. Respondents in the group up to 34 years old reported the least fear of pain (15.8%), while the greatest fear of pain was found in the group aged 50–64 years (32.0%).

Education was also a crucial factor influencing knowledge about palliative care. The more educated participants were, the more likely they were to know the main aim of palliative care. There were also education-related differences in answers to other questions, such as where terminally ill patients should best be cared for. More than 50% of respondents that had only completed compulsory schooling thought it best to be cared for at home by relatives, an opinion that was shared by only 37.1% of respondents with a university degree. There is also evidence in the literature that wealthier people and women were more likely to receive palliative care from specialists [21]. This attitude is also reflected in our survey, as it became apparent that the different groups of people had different levels of knowledge and different perceptions, fears and expectations with respect to palliative care. In an ageing society, in which more and more people will need looking after and require palliative care, targeted information is necessary. Furthermore, when providing such information, it is important to take into account that there are social group-related differences in knowledge about palliative care. In addition, age-, gender- and education-related differences exist in attitudes, fears and expectations with regard to palliative care and ageing in general.

Based on these results, it would make sense to avoid blanket information campaigns but rather tailor them according to the audience. For example, it is well known that people from socially disadvantaged population groups in Austria tend to gather information via social media [22]. As the results of this survey also confirm what we know about the distribution of health literacy, namely that people with little education, in financially precarious situations or who are looking for work tend to have limited health literacy [22], it is necessary to investigate the various possibilities to reach out to and inform these groups of people. A good example of targeted information and training in the field of palliative care for lay people are the Last Aid Courses, which are successfully held in various countries [23,24].

In order to support those that bear the greatest burden of care and thus to relieve society as a whole, information campaigns are required that target groups of people that know little about palliative care, so that they become more aware of, and take advantage of, available services. In this way, the quality of life of terminally ill patients and their caregivers in these groups may be increased.

Limitations of the Study

There may have been some bias in the sample, as the participants were recruited in medical practices and therefore do not include people that never consult a doctor. Another limitation is that the questionnaire was only distributed in a printed version and not as an online version and may therefore not have appealed to tech-savvy people, who may have a different level of awareness of palliative care than those in our sample and may know about different aspects of it. A limitation is also that all but one of the questions were closed-ended, and that only one question provided the opportunity to give an additional response over and above existing options. Thus, participants may have been unable to give the answers they would like. However, we were constrained in our ability to change the structure of the questionnaire by our interest in ensuring the international comparability of the results.

5. Conclusions

To facilitate the care of severely ill patients at home, it would make sense to develop targeted information campaigns in Western industrialized countries. This would also make it possible to reach out to groups, such as women, that bear the greatest burden of caregiving and to inform them of available support options. Such campaigns should also attempt to deliver information to less informed groups of people, such as young, poorly educated men, in order to raise their awareness of the difficulties and challenges of providing care to terminally ill patients.

Author Contributions: Conceptualization, U.S.-K. and E.Z.; methodology, A.A.; software, A.A.; validation, N.P. and M.P.-A.; formal analysis, A.A.; investigation, M.L.; data curation, A.A.; writing—original draft preparation, U.S.-K.; writing—review and editing, N.P. and M.P.-A.; visualization, N.P.; supervision, A.S.; project administration, A.S. All authors have read and agreed to the published version of the manuscript.

Funding: This research received no external funding.

Institutional Review Board Statement: Ethics approval was granted by the Medical University of Graz (EK Nr: 1382/2019 Version 1).

Informed Consent Statement: Written informed consent has been obtained from the patients to publish this paper.

Data Availability Statement: The datasets used and/or analyzed for the current study are available from the corresponding author on reasonable request.

Acknowledgments: We would like to thank all participants who took part in this cross-sectional study. We are most grateful to Phillip Elliott for editing the final manuscript.

Conflicts of Interest: The authors declare no conflict of interest.

Appendix A

Full questionnaire
WISSEN DER BEVÖLKERUNG ÜBER DIE PALLIATIVMEDIZINISCHE BETREUUNG IN DER STEIERMARK
1. Was sind Ihrer Meinung nach die größten Ängste einer Patientin/eines Patienten, bei der/dem eine unheilbare Krankheit diagnostiziert wurde? (Bitte wählen Sie aus den folgenden Möglichkeiten drei aus und ordnen Sie sie nach Relevanz—1., 2., 3.)
___ Angst vor Schmerzen.
___ Angst vor dem Tod.
___ Angst davor, nicht mehr selbstständig zu sein.
___ Angst vor dem Verlust der geistigen Fähigkeiten.
___ Angst vor Einsamkeit.
___ Angst davor, behindert/unbeweglich zu werden.
___ Angst vor finanziellen Belastungen.
___ Angst davor, jemandem zur Last zu fallen.
___ Ich weiß es nicht.

2. Was müsste Ihrer Meinung nach Betroffenen mit einer unheilbaren Krankheit und ihren Familien geboten werden? *(Sie können mehrere Antworten kennzeichnen.)*

(a) Hilfe bei Schmerzen und anderen Symptomen zu Hause.
(b) Häusliche Pflege der Patientin/des Patienten tagsüber.
(c) Häusliche Pflege der Patientin/des Patienten nachts.
(d) Komplementärmedizinische Therapien.
(e) Ein/e Seelsorger/in.
(f) Ein/e Sozialarbeiter/in, die/der bei Bedarf für die Patientin/den Patienten und die Familie telefonisch erreichbar wäre.
(g) Unterstützung bei Haushaltsaufgaben, Einkäufen, Transporten usw.
(h) Zusätzliche Unterstützung zu Hause, sodass die pflegenden Angehörigen Freizeit bzw. Zeit für sich haben.
(i) Informationen und Ratschläge über finanzielle Hilfe.
(j) Medizinische Versorgung im Hospiz.
(k) Medizinische Versorgung im Krankenhaus.

3. Was denken Sie, wie viel wird in der Gesellschaft über den Tod und das Sterben gesprochen? *(Bitte wählen Sie nur eine Antwort aus.)*

(a) Zu wenig.
(b) Ungefähr ausreichend.
(c) Zu viel.

4. Wo würden Sie den letzten Zeitraum Ihres Lebens verbringen wollen, wenn Sie an einer unheilbaren Krankheit erkranken würden? *(Bitte wählen Sie nur eine Antwort aus.)*

(a) Zu Hause.
(b) Im Krankenhaus.
(c) Im Pflegeheim.
(d) Diese Frage kann ich nicht beantworten.

5. Wissen Sie was eine Patientenverfügung ist?

(a) Ja.
(b) Nein.

6. Wie schätzen Sie Ihre Kenntnisse über die palliativmedizinische Betreuung in unserem Bundesland ein? *(Bitte wählen Sie nur eine Antwort aus.)*
(a) Über die palliativmedizinische Betreuung weiß ich nichts.
(Wenn Sie „a" ankreuzen, fahren Sie bitte mit Frage 15 auf Seite 5 fort.).
(b) Über die palliativmedizinische Betreuung habe ich schon etwas gehört.
(c) Über die palliativmedizinische Betreuung weiß ich viel.
(d) Ich verfüge über umfangreiches Wissen über die palliativmedizinische Betreuung.

7. Wenn Sie von der palliativmedizinischen Betreuung bereits gehört haben: Woher haben Sie diese Informationen bekommen? ***(Sie können mehrere Antworten kennzeichnen.)***

(a) Ich habe persönlich palliativmedizinische Betreuung erhalten.
(b) Eine nähere Freundin/Angehörige oder ein näherer Freund/Angehöriger hat palliativmedizinische Betreuung erhalten.
(c) Eine fernere Angehörige/Bekannte oder ein ferner Angehöriger/Bekannter hat palliativmedizinische Betreuung erhalten.
(d) Ein/e Nachbar/in hat palliativmedizinische Betreuung erhalten.
(e) Ein/e Freund/in oder eine/ein Angehörige/r hat darüber erzählt.
(f) Ich arbeite mit Patientinnen/Patienten, die palliativmedizinische Betreuung erhalten.
(g) Ich arbeite im medizinischen Bereich.
(h) Radio/Fernsehen/Zeitung.
(i) Internet/soziale Netzwerke.
(j) Sammeln von Spenden/Wohltätigkeitsaktionen.
(k) Sonstiges: ____________________

8. Bitte wählen Sie aus den folgenden Sätzen den Satz aus, der Ihrer Meinung nach das Ziel der palliativmedizinischen Betreuung am besten beschreibt. ***(Bitte wählen Sie nur eine Antwort aus.)***

(a) Palliativmedizinische Betreuung beschleunigt das Sterben.
(b) Palliativmedizinische Betreuung verzögert den Tod.
(c) Palliativmedizinische Betreuung ermöglicht der Patientin/dem Patienten, ein aktives Leben fortzuführen.
(d) Palliativmedizinische Betreuung beruhigt die Patientin/den Patienten.
(e) Palliativmedizinische Betreuung verbessert die Lebensqualität der Patientin/des Patienten.
(f) Ich weiß es nicht.

9. Was sind Ihrer Meinung nach die größten Bedürfnisse der Patientinnen/Patienten mit einer unheilbaren Krankheit, wenn sie am Lebensende angelangt sind? ***(Bitte wählen Sie aus den folgenden Möglichkeiten nur drei aus und ordnen Sie sie nach Relevanz—1., 2., 3.)***

____ Minderung des körperlichen Leidens.
____ Fachärztliche medizinische Versorgung.
____ Häusliche medizinische Versorgung und Hauskrankenpflege.
____ Unterstützung für häuslich tätige Pflegekräfte.
____ Unterstützung durch eine Psychologin/einen Psychologen.
____ Spirituelle Unterstützung.
____ Ich weiß es nicht.

10. Was sind Ihrer Meinung nach die größten Bedürfnisse der Angehörigen, die ein Familienmitglied mit unheilbarer Krankheit betreuen? ***(Bitte wählen Sie aus den folgenden Möglichkeiten nur drei aus und ordnen Sie sie nach Relevanz—1., 2., 3.)***

____ 24-stündige fachärztliche Versorgung.
____ Hauskrankenpflege.
____ Zugänglichkeit/Verfügbarkeit von freiwilligen Betreuerinnen/Betreuern.
____ Speziell angepasste Wohnzentren—Hospize.
____ Psychologische Unterstützung.
____ Unterstützung für die Angehörigen während der Trauerzeit nach dem Tod der Patientin/des Patienten.
____ Ich weiß es nicht.

11. Wo ist Ihrer Meinung nach für die Betreuung von Patientinnen/Patienten mit einer unheilbaren Krankheit am besten gesorgt? ***(Bitte wählen Sie nur eine Antwort aus.)***

(a) Zu Hause versorgt durch die Familie/Angehörige.
(b) Zu Hause versorgt durch berufliche Pflegekräfte.
(c) Im Hospiz.
(d) Im Krankenhaus.
(e) Ich weiß es nicht.

12. Kennen Sie jemanden aus Ihrer Familie, Ihrem Freundes- oder Bekanntenkreis, die/der eine persönliche Erfahrung mit palliativmedizinischer Betreuung gemacht hat? ***(Bitte wählen Sie nur eine Antwort aus.)***

(a) Ja.
(b) Nein.

13. Wer von den Patientinnen/Patienten, die an den unten angeführten Krankheiten leiden, sollte eine palliativmedizinische Betreuung erhalten? ***(Bitte kennzeichnen Sie eine der Möglichkeiten bei jeder Krankheit.)***

	5 (Ich stimme vollkommen zu.)	4 (Ich stimme zu.)	3 (Ich stimme teilweise zu.)	2 (Ich stimme nicht zu.)	1 (Ich stimme überhaupt nicht zu.)	Ich weiß es nicht.	Ich kenne diese Erkrankung nicht.
Krebs							
Nierenversagen							
Amyotrophe Lateralsklerose (ALS)							
Demenz							
Schlaganfall							
Herzversagen							
HIV/AIDS							
Chronische Lungenerkrankungen							
Multiple Sklerose							

14. Zu welchem Zeitpunkt würden Sie sich Informationen über die palliativmedizinische Betreuung wünschen, wenn Sie an einer unheilbaren Krankheit erkranken würden? ***(Bitte wählen Sie nur eine Antwort aus.)***

(a) Ich würde mir keine Informationen wünschen.
(b) Ich würde mir wünschen, dass die Informationen allgemein verfügbar wären.
(c) Ich würde mir Informationen nur dann wünschen, wenn meine unheilbare Erkrankung lebensbedrohlich wird.
(d) Ich würde mir Informationen nur dann wünschen, wenn die lebensbedrohliche Erkrankung unweigerlich zum Tod führen würde.

15. Wie alt sind Sie?:

16. Geschlecht:

(a) Weiblich
(b) Männlich

17. Höchste abgeschlossene Ausbildung:

(a) Nicht abgeschlossene Pflichtschule
(b) Pflichtschule
(c) Lehre
(d) Fachschule oder Handelsschule
(e) Matura
(f) Fachhochschule
(g) Universität

18. Postleitzahl des Orts, in dem Sie leben:

Appendix B

Full questionnaire translated
QUESTIONNAIRE ON THE AWARENESS AND KNOWLEDGE OF PALLIATIVE MEDICAL CARE IN THE STYRIAN POPULATION
1. In your opinion, what are the greatest fears of a patient who has been diagnosed with a terminal illness? (Please select three of the following options and rank them in order of relevance—1st, 2nd, 3rd)
___ Fear of pain.
___ Fear of death.
___ Fear of no longer being independent.
___ Fear of losing mental capabilities.
___ Fear of loneliness.
___ Fear of becoming disabled/immobile.
___ Fear of financial burdens.
___ Fear of being a burden to someone.
___ I don't know.

2. What services do you think should be provided to people with a terminal illness and their families? (You may give several answers.)

(a) Help at home in case of pain and other symptoms.
(b) Domestic care for the patient during the day.
(c) Domestic care for the patient at night.
(d) Complementary therapies.
(e) Pastoral care.
(f) A social worker that the patient and family could reach on the phone if necessary.
(g) Assistance with household tasks, shopping, transportation etc.
(h) Additional support at home to allow the family caregivers to have some free time and time for themselves.
(i) Information and advice on financial aid.
(j) Medical care in a hospice.
(k) Medical care in hospital

3. How much do you think people generally speak about death and dying? (Please select one answer only.)

(a) Too little.
(b) About the right amount.
(c) Too much.

4. If you had a terminal illness, where would you like to spend the final stage of your life? (Please select one answer only.)

(a) At home.
(b) In a hospital.
(c) In a nursing home.
(d) I don't know.

5. Do you know what a patient decree is?

(a) Yes.
(b) No.

6. How do you rate your knowledge and awareness of palliative care in our federal state? (Please select one answer only.)
(a) I know nothing about palliative care.
(If "a" is true for you, please continue to question 15.)
(b) I have heard about palliative care.
(c) I know a fair amount about palliative care.
(d) I know a great deal about palliative care.

7. If you have already heard of palliative care, where did you find out about it? (You may give several answers.)

(a) I have received palliative care myself.
(b) A close friend/relative has received palliative care.
(c) A distant relative/acquaintance has received palliative care.
(d) A neighbor has received palliative care.
(e) A friend or relative has told me about it.
(f) I work with patients that receive palliative care.
(g) I work in the field of medicine.
(h) Radio/TV/newspaper.
(i) Internet/social media.
(j) Fundraising/charity drives.
(k) Other: ______________________________

8. Please select the following sentence that in your opinion best describes palliative care. (Please select one answer only.)

(a) Palliative care hastens death.
(b) Palliative care delays death.
(c) Palliative care permits the patient to continue living an active life.
(d) Palliative care calms the patient.
(e) Palliative care improves the patient's quality of life.
(f) I don't know.

9. What do you think are the greatest needs of patients with a terminal illness that have reached the end of their lives? (Please select three of the following options and rank them in order of relevance—1st, 2nd, 3rd)

____ Reduction in physical suffering.
____ Specialist medical care.
____ Home nursing care (medical and nursing services).
____ Support for home-based caregivers.
____ Professional psychological support.
____ Spiritual support.
____ I don't know.

10. What do you think are the greatest needs of family members that provide care to a patient with a terminal illness? (Please select three of the following options and rank them in order of relevance—1st, 2nd, 3rd)

____ 24-hour specialist care.
____ Home nursing care.
____ Access to and availability of voluntary caregivers.
____ Specially adapted residential facilities/hospices.
____ Psychological care.
____ Grief counseling.
____ I don't know.

11. Where and by whom do you think care is best provided to patients with a terminal illness? (Please select one answer only.)

(a) At home by family/relatives.
(b) At home by professional care workers.
(c) In a hospice.
(d) In hospital.
(e) I don't know.

12. Has anyone in your family or circle of friends and acquaintances had any personal experience of palliative care? (Please select one answer only.)

(a) Yes.
(b) No.

13. Among patients with the illnesses listed in the table below, which do you think should receive palliative care? (Please mark one of the options for each illness.)

	5 (I fully agree.)	4 (I agree.)	3 (I partly agree.)	2 (I don't agree.)	1 (I don't agree at all.)	I don't know	I don't know anything about this illness
Cancer							
Kidney failure							
Amyotrophic Lateral Sclerosis (ALS)							
Dementia							
Stroke							
Heart failure							
HIV/AIDS							
Chronic lung diseases							
Multiple Sclerosis							

14. If you were diagnosed with a terminal illness, when would you like to be provided with information on palliative care? (Please select one answer only.)

(a) I would not want any information.
(b) I would like the information to be publicly available.
(c) I would like to receive such information when my terminal illness became life-threatening.
(d) I would like to receive such information when it became clear that I was dying of my terminal illness.

15. How old are you? __

16. Gender:

(a) Female
(b) Male

17. Highest level of education:

(a) Compulsory schooling incomplete
(b) Compulsory schooling
(c) Apprenticeship
(d) Technical college/trade school
(e) High school (general qualification for university entrance)
(f) University of Applied Sciences
(g) University

18. Postal code of your home: ______________

Appendix C

Table A1. Differences in survey participants' views on the greatest needs of palliative care patients (table corresponding to Figure 1).

			(a) Age			
	18–34 Years	35–49 Years	50–64 Years	65+ Years	*p*-Value	
Spiritual support	1.4%	2.7%	0.0%	1.5%	0.505	
Reducing physical suffering	74.3%	76.0%	69.5%	73.5%	0.822	
Psychological care	10.1%	4.0%	3.7%	0.0%	0.031	
Medical specialist care	2.9%	8.0%	6.1%	8.8%	0.462	
Home nursing care	7.1%	8.0%	14.6%	7.4%	0.317	
Caregiver support	4.3%	0.0%	3.7%	5.9%	0.177	
			(b) Education			
	EL1: Compulsory School	EL2: Apprentice-ship	EL3: Trade School	EL4: High School	EL5: University	*p*-Value
Spiritual support	0.0%	0.0%	1.9%	2.3%	2.2%	0.581
Reducing physical suffering	71.4%	69.0%	75.9%	65.9%	79.8%	0.381
Psychological care	0.0%	2.3%	1.9%	9.1%	6.7%	0.241
Medical specialist care	4.8%	11.5%	7.4%	2.3%	3.4%	0.189
Home nursing care	9.5%	11.5%	9.3%	11.4%	6.7%	0.811
Caregiver support	4.8%	4.6%	3.7%	6.8%	0.0%	0.101
		(c) Sex				
	Female	Male	*p*-Value			
Spiritual support	1.6%	1.0%	1.000			
Reducing physical suffering	72.3%	75.0%	0.610			
Psychological care	5.8%	1.9%	0.149			
Medical specialist care	7.3%	4.8%	0.399			
Home nursing care	8.4%	11.5%	0.376			
Caregiver support	2.6%	4.8%	0.331			

Table A2. Differences in survey participants' views on the greatest needs of their relatives (table corresponding to Figure 2).

		(a) Age			
	18–34 Years	35–49 Years	50–64 Years	65+ Years	*p*-Value
Volunteer caregivers	5.7%	6.7%	6.1%	2.9%	0.774
Psychological care	27.1%	20.0%	14.6%	2.9%	0.001
Hospice	2.9%	10.7%	9.8%	11.8%	0.237
Home nursing	30.0%	26.7%	26.8%	20.6%	0.646
Grief counseling	8.6%	1.3%	2.4%	5.9%	0.145
24 h availability of specialist care	22.9%	33.3%	36.6%	48.5%	0.017

Table A2. *Cont.*

(b) Education						
	EL1: Compulsory School	**EL2: Apprentice-ship**	**EL3: Trade School**	**EL4: High School**	**EL5: University**	***p*-Value**
Volunteer caregivers	4.8%	5.7%	3.7%	6.8%	5.6%	0.974
Psychological care	0.0%	9.2%	16.7%	27.3%	21.3%	0.010
Hospice	0.0%	10.3%	11.1%	0.0%	12.4%	0.048
Home nursing	28.6%	23.0%	20.4%	22.7%	33.7%	0.360
Grief counseling	19.0%	1.1%	5.6%	9.1%	1.1%	0.002
24 h availability of specialist care	38.1%	47.1%	38.9%	34.1%	21.3%	0.010
(c) Sex						
	Female	**Male**	***p*-Value**			
Volunteer caregivers	5.2%	5.8%	0.847			
Psychological care	18.8%	11.5%	0.104			
Hospice	8.9%	8.7%	0.943			
Home nursing	22.0%	33.7%	0.029			
Grief counseling	5.2%	2.9%	0.554			
24 h availability of specialist care	35.6%	34.6%	0.865			

Table A3. Differences in survey participants' views on the fears of palliative care patients (table corresponding to Figure 3).

(a) Age						
	18–34 Years	**35–49 Years**	**50–64 Years**	**65+ Years**	***p*-Value**	
Pain	15.8%	22.2%	32.0%	27.8%	0.030	
Losing mental abilities	5.8%	4.0%	8.7%	12.4%	0.131	
Losing independence	16.7%	17.2%	13.6%	20.6%	0.623	
Loneliness	2.5%	0.0%	0.0%	1.0%	0.216	
Financial burdens	0.8%	0.0%	1.0%	0.0%	1.000	
Death	40.8%	47.5%	30.1%	11.3%	0.000	
Being a burden to someone	12.5%	6.1%	3.9%	14.4%	0.026	
Becoming disabled	4.2%	3.0%	7.8%	9.3%	0.195	
(b) Education						
	EL1: Compulsory School	**EL2: Apprentice-ship**	**EL3: Trade School**	**EL4: High School**	**EL5: University**	***p*-Value**
Pain	28.6%	26.3%	21.4%	14.5%	28.3%	0.200
Losing mental abilities	11.4%	5.9%	10.0%	11.8%	4.2%	0.222
Losing independence	20.0%	19.5%	17.1%	19.7%	11.7%	0.467
Loneliness	5.7%	0.8%	0.0%	1.3%	0.0%	0.038
Financial burdens	0.0%	0.0%	2.9%	0.0%	0.0%	0.034
Death	14.3%	32.2%	28.6%	36.8%	39.2%	0.067
Being a burden to someone	14.3%	4.2%	8.6%	9.2%	13.3%	0.137
Becoming disabled	5.7%	8.5%	10.0%	3.9%	2.5%	0.141

Table A3. *Cont.*

(c) Sex			
	Female	**Male**	***p*-Value**
Pain	27.5%	19.4%	0.058
Losing mental abilities	7.4%	8.0%	0.813
Losing independence	19.3%	13.7%	0.135
Loneliness	0.8%	1.1%	1.000
Financial burdens	0.4%	0.6%	1.000
Death	26.6%	41.7%	0.001
Being a burden to someone	10.7%	7.4%	0.262
Becoming disabled	5.7%	6.3%	0.815

Table A4. Differences in survey participants' views on the services that should be provided to palliative care patients and their relatives (table corresponding to Figure 4).

(a) Age						
	18–34 Years	**35–49 Years**	**50–64 Years**	**65+ Years**	***p*-Value**	
Time off for family caregivers	53.3%	59.6%	62.1%	57.7%	0.593	
Pastoral care	42.5%	16.2%	10.7%	8.2%	0.000	
Nightcare	40.0%	49.5%	44.7%	34.0%	0.150	
Information on financial support	45.0%	44.4%	34.0%	14.4%	0.000	
Home pain management	65.8%	73.7%	69.9%	71.1%	0.635	
Home assistance	49.2%	34.3%	37.9%	37.1%	0.109	
Daycare	57.5%	47.5%	47.6%	43.3%	0.181	
Complementary and alternative medicine	15.0%	30.3%	32.0%	13.4%	0.001	
Availability of social workers	34.2%	29.3%	30.1%	14.4%	0.009	
(b) Education						
	EL1: Compulsory School	**EL2: Apprentice-ship**	**EL3: Trade School**	**EL4: High School**	**EL5: University**	***p*-Value**
Time off for family caregivers	48.6%	61.0%	51.4%	64.5%	57.5%	0.370
Pastoral care	8.6%	12.7%	12.9%	30.3%	30.0%	0.000
Nightcare	37.1%	39.0%	38.6%	43.4%	47.5%	0.614
Information on financial support	25.7%	28.0%	32.9%	51.3%	35.8%	0.012
Home pain management	57.1%	68.6%	75.7%	73.7%	69.2%	0.346
Home assistance	40.0%	31.4%	35.7%	50.0%	45.0%	0.071
Daycare	51.4%	43.2%	45.7%	51.3%	55.8%	0.362
Complementary and alternative medicine	14.3%	20.3%	27.1%	25.0%	22.5%	0.590
Availability of social workers	11.4%	22.9%	21.4%	28.9%	39.2%	0.004

Table A4. *Cont.*

	(c) Sex		
	Female	**Male**	***p*-Value**
Time off for family caregivers	64.3%	49.1%	0.002
Pastoral care	23.0%	17.1%	0.147
Nightcare	45.5%	37.1%	0.088
Information on financial support	38.5%	30.3%	0.081
Home pain management	71.3%	68.0%	0.466
Home assistance	38.1%	42.9%	0.329
Daycare	50.0%	48.6%	0.773
Complementary and alternative medicine	25.4%	18.3%	0.085
Availability of social workers	29.5%	24.6%	0.264

References

1. World Health Organization (WHO). Palliative Care. Available online: https://www.who.int/news-room/fact-sheets/detail/palliative-care (accessed on 14 June 2023).
2. Bajwah, S.; Oluyase, A.O.; Yi, D.; Gao, W.; Evans, C.J.; Grande, G.; Todd, C.; Costantini, M.; Murtagh, F.E.; Higginson, I.J. The effectiveness and cost-effectiveness of hospital-based specialist palliative care for adults with advanced illness and their caregivers. *Cochrane Database Syst. Rev.* **2020**, *9*, CD012780.
3. Hui, D.; Hannon, B.L.; Zimmermann, C.; Bruera, E. Improving patient and caregiver outcomes in oncology: Team-based, timely, and targeted palliative care. *CA Cancer J. Clin.* **2018**, *68*, 356–376. [CrossRef] [PubMed]
4. May, P.; Garrido, M.M.; Cassel, J.B.; Kelley, A.S.; Meier, D.E.; Normand, C.; Smith, T.J.; Stefanis, L.; Morrison, R.S. Prospective cohort study of hospital palliative care teams for inpatients with advanced cancer: Earlier consultation is associated with larger cost-saving effect. *J. Clin. Oncol.* **2015**, *33*, 2745. [CrossRef]
5. McIlfatrick, S.; Hasson, F.; McLaughlin, D.; Johnston, G.; Roulston, A.; Rutherford, L.; Noble, H.; Kelly, S.; Craig, A.; Kernohan, W.G. Public awareness and attitudes toward palliative care in Northern Ireland. *BMC Palliat. Care* **2013**, *12*, 34. [CrossRef] [PubMed]
6. Kahveci, K.; Gökçınar, D. Knowledge about palliative care in the families of patients. *Acta Med.* **2014**, *30*, 1370–1372.
7. Huo, J.; Hong, Y.-R.; Grewal, R.; Yadav, S.; Heller, I.W.; Bian, J.; Wilkie, D.J. Knowledge of palliative care among American adults: 2018 health information national trends survey. *J. Pain Symptom Manag.* **2019**, *58*, 39–47.e33. [CrossRef] [PubMed]
8. Zelko, E.; Gašpar, D.; Gjuras, E.; Škvarč, N.K. Awareness and expectations of visitors to family medicine practices about palliative care in Slovenia. *Acta Med. -Biotech.* **2021**, *14*, 18–27. [CrossRef]
9. Maciasz, R.; Arnold, R.; Chu, E.; Park, S.; White, D.; Vater, L.; Schenker, Y. Does it matter what you call it? A randomized trial of language used to describe palliative care services. *Support Care Cancer* **2013**, *21*, 3411–3419. [CrossRef] [PubMed]
10. Bandieri, E.; Borelli, E.; Gilioli, F.; Bigi, S.; Mucciarini, C.; Ferrari, U.; Eliardo, S.; Pinto, L.; Porro, C.A.; Efficace, F. Stigma of Palliative Care among Patients with Advanced Cancer and Their Caregivers on Early Palliative Care. *Cancers* **2023**, *15*, 3656. [CrossRef] [PubMed]
11. Steiermaerkische Krankenanstaltengesellschaft m.b.h. Koordination Palliativbetreuung. Available online: https://www.palliativbetreuung.at/ueber-uns#c38104 (accessed on 26 July 2022).
12. Farnik, M.; Pierzchała, W.A. Instrument development and evaluation for patient-related outcomes assessments. *Patient Relat. Outcome Meas.* **2012**, *4*, 1–7. [CrossRef] [PubMed]
13. Benini, F.; Fabris, M.; Pace, D.S.; Verno, V.; Negro, V.; De Conno, F.; Orzalesi, M.M. Awareness, understanding and attitudes of Italians regarding palliative care. *Ann. Dell'istituto Super. Sanità* **2011**, *47*, 253–259.
14. Spatuzzi, R.; Giulietti, M.V.; Ricciuti, M.; Merico, F.; Romito, F.; Reggiardo, G.; Birgolotti, L.; Fabbietti, P.; Raucci, L.; Rosati, G.; et al. Does Family Caregiver Burden Differ between Elderly and Younger Caregivers in Supporting Dying Patients with Cancer? An Italian Study. *Am. J. Hosp. Palliat. Med.* **2020**, *37*, 576–581. [CrossRef] [PubMed]
15. Dahlberg, L.; Demack, S.; Bambra, C. Age and gender of informal carers: A population-based study in the UK. *Health Soc. Care Community* **2007**, *15*, 439–445. [CrossRef]
16. Bueno, M.V.; Chase, J.-A.D. Gender Differences in Adverse Psychosocial Outcomes among Family Caregivers: A Systematic Review. *West. J. Nurs. Res.* **2023**, *45*, 78–92. [CrossRef] [PubMed]
17. Brazil, K.; Thabane, L.; Foster, G.; Bédard, M. Gender differences among Canadian spousal caregivers at the end of life. *Health Soc. Care Community* **2009**, *17*, 159–166. [CrossRef] [PubMed]
18. Tur-Sinai, A.; Teti, A.; Rommel, A.; Hlebec, V.; Lamura, G. How many older informal caregivers are there in Europe? Comparison of estimates of their prevalence from three European surveys. *Int. J. Environ. Res. Public Health* **2020**, *17*, 9531. [CrossRef]

19. Strupp, J.; Köneke, V.; Rietz, C.; Voltz, R. Perceptions of and Attitudes toward Death, Dying, Grief, and the Finitude of Life—A Representative Survey Among the General Public in Germany. *OMEGA J. Death Dying* **2021**, *84*, 157–176. [CrossRef] [PubMed]
20. Collins, A.; McLachlan, S.-A.; Philip, J. Community knowledge of and attitudes to palliative care: A descriptive study. *Palliat. Med.* **2020**, *34*, 245–252. [CrossRef]
21. Tanuseputro, P.; Budhwani, S.; Bai, Y.Q.; Wodchis, W.P. Palliative care delivery across health sectors: A population-level observational study. *Palliat. Med.* **2017**, *31*, 247–257. [CrossRef] [PubMed]
22. Griebler, R.; Straßmayr, C.; Mikšová, D.; Link, T.; Nowak, P. *Gesundheitskompetenz in Österreich: Ergebnisse Der Österreichischen Gesundheitskompetenzerhebung HLS19-AT*; Bundesministerium für Soziales: Vienna, Austria, 2021.
23. Zelko, E.; Bollig, G. *Report from the Third International Last Aid Conference: Cultural Diversity in Palliative Care*; SAGE Publications Sage UK: London, UK, 2023; Volume 17, p. 26323524231166932.
24. Bollig, G.; Brandt, F.; Ciurlionis, M.; Knopf, B. Last aid course. An education for all citizens and an ingredient of compassionate communities. *Healthcare* **2019**, *7*, 19. [CrossRef] [PubMed]

healthcare

MDPI

Article

Experiences of Primary Care Nurse Case Managers in Palliative Care Needs Identification and Complex Chronic Patients' Referral to Advanced Palliative Care Resources

María Inmaculada Herrera-Gómez [1], Luz María Iribarne-Durán [2,*], María Paz García-Caro [1,3,4], Manuel López-Morales [1,3,5], Ana Alejandra Esteban-Burgos [1,6] and Rafael Montoya-Juárez [1,3,4]

1 Instituto de Investigación Biosanitaria de Granada (ibs. GRANADA), 18012 Granada, Spain; mpazgc@ugr.es (M.P.G.-C.); malomorales@ugr.es (M.L.-M.); aesteban@ujaen.es (A.A.E.-B.); rmontoya@ugr.es (R.M.-J.)
2 Centro Nacional de Sanidad Ambiental, Instituto de Salud Carlos III (CNSA-ISCIII), 28222 Granada, Spain
3 Departamento de Enfermería, Universidad de Granada, 18016 Granada, Spain
4 Centro de Investigación Mente, Cerebro y Comportamiento, Universidad de Granada, 18071 Granada, Spain
5 Servicio de Urgencias de Atención Primaria, Sistema Andaluz de Salud, 18013 Granada, Spain
6 Departamento de Enfermería, Universidad de Jaén, 23071 Jaén, Spain
* Correspondence: luzmaria.iribarne@isciii.es; Tel.: +34-918-223-740

Abstract

Introduction: Palliative needs assessment and referral to advanced palliative care resources are fundamental aspects of complex chronic patients' care. Primary care Nurse Case Managers play a key role in the care of these patients. **Objective:** We aimed to describe the experiences of primary care Nurse Case Managers in palliative care needs identification and complex chronic patients' referral to advanced palliative care resources. **Method:** This is a qualitative descriptive study with a phenomenological approach. Semi-structured online interviews were conducted with primary care Nurse Case Managers. A thematic analysis was performed using ATLAS.ti software. **Results:** 20 nurses participated, 16 of whom were women, with a mean age of 52.3 years and an average of 15.9 years of experience in primary care. Regarding "Palliative care Needs Assessment", four sub-themes have been identified: "What do you understand?", "How do you assess?", "Difficulties" and "Alternatives" to current palliative care needs assessment. For the "Palliative Care Referral" theme four sub-themes have been identified: "Criteria", "Tools", "Difficulties" and "Alternatives" for referral. Discussion: Palliative needs are identified in patients with incurable diseases when there are no curative treatment options and when quality of life must be prioritized. Symptoms, general condition, progression, and comorbidity are assessed. Open interviews and home visits are essential for assessing the social and family context and the home resources available. Barriers identified include the conspiracy of silence, limited training in non-oncological palliative care, and a lack of staff and caregiver's understanding of illness situation. The presence of difficult symptoms and a limited life expectancy were identified as key criteria for referral to palliative care. The physician's assessment, the family's request, and consultation with specialized teams play a key role in prognosis. Barriers include late referrals, lack of a palliative background, inequity in access to resources, and low visibility of the palliative care needs of non-cancer patients. **Conclusions:** Significant challenges remain in identifying palliative needs and referral to specialized resources, highlighting the need to optimize resources, strengthen professional training, and improve coordination between levels of care to ensure quality palliative care.

https://doi.org/10.3390/healthcare14010085

Keywords: palliative care; palliative medicine; terminal care; primary care; prognosis; nursing

1. Introduction

Palliative care (PC) focuses on improving the quality of life of patients and families facing problems associated with life-threatening illnesses through the prevention and relief of suffering [1]. Although initially focused exclusively on the care of cancer patients, its current scope includes any chronic disease in advanced and terminal stages. According to the World Health Organization (WHO), palliative care should begin at the onset of any life-threatening illness and become more relevant as the patient progresses toward death [1].

The model of Care for People with Complex Needs in Catalonia [2] defines three situations related to the progression of chronic disease: the complex chronic patient (CCP), the advanced chronic patient, and the terminally ill patient. CCPs are chronic patients who have complex health needs arising from the coexistence of chronic diseases, organ or system dysfunction, and factors involving healthcare or social complexity [3]. In the case of advanced chronic patients, palliative care needs (PCN) arise, such as limited life expectancy and increased demands of symptom control, management of therapeutic futility, identification of patient values and preferences, attention to spirituality, and addressing the psychosocial needs of the patient and family [4–6].

Healthcare professionals, especially in primary care (PC), must be trained to identify CCPs with PCN. To improve the identification of PCN, it is necessary to have instruments that allow standardization of data collection and facilitate comparison over time, such as the NECPAL CCOMS-ICO [5]. The NECPAL CCOMS-ICO tool is a validated screening instrument designed to support the early identification of individuals with PCNs through a multidimensional, prognostic, and needs-based approach, developed by the Catalan Institute of Oncology. This tool integrates the Surprise Question (*"Would you be surprised if this patient died within the next 12 months?"*) as a screening tool to assess 14 indicators of PCN, including functional, cognitive, and nutritional decline, the presence of dependence, multimorbidity, healthcare resources, and specific indicators of advanced chronic diseases.

On the other hand, another fundamental characteristic of the integrated PC model proposed by both the WHO and the European Association for Palliative Care (EAPC) is the provision of care at two levels: basic and advanced PC [7,8]. Basic PC should be provided by all professionals, in any context (primary care, hospitals, nursing homes) to patients with non-complex PCN. In contrast, specialized PC is provided by specialized resources and services whose main activity is the provision of PC, aimed at patients with high palliative complexity. Some patients will only require basic PC, but others will need to be referred to specialized PC, in complex situations or on a continuous basis until their death. Referral to PC means that specialized PC team professionals must act in coordination with teams providing basic care, especially those in primary care, to provide continuity of care throughout the course of the disease [7]. In the context of the Andalusian Public Health System, the Palliative Care Complexity Diagnostic Tool (IDC-Pal) [9,10] allows the identification of patients who require referral to specialized PC, establishing the level of palliative complexity based on the clinical, psychological, and social factors of the patients.

The role of primary care healthcare professionals is fundamental in identifying palliative needs and referring patients with complex conditions to specialized PC resources. In this regard, primary care nurse case managers (NCM) in Andalusia have the necessary skills to participate in both functions [11]. Although NCMs do not have the competences to refer patients to specialized palliative care resources themselves, they can participate in the

https://doi.org/10.3390/healthcare14010085

discussion about which patients may need these resources and should help gather all the necessary information for this purpose. Nevertheless, the experience of these professionals regarding the identification of palliative care needs and the referral to specialized PC resources is crucial and has not been described in previous research.

This study is part of the INCOPAL project (AP-0209-2019), which aimed to determine the effectiveness of an intervention based on the standardized assessment of the PCN and complexity of CCPs, using the NECPAL CCOMS-ICO and IDC-Pal tools. At the end of the project, it was decided to conduct a qualitative study to describe the experiences of the NCM, both participating and non-participating in the INCOPAL project, regarding the identification of PCN and referral of CCP to specific PC resources.

2. Methods

2.1. Design

Descriptive qualitative study with a phenomenological approach. This methodological perspective allows for an in-depth exploration and comprehensive understanding of the participants' experiences in their professional practice, considering their accounts as a primary source of knowledge [12]. Qualitative descriptive studies produced findings closer to the data as given, (or data-near), and are linked to thematic analysis [13].

2.2. Selection of Participants

Primary care NCMs with more than three years of experience were selected from centres in all provinces of Andalusia. NCMs who had been part of the INCOPAL project participated were asked to recommend at least one other NCM who had not participated in the project and was not familiar with its objectives or results, using snowball sampling.

2.3. Data Collection Instruments and Procedure

A semi-structured interview script (Table 1) was used, developed ad hoc and organized into three blocks: PCN, Referral to PC, and evaluation of the INCOPAL project (this was only answered by project participants). The professionals were contacted by phone or email, agreeing with each one on a date for the interview. All interviews were conducted via Google Meet and recorded on video. The researchers who conducted the interviews had no professional relationship with the interviewees. Authorization for recording and subsequent transcription was obtained at the beginning of each interview. Participants were guaranteed the right to withdraw from the study at any time, without having to justify their decision or suffer any prejudice as a result. The recordings were accessible only to the research team and for the sole purpose of transcribing the results.

Table 1. Semi-structured interview questions.

	Questions
Palliative Care Needs	• What do you understand by palliative needs? • How do you assess palliative needs in your daily practice? • What difficulties do you face in assessing palliative needs? • What would you change? What alternatives would you have?
PC Referral	• When do you refer a case to palliative care? • What is that process like? • What difficulties do you face in referring to palliative care? • What would you change? What alternatives would you have?
INCOPAL Evaluation	• How has your view of palliative care needs assessment and referral to palliative care changed because of participating in the project?

https://doi.org/10.3390/healthcare14010085

2.4. Data Analysis

The interviews were transcribed verbatim. A thematic analysis was conducted, following a structured sequence. Prior the analysis, the researchers reflected of their positions and experiences on palliative care needs identification and complex chronic patients' referral to advanced palliative care resources. First, each transcript was read thoroughly to familiarize with the content. Subsequently, a second, more detailed reading was conducted, assigning codes to the most relevant pieces of information. The themes and sub-themes were determined by the interview questions, while the codes were identified inductively. Two researchers discussed and agreed on the codes. A third researcher participated in the discussion in case agreement could not be reached on the inclusion of a code. The researchers considered that theoretical saturation had been reached, given that no new codes appeared in the last interviews conducted. The entire analysis was performed using ATLAS.ti 9.1.3 software (Berlin, Germany). This study has been approved by the Research Ethics Committee of the Andalusian Public Health System.

3. Results

As shown in Table 2, 20 NCMs from Andalusia participated in the study. 9 NCMs (45%) participated in the INCOPAL project, while 11 (55%) did not. Of the total number of participants, 4 were men (20%) and 16 were women (80%). The mean age was 52.3 years (SD = 8.72), and the mean experience in PC was 15.9 years (SD = 12.09) (Table 2).

Table 2. Participants characteristics.

	INCOPAL	Age (Years)	Gender	Experience in Primary Care (Years)
1	Yes	46	Female	10
2	No	30	Male	7
3	Yes	61	Male	39
4	No	48	Male	9
5	No	46	Female	3
6	No	34	Female	4
7	Yes	61	Female	35
8	Yes	57	Female	18
9	No	57	Female	21
10	Yes	57	Male	35
11	No	60	Female	20
12	No	54	Female	3
13	Yes	61	Female	5
14	Yes	60	Female	22
15	Yes	60	Female	7
16	No	55	Female	3
17	No	50	Female	20
18	No	56	Female	34
19	No	49	Female	17
20	Yes	56	Female	6

The codes used in the analysis are illustrated by textual quotations from the participants (verbatims). Participants verbatims were identified by their code, age, sex (M = Men/W = Woman), and whether they had participated in the INCOPAL project (yes/no).

https://doi.org/10.3390/healthcare14010085

3.1. Palliative Needs

The codes, themes and sub-themes related to PCNs are shown in Figure 1.

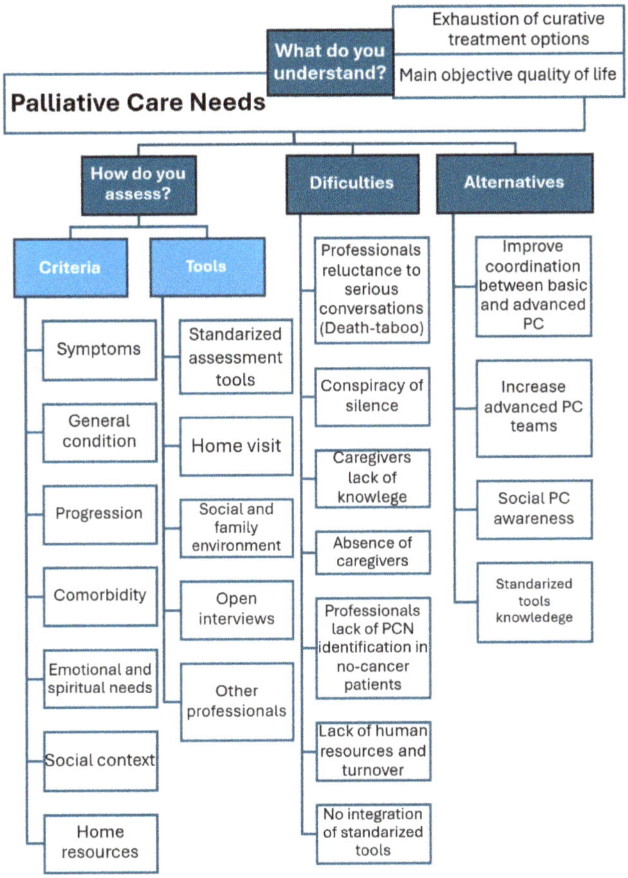

Figure 1. Palliative Care Needs codes, themes and sub-themes.

3.1.1. What Do You Understand by PCNs?

Although none of the participants clearly defined what they understood by PCN, most agreed that patients with PCN are those with cancer or non-cancer diseases who have *exhausted all curative treatment options*. At this point, the *main objective becomes the quality of life* of both the patient and their family. One interviewee emphasized that PC should begin as soon as an incurable disease is diagnosed, without waiting for the patient to reach the terminal stage.

"You are going to focus on comfort care, on care that does not go beyond simply making the patient feel as comfortable as possible." (19, 49 y, W, No INCOPAL)

"Above all, you have to provide care, comfort measures aimed more at their well-being, more at the intention of caring than at curing those diseases." (4, 48 y, W, No)

"Patients with complex chronic conditions that progress to the end and patients who have cancer, where the progression is much faster and more aggressive, and who may come to me at much more complex stages." (16, 55 y, W, No)

"Palliative care should be provided from the moment I am diagnosed with an incurable disease." (2, 30 y, M, No)

https://doi.org/10.3390/healthcare14010085

3.1.2. How Do You Assess PCNs?

The assessment of PCN involves a comprehensive evaluation of different *criteria*: clinical *symptoms*, the patient's *general condition*, their *progression*, and the presence of *comorbidities*. In this assessment, the *emotional and spiritual needs* of patients also become relevant.

"Assessing not only clinical and care aspects, but also emotional and spiritual aspects is essential because, at the end of the day, is what moves us, and what perhaps enables us to face these difficult moments." (10, 57 y, W, yes)

"Above all, addressing those spiritual needs of how they are coping with the process, what strengths they have as internal resources when working through moments of crisis in their daily lives." (16, 55 y, W, No)

Regarding PCNs assessment tools, some interviewees use *standardized assessment tools* that are integrated into the computer system in their daily practice. The NCMs participating in the INCOPAL project mention that they use different instruments to identify PCN and the IDC-pal to determine the degree of complexity of the patient.

"At the clinical level, I assess palliative needs first according to clinical symptoms, clinical pathology, progression, patient dependence, and the complexity of that care." (1, 46 y, W, yes)

"Through the IDC-pal and the Barthel, Pfeiffer, social, and Gijón questionnaires. And if I see that the patient is in the final stage, the Karnofsky as well" (17, 50 y, W, No)

Some interviewees highlighted the importance of assessing not only the patient, but also their *social and family environment*, especially caregivers burden and the availability of resources in the home.

"Knowing what the family environment is like, what problems they have, what that patient means to the family, well, that's very important in order to care both, the patient and the family." (8, 57 y, W, yes)

"I don't just focus on the person. I also focus on the caregiver, the family surrounding the palliative patient, and what I do is an assessment of basic needs." (18, 56 y, W, No)

In this sense, *home visits* are essential for assessing PCN. *Open interviews* with the patient allow them to express their concerns and needs more freely, obtaining information that is not always revealed in a standard consultation with a structured interview.

"I usually try to listen a lot, listen carefully to what they tell me because sometimes it gives me much more information than when you are interrogating them." (7, 61 y, W, yes)

"I like it that way, directly with the patient and in a natural way, which is good. Which is part of the process, of course." (2, 30 y, M, No)

On the other hand, some interviewees point out that they do not have the opportunity to directly evaluate PCNs, as these are assessed in advance by *other healthcare professionals* before their intervention.

"They usually come already defined by the internist." (12, 54 y, W, No)

"I access palliative care patients through hospital NCMs and through my colleagues, so they practically come to me already assessed." (2, 30 y, M, No)

3.1.3. Difficulties in Assessing PCNs

Among the difficulties in assessing PCN, all participants highlighted the *conspiracy of silence*, which limits open communication about the reality of the disease and hinders informed decision-making. Healthcare professionals themselves contribute to this situation by avoiding difficult conversations about prognosis and limited treatment options.

"I try to make the family understand that I know that they want to protect their relative (. . .) But I also try to make them see that the patient has rights and we cannot deny them; Patients have the right to know or not to know." (18, 56 y, W, No)

https://doi.org/10.3390/healthcare14010085

"Often, this conspiracy of silence comes from professionals who do not dare to communicate the few therapeutic options available and show a difficult reality." (10, 57 y, M, yes)

Some interviewees acknowledge that *caregivers do not have the adequate knowledge* to take on the task of caregiving. One participant mentions the progressive decline in informal caregivers or *absence of caregivers* due to changes in family structure.

"Sometimes what I find is that you have to inform the family on how to use all the resources they may have." (12, 54 y, W, No)

"There are not as many caregivers available anymore. Caregivers are older, they are also very advanced in age." (10, 57 y, M, yes)

Almost all interviewees agree that *death remains a taboo* in society, which makes it difficult to accept PC. There is still *professionals' reluctance* to address this type of care, perceiving it as synonymous with failure. Family members and patients also share this perception.

"The society we live turns its back on death. It is a society that only seeks to extent life at any price." (16, 55 y, W, No)

"Culturally, when you reach palliative care, it is a failure. In fact, patients and family members experience it that way at first." (15, 60 y, W, yes)

On the other hand, the *lack of training in PC* is another significant barrier that hinders the identification and addressing of patients' needs. This lack of training particularly impacts professionals' ability to address patients' emotional and spiritual needs. In addition, there is a notable *lack of training in identifying PCN in non-oncology patients*, which contributes to many patients having delayed access to PC, limiting the interventions and support they can receive.

"There are areas that we tend to neglect, which, in the context of the end of life, need to be worked on, such as the emotional and spiritual spheres, which are difficult to work on with patients and which we find a little difficult to address." (4, 48 y, M, No)

"We all understand that when we cannot cure a cancer patient, they are palliative, but what about those frail elderly people, those with heart failure, those with COPD..." (6, 34 y, W, No)

"I see that these patients continue to attend consultations, follow-ups, and appointments with specialists, and no one makes the decision to say that at this point the patient is in a palliative situation." (19, 49 y, W, yes)

Participants also pointed out the *lack of healthcare personnel* and the continuous *turnover* of staff, especially nurses. Short-term contracts create instability in teams, which affects continuity of care and hinders specialization in PC. In addition, they cite a lack of time to perform a comprehensive assessment of patients, which leads them to prioritize the most obvious cases. All of this generates frustration and helplessness among professionals.

"The fundamental problem is the mobility we have had lately with professionals" (19, 49 y, W, yes)

"I don't know if in primary care, healthcare professionals are able to devote time, and perhaps that is what is failing us in identifying those patients who are not affiliated with palliative care." (6, 34 y, W, No)

The NCMs participating in the INCOPAL project indicated that essential tools, such as the IDC-Pal or NECPAL, are *not integrated into the computer system*, which makes it difficult to apply and record them in the medical record. Furthermore, the medical record is not always completed properly, and information regarding previous interventions, referrals, and home visits is not clearly reflected.

"The computer tool is used here in Andalusia, but it doesn't have many tools that facilitate that assessment." (4, 48 y, M, No)

https://doi.org/10.3390/healthcare14010085

"It's true that we have the IDC-Pal scale, but that scale, for example, is not registered in (the computer system). Since we don't have it registered, it's more complicated to register it." (11, 60 y, W, No)

3.1.4. Alternatives to Actual PCNs Assessment

As alternatives for assessing PCN, some interviewees highlighted the need to *improve coordination basic and advanced level of PC*, that might enhance continuity of care. Others, however, propose *increasing the number of specialized PC nurses and doctors*. One participant suggests implementing a "red button" in the computer system that would allow for early identification of patients with PCN, even before they are referred to specific resources.

"We should all work together so that the patient really benefits from my timely intervention, but also from the continuity of care provided by the palliative care unit and primary care." (6, 34 y, W, No)

"Provide palliative care with more staff so that they can care for patients entering the palliative process, regardless of the level of complexity." (17, 50 y, W, No)

"That you can really identify it in (computer system), medicine, and nursing, even if you can't refer it to the teams." (8, 57 y, W, yes)

Several interviewees highlighted the need to *raise awareness* among both professionals and society about the importance of PC. This involves ensuring access to PC training for all professionals. Some suggested that training should be mandatory during working hours. Interviewees who did not participate in the INCOPAL project emphasized the *need to know scales and instruments for assessing PCNs*, while those who collaborated in the project highlighted that it has allowed them to learn about and become familiar with many of these tools.

"End of life is part of the life cycle and that professionals have to be prepared to respond to that situation and also adapt and establish strategies for action." (6, 34 y, W, No)

"Perhaps offering some kind of more advanced course that people could take at a more affordable price and that would also be easier to attend in terms of work." (7, 61 y, W, yes)

3.2. *Referral to PC*

The themes and sub-themes related to referral to advanced PC resources are shown in Figure 2.

3.2.1. Criteria for Specialized PC Referral

One of the criteria for referral to PC most frequently mentioned by participants is the presence of *symptoms that are difficult to manage in primary care setting*. Participants emphasized that these patients require specialized management due to the complexity of their needs.

"When I make that assessment and find that the patient is highly complex and beyond the response we can give in primary care, that's when I refer them." (18, 56 y, W, No)

"Those complex chronic patients who are basically immobilized with almost 24-h home care. That's when I understand that it's time to move the person into the palliative care process." (10, 57 y, M, yes)

Other interviewees point out that referral to PC is considered when the patient is estimated to have a *short- or medium-term life expectancy*. Likewise, other interviewees state that, in their experience, referral to PC is usually made for cancer patients who cannot tolerate treatment and have *exhausted all therapeutic options*.

https://doi.org/10.3390/healthcare14010085

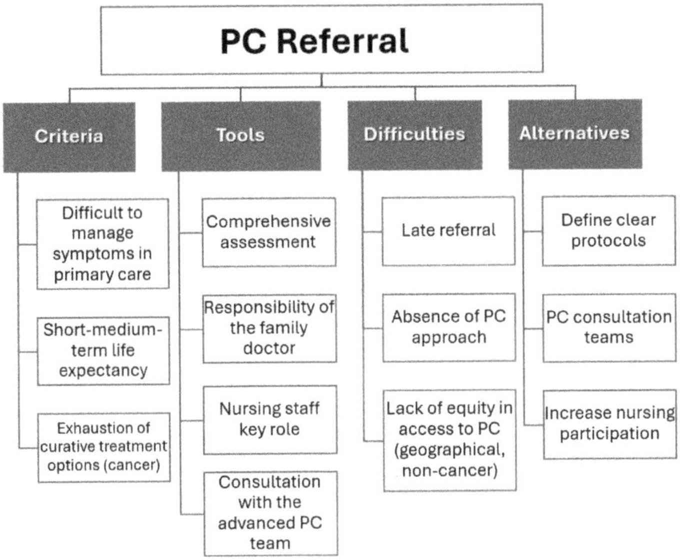

Figure 2. Referral to advanced PC resources codes, themes and sub-themes.

"If the person is in a palliative situation, undergoing palliative treatment, with no cure, and it is a matter of time and a short- to medium-term prognosis, then palliative care should be initiated." (9, 57 y, W, No)

"When I see that the situation is more complex and when the patient requires, let's say, a short-term prognosis." (11, 60 y, W, No)

"When the signs and symptoms treated by their family doctor do not resolve the situation or improve the patient's condition, we have exhausted all resources in terms of treatment, tests, and so on. Then we need more advanced resources." (13, 61 y, W, yes)

3.2.2. Tools for Specialized PC Referral

In relation to the referral process, the first step is to perform a *comprehensive assessment*. Half of the participants agreed that this assessment is the *responsibility of the family doctor*, although *nursing staff play a key role*. Several interviewees emphasized that this process requires close coordination with the multidisciplinary team.

" The doctor performs a physical examination and so on. While we make our assessment based on needs and also perform a physical examination." (18, 56 y, W, No)

"Talking to the care team: family doctor, family nurses, social worker at the healthcare centre, in order to communicate the situation of reversibility, worsening, poor prognosis, increased intensity of interventions and visits..." (10, 57 y, M, yes)

Many of the participants highlighted the *consultation with the specialized PC team*, emphasizing the need for fluid communication. Other NCMs stated that, in some cases, it is the family who requests PC when they perceive a deterioration in the patient's condition.

"If a patient is referred who is in a much more advanced stage and I want them to be seen soon, I speak to them (specialized PC team) directly and maybe they will see them the next day." (14, 60 y, W, yes)

"Often it is the family who contacts you, because sometimes you don't get to see all the patients, they are being seen by specialists." (20, 56 y, W, yes)

https://doi.org/10.3390/healthcare14010085

3.2.3. Difficulties for Specialized PC Referral

Among the difficulties in referral to PC, some interviewees pointed out that referral often occurs *too late*, when the patient is already in the last days of life. They mentioned that, in practice, it is difficult to refer patients in the early or intermediate stages of the process, due to the *reluctance of certain health professionals to adopt a palliative care approach*.

"They act when the patient is already in a very advanced or final stage, when it is time to sedate, while all the literature tells you is that these teams have to work intensively at the beginning of the process." (8, 57 y, W, yes)

"They want to be too clear when sending patients to palliative care. It has to be too obvious from the beginning to send them." (15, 60 y, W, yes)

On the other hand, participants highlighted the *lack of equity in access to PC*, depending on *geographical factors*. Some patients from rural areas die without receiving adequate PC, far from their families or without the possibility of staying at home, as they would wish. Several interviewees emphasized that *non-cancer patients* have more difficult access to PC.

"It is very sad that, depending on where you live, you may die with more or less dignity because if you want to die at home, if you don't have a home support and palliative care team, you may not be able to consider it." (14, 60 y, W, yes)

"I mean that it (PC) depends on the professional you get, it depends on which hospital you are in, it depends on which service, it depends on which health centre your home is in, it depends on whether you get the morning shift, the afternoon shift, the night shift..." (18, 56 y, W, No)

Some participants suggested the need to *define clear protocols* for referring patients to the hospital, avoiding unnecessary steps, and optimizing coordination between PC and hospital services. Other NCM suggested the creation of *PC consultation teams* within districts or hospital centres, to offer advice and continuous updating on the management of PC patients. Several interviewees recommended that referral to PC should not depend exclusively on the physician, but that the *nursing team should actively participate* in the referral and decision-making process. One interviewee proposed the creation of a specialized team for non-oncological diseases, and another the creation of a specific form in the computer system.

"Establishing this formal, well-known, and clear circuit, especially in the event that a patient needs to be referred to a hospital. Above all to avoid that initial hassle at the emergency room door." (4, 48 y, M, No)

"It would be great to have a unit or a team of highly trained people in the district or hospital or somewhere where we can ask for information or where we can always be up to date." (2, 30 y, M, No)

"There should also be an advanced support team to help us primary care professionals carry out this follow-up and approach work for non-cancer patients." (10, 57 y, M, yes)

"Nurses are the ones who are actually doing the work at home, and follow-up care for patients at home is mainly carried out by nurses, which means that nurses are the first to realize when a patient needs palliative care." (16, 55 y, W, No)

"If there was a questionnaire or form in the computer program that could be filled out and sent to palliative care at to be viewed, it would be much faster" (17, 50 y, W, No)

3.3. Evaluation of the INCOPAL Project

3.3.1. Changes in Participants' Understanding of PC

The INCOPAL project has generated changes in the perception and approach to PC by the participating NCMs. It has allowed them to *understand that the approach to PC* transcends physical symptoms, and they have adopted a *more holistic view* in their professional practice. One of the participants stated that his perception of which patients require PC has changed,

https://doi.org/10.3390/healthcare14010085

now *including non-oncology patients*. Another interviewee mentioned that the project has helped to highlight the *importance of early detection of PCN*, allowing for better care planning.

"What really needs to be identified is not just the symptoms, but much more than that, namely the families, the team, how to approach that patient with the entire team." (1, 46 y, W, yes)

"We always have the concept of palliative care for cancer patients, and really, with this participation, I have seen that this is not the case. Palliative patients involve many more pathologies than just cancer." (1, 46 y, W, yes)

"The project helps you to appreciate more or make more visible the palliative care needs at an earlier stage." (15, 60 y, W, yes)

Some NCM stated that the project has made them *more aware of the difficulties in PC*, such as the lack of resources or the difficulty of accessing the services. Others highlighted the *importance of scales and questionnaires* to assess patients in a more accurate and structured way.

3.3.2. Criticism of INCOPAL Project

In this regard, some of the participants recommended *reducing the number of questionnaires*, eliminating those that are redundant or irrelevant, or combining the questionnaires into one. On the other hand, one participant pointed out that he has missed *specific instruments to assess the situation of the primary caregiver*.

"It really reflects the gap between palliative needs and the response we provide." (8, 57 y, W, yes)

"Knowing some questionnaires and assessment scales that we could incorporate into that assessment to make it more complete." (13, 61 y, W, yes)

"There are questionnaires that I would remove because an assessment, an evaluation of the patient with all these questionnaires is practically impossible, so I would reduce them." (1, 46 y, W, yes)

"There are no scales aimed at assessing the caregiver's situation, the caregiver's emotions, the difficulty the caregiver has had or is having in caring for that complex chronic person in palliative care. I have missed them." (10, 57 y, M, yes)

4. Discussion

This is one of the first studies to describe the experience of NCM in palliative care needs identification and CCP referral to advanced PC resources.

The NCMs interviewed conduct a comprehensive assessment of PCN using standardized scales and open interviews as assessment tools. Among the criteria for referral to advanced PC resources, are difficult-management symptoms and limited prognosis. Barriers such as the conspiracy of silence, lack of training in specialist care, and scarcity of resources persist, leading to late referrals and inequality in access to specialist care.

Late identification of PCN is one of the main difficulties in providing PC. PCN are often recognized too late, limiting the possibility of early intervention in the course of the disease. In this regard, the participants in our study indicated that referral to PC takes place when the available therapeutic options have been exhausted. Only one of them pointed out that PC should begin at the onset of the life-threatening disease.

According to Van der Stap et al. [14], curative and disease-focused treatments are often prolonged excessively, delaying the initiation of PC and negatively impacting the quality of care. Conversely, the implementation of early palliative care improves the patient's understanding of their disease process and the quality of end-of-life care and reduces the use of excessive therapeutic measures during the last month of life [15]. The regular use of standardized tools such as NECPAL [5] in CCP can improve access to PC for these patients.

https://doi.org/10.3390/healthcare14010085

One of the problems pointed out by participants is the lack of attention to non-cancer patients. PC was originally designed for terminally ill cancer patients, so there is limited knowledge about when and how to transition to PC in non-cancer patients [16]. Bonares et al. [17] demonstrated, in a comparison between cardiologists, pulmonologists, and oncologists in Canada, that non-cancer patients are less likely to receive specialized palliative care and are referred later. In this regard, Jang et al. [18] show that non-cancer patients may experience levels of suffering equal to or even greater than cancer patients, due, among other factors, to the lack of identification of PCN in these patients.

The lack of human and material resources to perform a comprehensive assessment of the patient in PC negatively impacts the assessment of PCN. Pitzer et al. [19] identified in a mixed methods systematic review that lack of human resources is a main barrier in providing PC. These difficulties were supported by Jones et al. [20], who highlighted the shortage of nurses in PC, as well as geographical inequality in access to specialized PC services. Future studies should consider staffing levels and the geographical dispersion of the population as key factors of inequality in access to PC in cancer and non-cancer patients.

The healthcare professionals interviewed reported lack of training in PC, especially in addressing patients emotional and spiritual needs. A recent review [21] highlighted that PC professionals face a lack of training and insufficient preparation to deliver spiritual care. Pavlic et al. [22] supported this observation by pointing out that, while pain management is usually include in healthcare training, other fundamental aspects, such as non-physical symptoms and the psychosocial and spiritual dimensions of care, are often insufficiently addressed, especially in non-cancer patients.

This research shows that some professionals continue to perceive PC as synonymous with therapeutic failure. The focus on cure, the nonacceptance of terminal prognosis and the negative perceptions of palliative care was highlighted as a barrier in the provision of PC in Pitzer et al. review [19]. Shen and Wellman [23] pointed to the existence of a social stigma associated with PC, linking them to surrender, weakness, or the loss of hope, which influences people's willingness to accept them for themselves or their loved ones.

4.1. Strengths and Limitations

This study is one of the first studies conducted to explore the experience of NCMs in PCN identification and CCP referral to advanced PC resources. The inclusion of professionals from different parts of Andalusia is a strength, as it provides a diversity of perspectives; however, the uneven distribution of the sample across provinces may have influenced the results, given that working conditions and the organization of health services vary considerably across the region. The majority participation of female NCMs accurately reflects the feminization of the nursing profession, providing a realistic picture of the professional profile in PC. However, this overrepresentation may have partially conditioned the interpretation of the results, limiting the male perspective. Finally, although the cross-sectional design captures the perceptions of NCMs at a specific point in time, it offers an up-to-date snapshot of the impact of the INCOPAL project on clinical practice. As a qualitative study, the results should be considered carefully to extrapolate conclusions to other similar contexts. Nevertheless, qualitative research methodology does not aim for representativeness of the results, but rather for understanding the phenomena.

4.2. Clinical, Policies and Research Implications

From a clinical perspective, the systematic use of validated tools such as NECPAL [5] should be promoted to enhance the early detection of PCN and facilitate proactive care planning in CCP. Policymakers should prioritise the incorporation of standardized instruments into digital systems and ensure time for comprehensive assessment.

https://doi.org/10.3390/healthcare14010085

Furthermore, strengthening NCM competencies through structured PC education programs is crucial, particularly in areas such as psychosocial and spiritual care.

Clinical practice should also prioritize the inclusion of non-cancer patients, who continue to experience inequitable access to PC. Policies should promote disease-specific referral criteria and interprofessional protocols, particularly those that recognise nurses' competencies in initiating referrals, could mitigate this imbalance and ensure equitable PC delivery across diagnostic groups.

Research should explore interventions aimed at reducing professional barriers to PC implementation and examine their impact on clinical decision-making and patient satisfaction.

Finally, policymakers and managers should address structural determinants of inequality in PC, including workforce shortages, regional disparities, and limited service availability. Addressing these gaps will be essential to advancing equitable, holistic, and patient-centred PC for all individuals with life-limiting illnesses.

5. Conclusions

For NCMs, early comprehensive assessment of PCN in oncological and non-oncological patients and their families is a key element of PC in primary care. NCMs use standardized scales, home visits, and open interviews, and they face barriers such as the conspiracy of silence, death taboo, lack of training and human resources. Difficult-to-manage symptoms and limited prognosis are prominent factors in the referral of CCPs to PC. Late referral and inequity in access to advanced PC resources continue to occur due to geographical dispersion and limited visibility of the needs of non-oncological patients. It is necessary to strengthen coordination between levels of care, establish clear protocols, and enable digital tools that facilitate a more agile and equitable response to PC.

Author Contributions: Conceptualization, L.M.I.-D. and R.M.-J.; Methodology, R.M.-J.; Formal analysis, M.I.H.-G. and L.M.I.-D.; Investigation, M.P.G.-C. and A.A.E.-B.; Resources, M.L.-M. and R.M.-J.; Data curation, M.I.H.-G. and L.M.I.-D.; Writing—original draft, M.I.H.-G., L.M.I.-D., M.P.G.-C., A.A.E.-B. and R.M.-J.; Writing—review & editing, L.M.I.-D., M.P.G.-C., M.L.-M., A.A.E.-B. and R.M.-J. All authors have read and agreed to the published version of the manuscript.

Funding: This research was funded by grants from "Biomedical and Health Sciences Research, Development, and Innovation in Andalusia" by the Regional Government of Andalusia (AP-0209-2019). The authors also thank the Ministry of Science, Innovation, and Universities for the postdoctoral research contract (JDC2023-052607-I) awarded to L.M. Iribarne-Durán. The funders had no role in the study design, data collection or analysis, decision to publish, or preparation of the manuscript.

Institutional Review Board Statement: The study was conducted in accordance with the Declaration of Helsinki, and the protocol was approved by the Ethics Committee of Andalucía (approval no. 2d2d98a57bb6e00fb5a6e99969c7fcb7839c5cdc, approval date: 16 October 2019).

Informed Consent Statement: Informed consent was obtained from all subjects involved in the study.

Data Availability Statement: The database used and analyzed in this study is available from the corresponding author upon reasonable request. Access is restricted due to confidentiality, privacy, and ethical considerations, as the data contain sensitive personal information that could potentially identify study participants.

Conflicts of Interest: The authors declare no conflicts of interest.

https://doi.org/10.3390/healthcare14010085

References

1. Palliative Care-World Health Organization. Available online: https://www.who.int/es/news-room/fact-sheets/detail/palliative-care (accessed on 4 November 2025).
2. Blay, C.; Limón, E. *Bases Para un Modelo Catalán de Atención a las Personas con Necesidades Complejas: Conceptualización e Introducción a los Elementos Operativos. Programa de Prevenció i Atenció a la Cronicitat*; Departament de Salut, Generalitat de Catalunya: Barcelona, Spain, 2017; Available online: https://hdl.handle.net/11351/3305 (accessed on 4 November 2025).
3. Ministerio de Sanidad, Servicios Sociales e Igualdad. *Estrategia Para el Abordaje de la Cronicidad en el Sistema Nacional de Salud*; Ministerio de Sanidad, Servicios Sociales e Igualdad: Madrid, Spain, 2012.
4. Amblàs-Novellas, J.; Murray, S.A.; Oller, R.; Torné, A.; Martori, J.C.; Moine, S.; Latorre-Vallbona, N.; Espaulella, J.; Santaeugènia, S.J.; Gómez-Batiste, X. Frailty degree and illness trajectories in older people towards the end-of-life: A prospective observational study. *BMJ Open* **2021**, *11*, e042645. [CrossRef] [PubMed]
5. Gómez-Batiste, X.; Martínez-Muñoz, M.; Blay, C.; Amblàs, J.; Vila, L.; Costa, X.; Espaulella, J.; Villanueva, A.; Oller, R.; Martori, J.C.; et al. Utility of the NECPAL CCOMS-ICO© tool and the Surprise Question as screening tools for early palliative care and to predict mortality in patients with advanced chronic conditions: A cohort study. *Palliat. Med.* **2017**, *31*, 754–763. [CrossRef] [PubMed]
6. Calsina-Berna, A.; AmblàsNovellas, J.; González-Barboteo, J.; Bardés Robles, I.; Beas Alba, E.; Martínez-Muñoz, M.; Madariaga Sánchez, R.; Gómez Batiste Alentorn, X. Prevalence and clinical characteristics of patients with Advanced Chronic Illness and Palliative Care needs, identified with the NECPAL CCOMS-ICO© Tool at a Tertiary Care Hospital. *BMC Palliat. Care* **2022**, *21*, 210. [CrossRef] [PubMed]
7. World Health Organization. *Integrating Palliative Care and Symptom Relief into Primary Health Care: A WHO Guide for Planners, Implementers and Managers*; World Health Organization: Geneva, Switzerland, 2018.
8. Radbruch, L.; Payne, S. White paper on standards and norms for hospice and palliative care in Europe: Part 1. *Eur. J. Palliat. Care* **2009**, *16*, 278–289.
9. Martín-Roselló, M.L.; Fernández-López, A.; Sanz-Amores, R.; Gómez-García, R.; Vidal-España, F.; Cía-Ramos, R. *IDC-Pal: Instrumento Diagnóstico de la Complejidad en Cuidados Paliativos. Documento de Apoyo al PAI Cuidados Paliativos*; Junta de Andalucía, Consejería de Igualdad, Salud y Políticas Sociales: Sevilla, Spain, 2014.
10. Carrasco-Zafra, M.I.; Gómez-García, R.; Ocaña-Riola, R.; Martín-Roselló, M.L.; Blanco-Reina, E. Level of Palliative Care Complexity in Advanced Cancer Patients: A Multinomial Logistic Analysis. *J. Clin. Med.* **2020**, *9*, 1960. [CrossRef] [PubMed]
11. Junta de Andalucía, Consejería de Salud y Consumo. *Proceso Asistencial Integrado: Cuidados Paliativos*, 3rd ed.; Junta de Andalucía, Consejería de Salud y Consumo: Sevilla, Spain, 2019.
12. Husserl, E. *Invitación a la Fenomenología*; Paidós: Barcelona, Spain, 1998.
13. Sandelowski, M. What's in a name? Qualitative description revisited. *Res. Nurs. Health* **2010**, *33*, 77–84. [CrossRef] [PubMed]
14. Van der Stap, L.; de Nijs, E.J.M.; Oomes, M.; Juffermans, C.C.M.; Ravensbergen, W.M.; Luelmo, S.A.C.; Horeweg, N.; van der Linden, Y.M. The self-perceived palliative care barriers and educational needs of clinicians working in hospital primary care teams and referral patterns: Lessons learned from a single-center survey and cohort study. *Ann. Palliat. Med.* **2021**, *10*, 2620–2637. [CrossRef] [PubMed]
15. Hui, D.; Heung, Y.; Bruera, E. Timely Palliative Care: Personalizing the Process of Referral. *Cancers* **2022**, *14*, 1047. [CrossRef] [PubMed]
16. Kim, S.; Lee, K.; Kim, S. Knowledge, attitude, confidence, and educational needs of palliative care in nurses caring for non-cancer patients: A cross-sectional, descriptive study. *BMC Palliat. Care* **2020**, *19*, 105. [CrossRef] [PubMed]
17. Bonares, M.; Le, L.W.; Zimmermann, C.; Wentlandt, K. Specialist Palliative Care Referral Practices Among Oncologists, Cardiologists, Respirologists: A Comparison of National Survey Studies. *J. Pain Symptom Manag.* **2023**, *66*, e1–e34. [CrossRef] [PubMed]
18. Jang, H.; Lee, K.; Kim, S.; Kim, S. Unmet needs in palliative care for patients with common non-cancer diseases: A cross-sectional study. *BMC Palliat. Care* **2022**, *21*, 151. [CrossRef] [PubMed]
19. Pitzer, S.; Kutschar, P.; Paal, P.; Mülleder, P.; Lorenzl, S.; Wosko, P.; Osterbrink, J.; Bükki, J. Barriers for Adult Patients to Access Palliative Care in Hospitals: A Mixed Methods Systematic Review. *J. Pain Symptom Manag.* **2024**, *67*, e16–e33. [CrossRef] [PubMed]
20. Jones, R.; Dale, J.; MacArtney, J. Challenges experienced by NCMs when providing palliative care in the UK: A systematic qualitative literature review. *BJNCM Open* **2023**, *7*, BJNCMO.2022.0159. [CrossRef]
21. Costeira, C.; Querido, A.; Ventura, F.; Loureiro, H.; Coelho, J.; Benito, E.; Nabal, M.; Dones, M.; Specos, M.; Laranjeira, C. Spiritual Care [Givers] Competence in Palliative Care: A Scoping Review. *Healthcare* **2024**, *12*, 1059. [CrossRef] [PubMed]

https://doi.org/10.3390/healthcare14010085

22. Rotar Pavlič, D.; Aarendonk, D.; Wens, J.; Rodrigues Simões, J.A.; Lynch, M.; Murray, S. Palliative care in primary care: European Forum for Primary Care position paper. *Prim. Health Care Res. Dev.* **2019**, *20*, e133. [CrossRef] [PubMed]
23. Shen, M.J.; Wellman, J.D. Evidence of palliative care stigma: The role of negative stereotypes in preventing willingness to use palliative care. *Palliat. Support. Care* **2019**, *17*, 374–380. [CrossRef] [PubMed]

https://doi.org/10.3390/healthcare14010085

healthcare

MDPI

Review

Last Aid Courses as a Means for Public Palliative Care Education—A Narrative Review of the Literature and 10 Years of Experience Around the World with Implications for Future Research

Georg Bollig [1,2,3,4,*,†], Jason Mills [3,5,*,†], Sindy Müller-Koch [3,6], Pandeli Pani [3,7], Bianca Neumann [8,9] and Erika Zelko [3,10,11]

1 Department of Anesthesiology, Intensive Care, Palliative Medicine and Pain Therapy, Helios Klinikum Schleswig, 24837 Schleswig, Germany
2 Department of Palliative Medicine, Faculty of Medicine and University Hospital, University of Cologne, 50937 Cologne, Germany
3 Last Aid Research Group International (LARGI), 24837 Schleswig, Germany
4 Letzte Hilfe Deutschland gGmbH, 24837 Schleswig, Germany
5 Research Centre for Palliative Care, Death, and Dying (RePaDD), College of Nursing and Health Science, Flinders University, Adelaide 5042, Australia
6 Nursing Home am Lerchenberg, 06886 Wittenberg, Germany
7 Deutsche Welle, 53113 Bonn, Germany
8 Sue Ryder, London NW1 1BU, UK
9 International Observatory on End of Life Care, Division of Health Research, Faculty of Health and Medicine, Health Innovation One, Sir John Fisher Drive, Lancaster University, Lancaster LA1 4AT, UK
10 Institute for Palliative Medicine, Medical Faculty, University Maribor, 2000 Maribor, Slovenia
11 Institute for General Medicine, Medical Faculty, Johannes Keppler University, 4040 Linz, Austria
* Correspondence: georg.bollig@helios-gesundheit.de (G.B.); jason.mills@flinders.edu.au (J.M.)
† These authors contributed equally to this work.

Abstract

Objective: To provide a narrative overview of the scientific knowledge on Last Aid Courses and experiences from different countries. **Background**: The levels of death literacy, grief literacy, and knowledge about palliative care are low in many countries around the world. For many people, dying, death, and grief are still a taboo. Public Palliative Care Education (PPCE), the public knowledge approach, and the Last Aid Course (LAC) aim to increase death literacy, grief literacy, and public knowledge about palliative care. **Methods**: A literature search in the databases PubMed/Medline, CINAHL, and PsycInfo was undertaken. Other additional sources were found by hand searching, books, reference lists, and the internet. A narrative overview of the existing literature on LAC and Public Palliative Care Education (PPCE) is provided. Experiences with PPCE and LAC from different countries are presented. Based on the findings, a future agenda for research on PPCE and LAC is presented. **Results and Discussion**: PPCE and LAC have been introduced in 23 countries. A total of 17 articles and reviews on Last Aid were included. Research on the effects of LAC in different countries and cultural issues connected to LAC are ongoing. **Conclusions**: Since 2015, LACs have been introduced in 23 different countries. The LAC, the LAC-KT, and PPCE may enhance the public debate on dying, death, grief, and palliative care and may empower people to contribute to end-of-life care in the community. Future research on PPCE, the LAC, and the LAC-KT should focus on retention over time and the long-term effects of the courses.

Keywords: palliative care; public palliative care education; end-of-life care; compassionate communities; Last Aid Course; health literacy; death literacy; grief literacy; education

1. Introduction

The global demand for palliative and end-of-life care is expected to rise in the coming decades due to the growing number of chronically ill, elderly, and frail individuals worldwide [1–8]. Moreover, as most people express a preference for spending their final days at home, the need for home-based palliative care will also continue to increase around the world [9–12]. Due to the limited resources of the health care services in communities, several authors have recommended a public health palliative care approach, including citizens in palliative care provision in the community [13–16]. Kellehear posed the statement that "end-of-life care is everyone's business", meaning that everyone in the community should be engaged in palliative care provision in the community in cooperation with health care professionals [14,15]. A key problem and barrier for palliative care provision by lay persons in the community is the lack of public awareness around palliative care, death literacy, and grief literacy [17–28]. The first step for people to engage in palliative care provision in the community is awareness and the acquisition of basic knowledge on palliative care, which can be obtained from Last Aid Courses (LACs) for both lay people and professionals from healthcare and social services, as described by Bollig as the public knowledge approach to palliative care. This approach includes health, death, and grief literacy as parts of Public Palliative Care Education (PPCE) for everyone that ideally should already start in childhood [13,29].

Across many countries, broader social and demographic shifts are influencing how people understand and engage with death, dying, and care at the end of life. Many countries are also grappling with the realities of an ageing population, where growing numbers of older people are living with long-term conditions while health and social care services face increasing pressure [30]. At the same time, it has been shown how everyday caring roles have gradually moved from families and neighbourhoods into professional services, leaving many people feeling uncertain about how to help when someone is dying [31,32]. These changes sit alongside persistent gaps in public preparedness for dying and bereavement, with population studies reporting low levels of death literacy and limited awareness of palliative care or advance planning [33]. Research also suggests that people who have direct experience of caregiving or community involvement often develop a stronger sense of confidence and readiness around end-of-life issues, pointing to the value of experiential learning [34,35]. Hospices have increasingly responded to these needs by expanding their educational role. Hospices today are not only training health and social-care professionals but also offering outreach to schools, community groups, and local organisations to strengthen public confidence, communication, and practical skills around serious illness and bereavement. While such hospice-led programmes reflect well-established local approaches, recent international evidence highlights that low public and professional literacy about end-of-life care remains a major global barrier to equitable palliative care access, and that basic education for the wider health and social-care workforce is an urgent priority [8]. Due to a lack of awareness for palliative care and low death and grief literacy in the public, a number of experts have recommended education of the public [13,17–22]. Different experts and the Lancet Commission on the Value of Death have recommended improved death literacy, knowledge, and skills in end-of-life care for everyone [13,17,28,29]. In 1986, the World Health Organization's Ottawa Charter for Health Promotion recommended that the collaboration between health care services and communities should be an essential part of public health, including end-of-life care [36]. The long-established community-owned palliative care model in Kerala [37] demonstrates that when education and basic training are widely available, community-based approaches to end-of-life care can be implemented

https://doi.org/10.3390/healthcare14010096

at scale, with volunteers, families, and local organisations taking on meaningful roles in awareness-raising, practical support and care. In several European countries, nationally coordinated Public Palliative Care Education initiatives, such as Last Aid, have been developed to address similar challenges by providing accessible, standardised education for the general population. (Inter)national programmes like these can complement and strengthen local efforts by offering consistent, population-level learning opportunities that help bridge the gaps created by uneven resources, geographical variation, and differing levels of community engagement. Because these programmes are led by international steering groups that review and update course content on a regular basis, they can also help reduce bias and guard against knowledge inertia, ensuring that public education remains consistent with current evidence and diverse cultural perspectives. These wider insights offer an important foundation for understanding why Public Palliative Care Education has an increasingly significant role in strengthening community capacity and supporting shared involvement in end-of-life care. These international programmes can also help sustain public engagement and learning in settings where local resources are limited, offering a level of continuity that can be difficult for individual hospices or community organisations to maintain. When funding, staffing, or organisational capacity fluctuate, it is often the more resource-intensive activities, such as research, ongoing curriculum development, and publication, that are hardest to continue. Broader international initiatives can act as a stable framework that complements and supports local provision during these periods of strain.

Last Aid Courses (LACs), Last Aid Courses for kids and teens (LAC-KTs), and the public knowledge approach suggested by Bollig aim to enhance the public discussion on serious illness, dying, death, and grief and to provide the public with basic knowledge and skills in palliative care [13,29]. Last Aid Courses can be seen as building the knowledge base for compassionate communities to enable and empower the public for palliative care provision in the community [13,29]. LACs are standardized courses with four teaching modules with 45 min each that are taught by two certified Last Aid Course instructors with experience in the field of palliative care. The LAC is usually provided in a classroom setting with six to twenty participants but can also be held as an online course. It includes presentations, discussions, and practical training. An international Last Aid working group is responsible for a consensus on the standardized course curriculum and the course contents. National differences that need to be addressed and included in the national slide presentation are topic legislation, advance care planning, and the national organisation of palliative care provision [13]. Table 1 provides an overview of the four modules of the LAC and their contents.

Since the first introduction of the Last Aid Courses in Norway, Denmark, and Germany in 2014/2015, standardized LACs have been started in 23 countries in Europe, Canada, Brazil, Australia, and Singapore. In 2019, the Last Aid Research Group International (LARGI) was founded during the First International Last Aid Conference in Sønderborg in Denmark. The LARGI is a cooperation of international researchers and works on research on the views of participants and LAC instructors as well as the effects of the LAC worldwide. The German NGO Letzte Hilfe Deutschland gGmbH celebrated the 10th anniversary of Last Aid Courses for the public in Germany with a symposium in Schleswig in May 2025. After a decade of implementing the public knowledge approach for palliative care and LACs across multiple countries, it is appropriate to reflect on and synthesize the accumulated experience.

Aim of the study: To provide a narrative overview of the scientific knowledge on Last Aid Courses and the experiences from different countries using Public Palliative Care Education (PPCE) as framework.

https://doi.org/10.3390/healthcare14010096

Table 1. Contents of the Last Aid Course.

Module Nr.	Topic	Course Content
Module 1	Dying as a normal part of life	• Welcome and introductions • First aid and last aid • What you can do to care • The process of dying
Module 2	Planning ahead	• Networks of Support • Making decisions • Medical and ethical aspects • Advance care planning • Advance Directive • Medical power of attorney
Module 3	Relieving suffering	• Typical problems and symptoms • Caring/relieving suffering • Nutrition at the end of life • How to comfort
Module 4	Final goodbyes	• Saying goodbye/final farewell rituals • Funeral and various forms of burials • Grieving is normal • Grief and ways of grieving • Questions and comments

Duration of the LAC: 3.5 h including four modules with 45 min each plus a break of 30 min.

2. Materials and Methods

The current narrative review builds on a review that was previously published four years ago in 2021 [13]. To update and advance knowledge with a more precise context, the focus of this narrative review is on scientific publications about Last Aid and Public Palliative Care Education published between January 2015 and September 2025. First, a systematic search of the peer-reviewed literature was conducted using a predefined search strategy. PubMed, Medline, CINAHL, and PsycInfo databases were searched using the keyword "last aid" and MeSH (Medical Subject Heading) terms "palliative care education" and "public". All searches were limited to full-text articles published between 2015 and September 2025 in English language peer-reviewed journals. In addition to this, other sources were found by searching the internet, hand searching, books, and reference lists of papers and book chapters on the above-mentioned topics. Sources that were searched for this narrative review included the following:

- Searches in the databases PubMed and Medline, CINAHL, and PsycInfo;
- Internet searches;
- Hand searches from reference lists of retrieved literature;
- Written and oral reports of personal experiences from members of the International Last Aid working group, international experts, and the first author from the implementation of Public Palliative Care Education using Last Aid Courses in different countries.

Selection criteria for inclusion in the review were as follows: only articles in English published in scientific journals that fulfilled the inclusion criteria were included. The inclusion criteria used were as follows: publications focused on Last Aid Courses or Public Palliative Care Education for citizens. All other publications were excluded. Screening was undertaken by multiple reviewers to ensure that only those papers meeting inclusion criteria were included, and agreement was reached by discussion if differences were identified. Assessment of the presented articles included type of publication (original article,

https://doi.org/10.3390/healthcare14010096

review, etc.), main topic of the paper, evaluation method used (quantitative, qualitative, etc.), informants and response rate, main findings, and involved countries. The included articles are presented in Table 2 based on the above-mentioned criteria. An overview of the findings from the literature search and experiences from the implementation process will be presented under thematically arranged subthemes in the results. The methods used for data collection, analysis, and reporting follow the recommendations for narrative literature reviews proposed by Green, Johnson, and Adams [38]. In addition, the narrative review checklist was used for reporting the findings from the literature search [38]. Public Health Palliative Care (PHPC) and Public Palliative Care Education (PPCE) were used as a guiding framework to inform the review. PPCE is an approach to teach the public about dying, death, grief, and palliative care [39] and combines different literacies including health, death, and grief literacy. Through this combined approach, societies shall be empowered to talk openly about these topics and encouraged to participate in the care of people in need of palliative care in the community.

https://doi.org/10.3390/healthcare14010096

Table 2. Overview of Last Aid studies and reviews.

Articles: Authors, Journal, and Publication Year	Main Topic	Type of Study	Evaluation Method	Informants and Response Rate	Involved Countries	Main Findings
Bollig G, Mainzer K, Fiedler H, Pothmann R. The Last Aid Course for kids and teens from 8–14 years: Preliminary results from the first pilot test. *Hospice & Palliative Medicine International Journal*. 2020 Jan 14;4(1):1–3. [40]	First LAC-KT pilot course	Pilot study	Oral feedback from a group discussion	- Ten kids and teens from 9 to 14 years - 100% participated in an oral feedback round after the course	Germany	• LAC-KT is feasible and very well accepted by children and teenagers from 9 to 14 years of age. • Children and teenagers want to talk and learn about dying, death, and grief.
Bollig G, Knopf B, Meyer S, Schmidt M. A new way of learning end-of-life care and providing public palliative care education in times of the COVID-19 pandemic: Online Last Aid Courses. *Archives of Health Sciences*. 2020 Sep;4(1):1–2. [41]	Online Last Aid course (OLAC) started during the COVID-19 pandemic	Opinion article	Description of the work to establish an OLAC and proposal for implementation and research	Description of the process of establishing an OLAC by a working group and the very first experiences of the instructors	Germany	• Suggestions for implementation of OLAC are provided. • The first experiences with both Last Aid courses for citizens and the training of Last Aid Course instructors using online meetings are very encouraging. • Scientific evaluation of the OLAC is ongoing.
Bollig G, Meyer S, Knopf B, Schmidt M, Bauer EH. First experiences with online Last Aid Courses for public palliative care education during the COVID-19 pandemic. *Healthcare*. 2021 Feb 5;9(2). 172. [42]	Online Last Aid course (OLAC) started during the COVID-19 pandemic	Prospective mixed methods multicentre study	Questionnaire after course participation and focus group discussions of German Last Aid course instructors	A total of 92 of 156 participants (response rate 59%) from 15 online Last Aid Courses from Germany and Brazil	Germany Brazil	• Online Last Aid Courses are feasible and well accepted by the participants. • The online format increased the number of participants who are caregivers and younger people. • Many participants and instructors prefer classroom teaching, thus the online course was described as the second-best choice only.
Bollig G, Brandt Kristensen F, Wolff DL. Citizens appreciate talking about death and learning end-of-life care: A mixed-methods study on views and experiences of 5469 Last Aid Course participants. *Progress in Palliative Care*. 2021;29(3):140–148. [29]	Evaluation of LAC from Germany, Switzerland and Austria	Prospective mixed-methods multicentre study from three countries	Questionnaire after course participation	A total of 5469 of 6014 Last Aid Course participants from 408 courses in Germany, Switzerland, and Austria (response rate 91%)	Germany Switzerland Austria	• The median age of participants was 56 years. • A total of 88% were female. • A total of 76% of participants rated the course as very good. • A total of 99% would recommend the course to others. • Last Aid Courses are both feasible and accepted by citizens from different countries and backgrounds. • A total of 9.4% of participants had a medical profession.

https://doi.org/10.3390/healthcare14010096

Table 2. *Cont.*

Articles: Authors, Journal, and Publication Year	Main Topic	Type of Study	Evaluation Method	Informants and Response Rate	Involved Countries	Main Findings
Mueller E, Bollig G, Becker G, Boehlke C. Lessons learned from introducing Last Aid Courses at a university hospital in Germany. *Healthcare*. 2021 Jul 16;9(7). 906. [43]	LAC for employees of a tertiary university hospital	Prospective study using questionnaires	Pre- and post-survey questionnaire before and after LAC participation	A total of 55 of 56 participants completed an evaluation survey (response rate 98%)	Germany	• The most prevalent learning goals were preparation for emotional aspects of care for the dying and for medical/care aspects of care for the dying, and knowledge of supportive services and facilities. • Last Aid Courses were more suitable to educate non-medical hospital staff about care for the dying. • Medical staff requested courses with an extended curriculum in order to meet their learning goals. • Last Aid Courses were well accepted and helped to reduce information deficits on care for the dying.
Bollig G, Safi M, Schmidt M, Ewald H. Is there a need for cultural adaptation of the Last Aid Course? A mixed-methods study across the Danish-German Border. *Healthcare* 2022, *10*(4),658. [44]	LAC for German and Danish participants in the border region	Prospective mixed-methods study	Questionnaire after the LAC and focus group discussions	- A total of 53 of the 79 participants returned a questionnaire (response rate 67%). - A total of 49 of the 79 participants (response rate 62%) joined one of seven focus group discussions in Danish (three focus groups) or German (four focus groups)	Denmark Germany	• Almost all participants appreciated the LAC as an option to talk and learn about death and end-of-life care. • The informants found individual differences more important than cultural differences in end-of-life care but described differences connected to regulations and organization of services across the border. • Suggestions for adaptation and improvement of the LAC included the topics of organization and support across the border, religions, and cultures, and supporting people in grief. • The findings of the study will inform a revision of the Last Aid curriculum and future projects across the border and will help to include the views of minorities.

https://doi.org/10.3390/healthcare14010096

Table 2. *Cont.*

Articles: Authors, Journal, and Publication Year	Main Topic	Type of Study	Evaluation Method	Informants and Response Rate	Involved Countries	Main Findings
Zelko E, Vrbek L, Koletnik M. Last Aid Course—the Slovenian experience. *Healthcare* 2022, *10*(7), 1154. [45]	Experiences with LAC in Slovenia	Prospective mixed-methods study	Questionnaire after LAC participation	- A total of 386 LAC participants received a questionnaire personally or by e-mail. - A total of 250 questionnaires were returned (response rate 64.7%)	Slovenia	• The Slovenian Last Aid experience is comparable to that reported by countries where the course had been previously organized. • In Slovenia, the courses were extremely well-received and favourably rated. • The adaptation to Slovenian cultural requirements with information from the local communities was supported by materials prepared by the PO-LAST project.
MacAden L, Broadfoot K, Carolan C, Muirhead K, Neylon S, Keen J. Last Aid training online: Participants' and facilitators' perceptions from a mixed-methods study in rural Scotland. *Healthcare* 2022, *10*(5), 918. [46]	Evaluation of online Last Aid Courses in Scotland	Prospective mixed-methods study	Combination of online survey of OLAC participants followed by individual semi-structured qualitative interviews with both LAT participants and facilitators	- Of 68 LAC participants, 26 participants completed the survey (response rate of 38%) - Five LAC instructors participated in interviews	Scotland	• Provision of foundational death literacy education in social contexts enhances the personal knowledge, skills, and confidence of individual community members and supports the notion that this personal growth could lead to strengthened community action. • There is potential to include LAC as the foundational core training to promote death literacy in communities.
Giehl C, Chikradze N, Bollig G, Vollmer HC, Otte I. "I needed to know, no matter what I do, I won't make it worse"—expectations and experiences of Last Aid Course participants in Germany—A qualitative pilot study. *Healthcare* 2023, *11*(4), 592. [47]	Experiences of LAC participants with caring for seriously ill and dying people	Qualitative pilot study	Semi-structured interviews of LAC participants	Five LAC participants participated in telephone interviews	Germany	• Overall, the interviewed participants have a positive attitude toward Last Aid Courses. • They perceive the courses as helpful as they provide knowledge, guidance, and recommendations of action for concrete palliative situations. • Eight main topics emerged during analysis: expectations regarding the course, transfer of knowledge, reducing fear, the Last Aid Course as a safe space, support from others, empowerment and strengthening of own skills, and the improvement needs of the course. • The pilot interviews show initial indications that the impact, as well as supportive and challenging factors regarding the ability to care for relatives to cope, should be explored in further research.

https://doi.org/10.3390/healthcare14010096

Table 2. *Cont.*

Articles: Authors, Journal, and Publication Year	Main Topic	Type of Study	Evaluation Method	Informants and Response Rate	Involved Countries	Main Findings
Woodworth J. Building death literacy through Last Aid: An examination of agency, ambivalence and gendered informal caregiving within the Swedish welfare state. *NORA-Nordic Journal of Feminist and Gender Research* 2023. [48]	Evaluation of the implementation of the LAC as an initiative for health-promoting palliative care in Sweden	Case study	Case study with focus on the work of four course instructors in organizing and teaching Last Aid and the experiences of course participants; combination of personalistic observation and verbatim quotation incorporating a mixed-methods approach comprising action research (AR), focus groups, and participant observation	Four course instructors (including the first author) participated in the collection of the qualitative data	Sweden	• Participants articulated Last Aid as a tool which helped them reclaim agency amidst the inertia of competing norms and expectations of informal caregiving. • The findings indicate that the implementation of Last Aid into the Swedish context is characterized by a tension between norms of institutional caregiving versus community caregiving, representing a case of sociological ambivalence. • Women disproportionately perform informal caregiving for seriously ill significant others in an institutional context where state care services are diminishing.
Bollig G, Gräf K, Gruna H, Drexler D, Pothmann R. "We want to talk about death, dying and grief and to learn about end-of-life care"—lessons learned from a multi-center mixed-methods study on Last Aid Courses for kids and teens. *Children*. 2024 Feb 9;11(2):224. [49]	Evaluation of the implementation of LAC-KT and the experiences with the course	Prospective mixed methods study	Questionnaires and focus group interviews	A total of 2534 valid questionnaires were received from 2996 LAC-KT participants aged 7–17 years (response rate 85%). In addition, two focus group interviews of 22 LAC-KT instructors were performed.	Germany	• A total of 84% of the participants already had experience with death and dying. • A total of 91% found the LAC-KT helpful for everyone. • The majority of the participants appreciated the opportunity to talk and learn about death, dying, grief, and palliative care. • The LAC-KT is feasible, very well accepted, and a welcome opportunity for exchanging and obtaining information about dying, grief, and palliative care. • Further research on the effects and the implementation of the LAC-KT throughout the school curricula and the long-term effects of the training are needed.
Bollig G, Mueller-Koch S, Zelko E. Instructors' views on and experiences with Last Aid Courses as a means for public palliative care education—A longitudinal mixed-methods study. *Int. J. Environ. Res. Public Health* 2025, 22, 1117. [50]	Instructors' views on and experiences with Last Aid Courses	Prospective mixed methods study	Questionnaires and focus group interviews	Longitudinal study over 5 years	Germany	• The LAC participants felt empowered after the LACs. • Continuing development is a characteristic of the LAC project. • The positive effects of the LACs included empowerment and positive interactions between the instructors and participants. • LACs had a positive impact on all five principles of social space orientation.

Table 2. *Cont.*

Articles: Authors, Journal, and Publication Year	Main Topic	Type of Study	Evaluation Method	Informants and Response Rate	Involved Countries	Main Findings
Bollig G, Heller A. The Last Aid Course—A simple and effective concept to teach the public about palliative care and to enhance the public discussion about death and dying. *Austin Journal of Palliative Care*. 2016;1(2). [51]	Description of the LAC concept and first experiences with the implementation	Mini review	Review of the literature from a PubMed search and description of the Last Aid concept and the first experiences in practice from three countries	Results from the first German pilot study and general experiences with the course in Germany, Denmark, and Norway are described	Germany Denmark Norway	• Public Palliative Care Education is needed. • First experiences show that the Last Aid Course is feasible in different countries. • The LAC is very well accepted by the participants. • The LAC is a simple and effective concept to teach the public about palliative care.
Bollig G, Hjelm Brandt Kristensen F, Ciurlionis M, Knopf B. Last Aid Course. An education for all citizens and an ingredient of compassionate communities. *Healthcare*. 2019 Jan 28;7(1). 19. [52]	Description of the experiences with LAC and review of the literature	Review	Review of the literature on educational efforts regarding palliative care for non-professionals in PubMed/Medline and the existing literature on Last Aid courses	A literature search in PubMed and Medline led to 47 papers with accessible abstracts. Of these 47 papers, only 7 papers included palliative care education for the public as a major topic. Additional sources were found by hand searches in books and reference lists or the Internet.	n.a.	• The public requires more information and education about palliative care. • The Last Aid Courses are accepted by many people and have an enormous potential to spread information about palliative care throughout the public and can contribute to enhanced public discussion about end-of-life care. • More research on the education of non-professionals in palliative care, end-of-life care, and the compassionate community approach is necessary. • Research on the implementation of the Last Aid course is ongoing in different countries.
Bollig G, Bauer EH. Last Aid Courses as measure for public palliative care education for adults and children: A narrative review. *Annals of Palliative Medicine*. July 2021;10(7):8242–8253. [13]	A narrative overview of the current knowledge on Last Aid Courses (LACs) and experiences from the implementation process in different countries	Narrative review	A literature search in PubMed/Medline was performed and a narrative overview of the existing literature on LAC and PPCE is provided	A literature search in PubMed using "last aid" led to 6 results only. A search strategy combining "palliative care education" and "public" led to 69 results in PubMed. Fifty-six of these were published within the last 5 years.	n.a.	• Measures to raise awareness of palliative care, to improve the public discussion about death and dying, and to empower citizens to participate in end-of-life care in the community are needed and should be offered more widely. • LACs are one example of a feasible and well-accepted approach to PPCE in different countries. • The LAC can contribute to a public debate on death, dying, and palliative care and may contribute to the empowerment of citizens in the provision of end-of-life care. • Further research on PPCE and the LAC is necessary to add to the body of knowledge in this emerging field and is ongoing at present.

https://doi.org/10.3390/healthcare14010096

Table 2. *Cont.*

Articles: Authors, Journal, and Publication Year	Main Topic	Type of Study	Evaluation Method	Informants and Response Rate	Involved Countries	Main Findings
Elder AB. A narrative review—characterizing palliative care curriculum aimed at high school adolescents and young adults. *Illness, Crisis & Loss*. Online first 15 April 2025. [53]	Exploration of the characteristics of palliative care curriculum developed for high school adolescent and young adults	Narrative review	Literature search using the databases ERIC, PubMed, and CINHAL	A total of 202 articles were included. These articles were screened using strategic exclusion criteria, resulting in five relevant literature works in the analysis.	n.a.	• Studies including a variety of designs, methods, and strategies all resulted in positive participation, feedback, and experiences from high school AYA provided with palliative care curriculum. • The literature indicates that the use of subject matter experts within palliative care curriculum for high school students is a core characteristic in meeting the World Health Organizations recommendation to embed palliative care curriculum into public awareness strategies.
Seckin M, Tiwana R, Fry D, Bailey C. Key themes and approaches in palliative and end-of-life care education for the general public: A systematic review. *BMC Palliative Care* 2025 24:219. [54]	Identification of key educational components related to palliative and end-of-life care for citizens, volunteers, and the general public	Mixed-method systematic review	A mixed-methods systematic review was conducted, incorporating four electronic databases (MEDLINE, PsycINFO, CINAHL, and the Cochrane Library) and grey literature searches, and quality was assessed using Hawker et al.'s (2002) critical appraisal checklists	A total of 20 studies with 10.037 participants were included in the systematic review	n.a.	• The analysis revealed six main themes: foundational concepts and philosophies, communication and decision-making, planning and preparation, symptom management, end-of-life care practices, and caregiving support. • The review highlights the importance of training programmes to improve community involvement in caregiving and enhance the quality of care for individuals with life-limiting conditions. • Expanding access to such educational resources can empower more people to contribute confidently to end-of-life care in their communities. • The LAC is one the concepts that includes all six main themes (out of 16 different educational programs).

LAC = Last Aid Course (for adults), OLAC = online Last Aid Course (for adults), LAC-KT = Last Aid Course for kids and teens, PPCE = Public Palliative Care Education, and n.a. = not applicable.

https://doi.org/10.3390/healthcare14010096

3. Results and Discussion

The search strategy retrieved numerous publications on the topics of Last Aid Courses and/or Public Palliative Care Education. The first step of the assessment of the search results was the removal of duplicates. In addition to the literature search in scientific databases, a list of Last Aid publications from the homepage of Last Aid Germany [55], updated 27 September 2025 and including 65 publications on Last Aid (47 articles in journal, 13 books or book chapters and 5 other publications), was assessed and led to the inclusion of 12 articles reporting scientific studies and 5 reviews in Table 2 as well as other publications in journals and book chapters in the current review. Of the 65 listed publications, 62 were published in 2015 or later. This shows that there is a large interest in Last Aid Courses, resulting in a large number of publications on Last Aid Courses that have been published within the last 10 years, after the first Last Aid Courses were started in Norway in November 2014 and Germany in January 2015.

The literature search identified several articles on Last Aid studies and reviews. Table 2 provides an overview of 17 Last Aid studies and reviews published in English in scientific journals [13,29,40–54]. The presented articles are ordered by publication year with scientific articles first (n = 12) followed by reviews (n = 5).

The main results from the included studies were that LACs, LAC-KTs, and online Last Aid Courses (OLACs) are feasible and well accepted by different populations from different countries. Many participants feel encouraged to talk more openly about death and dying and to engage in end-of-life care provision in their community in the future. The first multicentre study on the LAC published in 2021 showed that 88% of the participants were female with a median age of 56 years [29]. Most participants (76%) rated the course as very good and 99% would recommend the course to others [29]. These findings are similar to the results of a scoping review on different death education programs that concluded that death education leads to "a higher willingness to discuss end-of-life decisions and decreased death anxiety, death avoidance, and fear of death" [56]. Interestingly, 9.4% of the 5469 participants of the above-mentioned study [29] had a medical profession, indicating an interest in talking about dying, death, and grief although belonging to a medical profession that may implicate a closer relationship to these topics than for the public. The reason for this need could be a lack of these topics during medical training.

A study on an LAC for employees of a German university hospital revealed that a number of members of the medical staff found the LAC more suitable for educating non-medical hospital staff about care for the dying and requested courses with an extended curriculum in order to meet their learning goals [43]. Based on these findings and wishes, a working group in Germany established a one-day Last Aid Course Professional for workers from health and social care. The first results of the pilot study have been published in German and received a prize for the best publication in the German Journal of Palliative Medicine in the year 2023, showing the recognition and impact within the scientific field of palliative medicine [55]. The results showed that the course is feasible, and that many of the participants rated the course as useful for healthcare personnel and appreciated new perspectives, reflections, and the interactive work on different options for action in palliative care.

A study on cultural differences across the German–Danish border showed that the informants found individual differences more important than cultural differences in end-of-life care but they described differences connected to regulations and organization of services across the border [44]. The informants suggested including the topics of organization and support across the border, religions, and cultures, and especially, advice on how to support people in grief [44]. LACs are welcome and useful in different countries and cultures [29,42–46,48].

https://doi.org/10.3390/healthcare14010096

A qualitative pilot study of caring relatives suggests that the LAC is seen as a safe place for discussion, empowers caring relatives, and strengthens their skills [47]. The LAC may also contribute to reclaiming agency [48]. Furthermore, the research on LAC indicates that informal caring for relatives is often provided by women [29,48]. The continuing development, quality assurance, and improvement of the course content through research is an important characteristic of the Last Aid project [50]. In addition to empowering LAC participants to engage in palliative care, the LAC influences all five principles of social space orientation and may thus contribute to improved palliative care in the community in the long term [50]. This impact includes effects on the framework of social space and its five principles of resource orientation, participation, networking, sustainability, and contextuality [50]. LAC can, e.g., lead to improved participation of lay people in end-of-life care in the community and the connection and adaptation of local networks of care [50]. Children and teenagers are also interested in talking about dying, death, and grief and appreciate the LAC-KT as an opportunity to talk and learn more about these topics [40,49]. Most of the participating children and teenagers aged 7 to 17 years (84%) already had experience with death and dying before taking the course and 91% found the LAC-KT helpful for everyone [49]. OLACs were introduced in Germany, Brazil, and Scotland during the COVID-19 pandemic in order to keep up with teaching despite meeting restrictions [41,42,46]. The results showed that although the online format is often only seen as the second-best option, it is possible to implement, meaningful, and even led to an increased participation of people who care for others at home and younger people [42]. According to MacAden et al., "Provision of foundational death literacy education in social contexts enhances the personal knowledge, skills, and confidence of individual community members and supports the notion that this personal growth could lead to strengthened community action.", and they suggested "to include LAC as the foundational core training to promote death literacy in communities." [46].

Since the start of the implementation of the first Last Aid Courses in Norway, Germany, and Denmark in 2014/2015, three reviews on LACs have been performed and published by Bollig et al. [13,51,52]. The main findings from these reviews were that the LAC as a simple approach to PPCE is feasible and well accepted in different countries. Both research and practical experience from the implementation indicate that the LAC can assist in improving the public debate on death, dying, and palliative care and may also contribute to the empowerment of citizens in the provision of end-of-life care. Two recent reviews published in 2025 have focused on PPCE for the general public [53,54]. One of them, published by Elder, about education for adolescents and young adults concluded that "a variety of designs, methods, and strategies were all identified to have positive participation, feedback, and experiences from high school AYA being provided palliative care curriculum" and that "the use of subject matter experts within palliative care curriculum for high school students is a core characteristic in meeting the World Health Organizations recommendation to embed palliative care curriculum into public awareness strategies" [53]. Seckin et al. [54] describe six main themes of palliative and end-of-life education for the public. These include foundational concepts and philosophies, communication and decision-making, planning and preparation, symptom management, end-of-life care practices, and caregiving support. Interestingly, only three educational concepts for the public include all six themes, one of them being the LAC [54].

In addition to the papers described in Table 2, other publications connected to Last Aid Courses included reports on international Last Aid conferences [55], editorials, comments, opinions, and letters on PPCE and LAC [55,57,58]. The experiences from different countries with the implementation of the LAC show that the LAC is feasible in different settings and across different cultures and ethnicities [13,29,45,46,48]. It has also been shown that

https://doi.org/10.3390/healthcare14010096

different organisations, e.g., palliative care organisations, universities, or the church, are possible national cooperating organisations for the implementation and organisation of LACs in different countries [55]. It has been stated that cultural beliefs and rituals may help to alleviate grief [59]. These topics are addressed in both the LAC and the LAC-KT and are introduced and discussed with the participants [13]. First Aid training for the public, including adults, elderly people, teenagers, and children, is a useful public health initiative and experts recommend it even as mandatory in schools or workplaces [60–65]. Some articles on Last Aid recommend implementing Last Aid Courses in an analogous fashion to First Aid courses in the public sphere [13,29,43,49,50]. Thus, Last Aid Courses are an essential part of Public Health Palliative Care. To raise the public awareness for palliative care is very important as the general public is lacking a detailed understanding of palliative care [66] and education and training have been suggested to raise awareness and to improve participation of the local communities in palliative care provision [67]. Talking about death and dying may support the grieving process of teenagers [68]. These findings are similar to the findings from the LAC-KT for teenagers that show that 84% of them have already had experience with dying and death and they want to talk about death and dying [13,49]. Importantly, however, there are apparent gaps in the literature and evidence base for Public Palliative Care Education, and these should be addressed in line with the recommendations made below.

3.1. Need for Future Research

The research on LACs, including different course formats and the effects of the LAC, is part of the international Last Aid project and is coordinated by the Last Aid Research Group International (LARGI) that was founded in Sønderborg, Denmark during the first International Last Aid Conference, 2019. LARGI is led by Erika Zelko and Georg Bollig.

3.1.1. Areas and Topics for Future Research on Last Aid

Based on the findings of the current review and discussions of the experts from the International Last Aid working group and the members of LARGI, Figure 1 presents the topics that are most important for future research on the international Last Aid Course project. Three areas are of outmost importance for Last Aid research in the future: LAC for adults, LAC for different groups, and the interaction between LAC and compassionate communities. In addition to the research on LAC for adults in different countries, the effect on caring relatives and the long-term effects of LAC demand further research—as does the investigation of knowledge retention over time. An international Delphi study on the contents of PPCE and the LAC with the participation of international experts would be useful for the further development of the LAC. As different LAC course formats for different groups have been developed in recent years, these also need a scientific evaluation to support the future improvement and wide implementation of these formats. A prototype of international cooperation and the need for cultural adaptation will be a planned project to translate the LAC-KT into different languages and for its implementation in different countries and across different groups and cultures. In order to improve community-based palliative care, education of the public is needed [21,28,29]. Therefore, the interaction between educational initiatives as the LAC and compassionate communities needs more research. Of special interest, is the evaluation of possible positive effects of the LAC on the death and grief literacy of the public and public awareness of dying, death, grief, and palliative care in general. Other interesting topics are the higher percentage of female LAC participants [29] and thus, future strategies to recruit more men to participate in the LAC. It has been shown that informal carers face many burdens at the end-of-life and that ways to address grief and bereavement and support employees who are informal

https://doi.org/10.3390/healthcare14010096

carers are needed in the workplace [69–71]. This is also described for employees who have experienced perinatal loss [72]. The European project EU-CoWork is currently trying to develop compassionate workplace programs to address the above-mentioned topics in the workplace [73]. The need to address dying, death, and grief in the workplace has also been found in a project by the Center for Palliative Medicine at the University of Cologne [74]. The next step of this project shall be the implementation of Lastaiders in the workplace, similarly to Firstaiders. A very interesting question is whether the LAC may contribute to an increased number of people who will die at their preferred place of death, for example, due to an improved possibility of home death that may be enabled through more support from the public after LAC training.

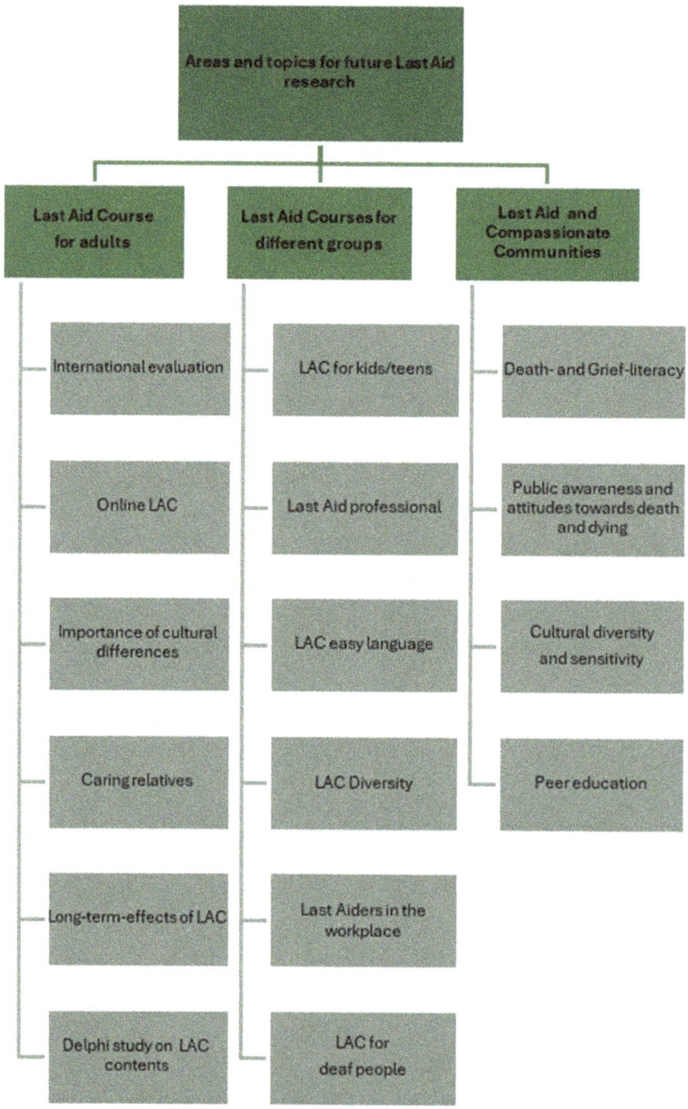

Figure 1. Areas and topics for future Last Aid research.

https://doi.org/10.3390/healthcare14010096

3.1.2. Last Aid as Part of Public Health Palliative Care and Compassionate Communities

An explanatory lens for understanding public reluctance to engage with end-of-life care thoughts and initiatives such as Last Aid is provided by Terror Management Theory [75]. It posits that human awareness of mortality provokes deep existential anxiety, which individuals and societies manage through cultural systems that offer meaning and a sense of symbolic immortality. In contemporary Western contexts, this often takes the form of the medicalisation and professionalisation of death, where dying is displaced into institutional settings and managed by experts, reducing direct and normal confrontation with mortality. This psychological mechanism reinforces a service-seeking culture, in which people defer responsibility for dying and grief to healthcare systems rather than viewing them as shared social experiences. From a critical realist perspective, such mortality-defence processes operate as underlying generative mechanisms that constrain participation in Public Palliative Care Education while simultaneously highlighting its necessity. Last Aid Courses, by normalizing discussion about death and re-embedding care within community life, can be seen as gentle counter-measures to these cultural defences, supporting both personal death awareness and collective capacity to care [13,29,50]. Within the United Kingdom, for example, these psychological and cultural mechanisms intersect with the structural realities outlined in Professor Chris Whitty's Chief Medical Officer's Annual Report 2023 [30]. He emphasises that the central public health challenge of ageing is not simply extending lifespan but enhancing independence, quality of life, and community capacity in the later years of life. From a critical realist standpoint, this vision reveals how macro-level structures, including health and social care integration, local infrastructure, and socioeconomic inequalities mediate the possibilities for community engagement at the end of life. While the service-seeking orientation and mortality-defence mechanisms described above may inhibit public participation, Whitty's framework points to potential enabling conditions for change: strengthening community assets, reducing isolation, and supporting intergenerational engagement. Building on these insights, Last Aid as an option for Public Palliative Care Education can be understood as a practical expression of Public Health Palliative Care (PHPC) principles, translating the values of participation, empowerment, and equity into accessible community education. Yet, the literature to date has focused primarily on feasibility and satisfaction, leaving underexplored the social infrastructure that Last Aid helps to create, encompassing the networks, norms, and shared vocabularies that enable collective care. Equally, questions of equity and access remain largely unexamined—particularly who remains excluded from participation due to socioeconomic, cultural, or geographical barriers. Increasing access through a variety of practical means will be important. For example, the use of novel educational approaches such as immersive simulation, gaming, or escape rooms may assist in improving accessibility and engagement around end-of-life issues. Addressing these gaps will be essential to ensure that Last Aid realises its PHPC potential as an inclusive, community-empowering intervention. In addition to the proposals for future research described above, future research should therefore also move beyond individual-level outcomes, to examine how Last Aid contributes to sustainable community capacity and long-term cultural change. Conceptually, this may be understood as a double-loop process [76], in which the first loop enhances individual health, death, and grief literacy, while the second loop reshapes the social norms and institutional arrangements that govern how dying and bereavement are collectively managed. In this way, Last Aid Courses could act as meso-level mechanisms linking individual reflection with community action, translating policy aspirations for compassionate, age-friendly societies into practice, and exemplifying how PHPC can be lived in everyday life. In conclusion, Last Aid Courses can be seen as building the knowledge base for compassionate communities to enable and empower the public for palliative care provision in the community [13,29].

https://doi.org/10.3390/healthcare14010096

4. Limitations

The most important limitation of this review is the limited number of publication on the LAC and LAC-KT. Most articles on the LAC and LAC-KT have been published by Bollig and/or other authors who are participants of the Last Aid Research Group International (LARGI) that was established during the First. International Last Aid Conference in Sønderborg in Denmark and which is led by Zelko and Bollig. Therefore, this article has a relatively high number of self-citations, which are not avoidable due to the limited number of scientific articles on the topic. The personal experiences of most of the authors can also be seen as a strength of the study as they have both personal experiences with LAC and an in-depth knowledge of the background, practice, and research in the field of PPCE. Further, there is potential for publication bias within the literature reviewed, largely originating from European/Western populations, and findings may not necessarily be generalizable to other geographical contexts and populations. Other possible limitations may be connected to the fact that most LAC participants are female, as shown by Bollig et al. [29], and missing information on the participants' backgrounds in terms of culture and diversity. Information about the recruiting strategies in different regions and countries is lacking or not reported in most articles. As the strategies used are very different and include school classes and preexisting groups of people as well as LACs that are open for all members of the public, this may be an area of interest for the future. These limitations could be addressed in future research on Last Aid.

5. Conclusions

Last Aid Courses have been introduced in 23 different countries since 2015. The LAC, the LAC-KT, and PPCE may enhance the public debate on dying, death, grief, and palliative care and may empower people to contribute to end-of-life care in the community. Future research should explore three main topics: 1. Last Aid Courses for adults including the long-term effects of the courses and a Delphi-study on the contents; 2. LACs for different groups including, e.g., LAC diversity and Lastaiders in the workplace; and 3. LACs and compassionate communities including, e.g., the effects on death literacy and grief literacy as well as participation of the public in education via peer education. Future research on PPCE, the LAC, and the LAC-KT should also focus on retention of skills and knowledge over time and long-term effects of the courses.

Author Contributions: G.B. and J.M. contributed equally to this paper and share the first authorship. Conceptualization and methodology, G.B., J.M., S.M.-K., P.P., B.N. and E.Z.; literature research and formal analysis, G.B. and J.M.; writing—original draft preparation, G.B. and J.M.; writing—review and editing, all authors; visualization, all authors; project administration, G.B. and J.M. All authors have read and agreed to the published version of the manuscript.

Funding: This research received no external funding.

Institutional Review Board Statement: Not applicable.

Informed Consent Statement: Not applicable.

Data Availability Statement: No new data were created or analyzed in this study. Data sharing is not applicable to this article.

Conflicts of Interest: G.B. is a board member of Letzte Hilfe Deutschland gGmbH. G.B. and S.M.K. receive financial compensation for giving Last Aid Instructor courses. G.B. owns the trademark Last Aid. Author P.P. is employed by the company Deutsche Welle. The remaining authors declare that the research was conducted in the absence of any commercial or financial relationships that could be construed as a potential conflict of interest.

https://doi.org/10.3390/healthcare14010096

Abbreviations

The following abbreviations are used in this manuscript:

gGmbH	gemeinnützige Gesellschaft mit beschränkter Haftung (non-profit non-governmental organization in Germany)
LAC	Last Aid Course
LAC-KT	Last Aid Course Kids and Teens
LARGI	Last Aid Research Group International
OLAC	Online Last Aid Course
NGO	Non-governmental Organization
PHPC	Public Health Palliative Care
PPCE	Public Palliative Care Education
n.a.	Not Applicable

References

1. Etkind, N.; Bone, A.E.; Gomes, B.; Lovell, N.; Evans, C.J.; Higginson, I.J.; Murtagh, F.E.M. How many people will need palliative care in 2040? Past trends, future projections and implications for services. *BMC Med.* **2017**, *15*, 102. [CrossRef] [PubMed]
2. Gomes, B.; Higginson, I.J.; Calanzani, N.; Cohen, J.; Deliens, L.; Daveson, B.A.; Bechinger-English, D.; Bausewein, C.; Ferreira, P.L.; Toscani, F.; et al. Preferences for place of death if faced with advanced cancer: A population survey in England, Flanders, Germany, Italy, The Netherlands, Portugal and Spain. *Ann. Oncol.* **2012**, *23*, 2006–2015. [CrossRef] [PubMed]
3. Clegg, A.; Young, J.; Iliffe, S.; Rikkert, M.O.; Rockwood, K. Frailty in elderly people. *Lancet* **2013**, *381*, 752–762. [CrossRef] [PubMed]
4. Salikhanov, I. Beyond high-income models: Effective palliative care for LMICs. *Support. Care Cancer* **2025**, *33*, 1022. [CrossRef]
5. Rodin, G.; Feldman, A.; Trapani, D.; Skelton, M.; Unger-Saldaña, K.; Essue, B.; Pihlak, R.; Walshe, C.; E Rosa, W.; Banegas, M.P.; et al. The human crisis in cancer: A Lancet Oncology Commission. *Lancet Oncol.* **2025**, *26*, e628–e670. [CrossRef]
6. Marshall, C.; Virdun, C.; Philipps, J.L. Strengthening care for adults with palliative care needs in high-income rural communities: A global policy environmental scan. *BMC Palliat. Care* **2025**, *24*, 253. [CrossRef]
7. Connor, S.R.; Garralda, E.; Tripodoro, V.A.; Centeno, C. Estimating the Number of Services & Patients Receiving Specialized Palliative Care Globally in 2025. *J. Pain Symptom Manag.* **2025**, *70*, 422–426. [CrossRef]
8. Peeler, A.; Afolabi, O.A.; Sleeman, K.E.; Akoum, M.E.; Gafer, N.; Hammerich, A.; Harding, R. Confronting global inequities in palliative care. *BMJ Glob. Health* **2025**, *10*, e017624. [CrossRef]
9. Murtagh, F.E.; Bausewein, C.; Verne, J.; Groeneveld, E.I.; Kaloki, Y.E.; Higginson, I.J. How many people need palliative care? A study developing and comparing methods for population-based estimates. *Palliat. Med.* **2014**, *28*, 49–58. [CrossRef]
10. Scholten, N.; Gunther, A.L.; Pfaff, H.; Karbach, U. The size of the population potentially in need of palliative care in Germany-an estimation based on death registration data. *BMC Palliat. Care* **2016**, *15*, 29. [CrossRef]
11. Lin, H.; Huang, Y.; Wang, Y. Facilitators and barriers to palliative care delivery in rural China: A qualitative study of the perceptions and experiences of rural healthcare professionals. *BMC Palliat. Care* **2025**, *24*, 211. [CrossRef] [PubMed]
12. Sabar, R.; Hochwald, I.I.; Weiss, M.; Yakov, G. The Professional Guest: Conceptualizing home visits in palliative care settings. *Palliat. Care Soc. Pract.* **2024**, *18*, 26323524241293821. [CrossRef] [PubMed]
13. Bollig, G.; Hayes Bauer, E. Last Aid Courses as measure for public palliative care education—A narrative review. *Ann. Palliat. Med.* **2021**, *10*, 8242–8253. [CrossRef] [PubMed]
14. Kellehear, A. Compassionate communities: End-of-life care as everyone's responsibility. *QJM Int. J. Med.* **2013**, *106*, 1071–1075. [CrossRef]
15. Kellehear, A. Compassionate Cities. In *Public Health and End-of-Life Care*; Routledge: Oxfordshire, UK, 2005.
16. Chan, W.S.; Funk, L. Developing Compassionate Community: Insights from the International Standards for Community Development. *Health Open Res.* **2024**, *6*, 17. [CrossRef]
17. McIlfatrick, S.; Hasson, F.; McLaughlin, D.; Johnston, G.; Roulston, A.; Rutherford, L.; Noble, H.; Kelly, S.; Craig, A.; Kernohan, W.G. Public awareness and attitudes toward palliative care in Northern Ireland. *BMC Palliat. Care* **2013**, *12*, 34. [CrossRef]
18. McIlfatrick, S.; Noble, H.; McCorry, N.K.; Roulston, A.; Hasson, F.; McLaughlin, D.; Johnston, G.; Rutherford, L.; Payne, C.; Kernohan, G.; et al. Exploring public awareness and perceptions of palliative care: A qualitative study. *Palliat. Med.* **2014**, *28*, 273–280. [CrossRef]
19. Gopal, K.S.; Archana, P.S. Awareness, knowledge and attitude about palliative care, in general, population and health care professionals in tertiary care hospital. *Int. J. Sci. Study* **2016**, *3*, 31–35.

https://doi.org/10.3390/healthcare14010096

20. Kozlov, E.; McDarby, M.; Reid, M.C.; Carpenter, B.D. Knowledge of Palliative Care Among Community-Dwelling Adults. *Am. J. Hosp. Palliat. Care* **2018**, *35*, 647–651. [CrossRef]
21. Boucher, N.A.; Bull, J.H.; Cross, S.H.; Kirby, C.; Davis, J.K.; Taylor, D.H. Patient, Caregiver, and Taxpayer Knowledge of Palliative Care and Views on a Model of Community-Based Palliative Care. *J. Pain Symptom Manag.* **2018**, *56*, 951–956. [CrossRef]
22. Westerlund, C.; Tishelman, C.; Benkel, I.; Fürst, C.J.; Molander, U.; Rasmussen, B.H.; Sauter, S.; Lindqvist, O. Public awareness of palliative care in Sweden. *Scand. J. Public Health* **2018**, *46*, 478–487. [CrossRef]
23. Noonan, K. Death literacy—Developing a tool to measure the social impact of public health initiatives. *Ann. Palliat. Med.* **2018**, *7*, AB007. [CrossRef] [PubMed]
24. Cakmak, V.S.; Seven, A.; Sari, E.S. Death anxiety and death literacy among Turkish patients with chronic diseases: A cross-sectional study. *BMC Psychiatry* **2025**, *25*, 299. [CrossRef] [PubMed]
25. Dinther, K.V.; Noonan, K.; Leonard, R.; Javanparast, S. The Death Literacy Index: Testing the Death System Literacy of Unpaid Carers of Palliative Patients. *Omega* **2025**. [CrossRef]
26. Butola, S.; Gursahani, R. Advance care planning and the ethical obligation of death literacy as a public health initiative in India. *Indian J. Med. Ethics* **2024**, *IX*, 308–312. [CrossRef] [PubMed]
27. Breen, L.; Kawashima, D.; Joy, K.; Cadell, S.; Roth, D.; Chow, A.; Macdonald, M.E. Grief literacy: A call to action for compassionate communities. *Death Stud.* **2022**, *46*, 425–433. [CrossRef]
28. Sallnow, L.; Smith, R.; Ahmedzai, S.H.; Bhadelia, A.; Chamberlain, C.; Cong, Y.; Doble, B.; Dullie, L.; Durie, R.; Finkelstein, E.A.; et al. Report of the Lancet Commission on the Value of Death: Bringing death back into life. *Lancet* **2022**, *399*, 837–884. [CrossRef]
29. Bollig, G.; Brandt Kristensen, F.; Wolff, D.L. Citizens appreciate talking about death and learning end-of-life care—A mixed-methods study on views and experiences of 5469 Last aid Course participants. *Prog. Palliat. Care* **2021**, *29*, 140–148. [CrossRef]
30. Whitty, C. *Chief Medical Officer's Annual Report 2021: Health in Coastal Communities*; Department of Health and Social Care: London, UK, 2021. Available online: https://www.gov.uk/government/publications/chief-medical-officers-annual-report-2021-health-in-coastal-communities (accessed on 20 October 2025).
31. Bauman, Z. *The Individualized Society*; Polity Press: Cambridge, UK, 1998.
32. Braverman, H. *Labor and Monopoly Capital: The Degradation of Work in the Twentieth Century*; Monthly Review Press: New York City, NY, USA, 1998.
33. Graham-Wisener, L.; Toner, P.; Leonard, R.; Groarke, J.M. Psychometric validation of the death literacy index and benchmarking of death literacy level in a representative UK population sample. *BMC Palliat. Care* **2022**, *21*, 145. [CrossRef]
34. Noonan, K.; Horsfall, D.; Leonard, R.; Rosenberg, J.P. Developing death literacy. *Prog. Palliat. Care* **2016**, *24*, 31–35. [CrossRef]
35. Horsfall, D.; Noonan, K.; Leonard, R. Bringing our dying home: How caring for someone at end of life builds social capital and develops compassionate communities. *Health Sociol. Rev.* **2012**, *21*, 373–382. [CrossRef]
36. World Health Organization. *The Ottawa Charter for Health Promotion*; WHO: Geneva, Switzerland, 1986.
37. Kumar, S.K. A regional community-based palliative care model. *J. Pain Symptom Manag.* **2007**, *33*, 623–627. [CrossRef] [PubMed]
38. Green, B.N.; Johnson, C.D.; Adams, A. Writing narrative literature reviews for peer-reviewed journals: Secrets of the trade. *J. Chiropr. Med.* **2006**, *5*, 101–117. [CrossRef] [PubMed]
39. Bollig, G.; Rosenberg, J.P. Public Health Palliative Care and Public Palliative Care Education. *Healthcare* **2023**, *11*, 745. [CrossRef]
40. Bollig, G.; Mainzer, K.; Fiedler, H.; Pothmann, R. The last aid course for kids and teens from 8–14 years: Preliminary results from the first pilot test. *Hosp. Palliat. Med. Int. J.* **2020**, *4*, 1–3. [CrossRef]
41. Bollig, G.; Knopf, B.; Meyer, S.; Schmidt, M. A New Way of Learning End-of-Life Care and Providing Public Palliative Care Education in Times of the COVID-19 Pandemic: Online Last Aid Courses. *Arch. Health Sci.* **2020**, *4*, 1–2. [CrossRef]
42. Bollig, G.; Meyer, S.; Knopf, B.; Schmidt, M.; Bauer, E.H. First Experiences with Online Last Aid Courses for Public Palliative Care Education during the COVID-19 Pandemic. *Healthcare* **2021**, *9*, 172. [CrossRef]
43. Mueller, E.; Bollig, G.; Becker, G.; Boehlke, C. Lessons Learned from Introducing Last Aid Courses at a University Hospital in Germany. *Healthcare* **2021**, *9*, 906. [CrossRef]
44. Bollig, G.; Safi, M.; Schmidt, M.; Ewald, H. Is There a Need for Cultural Adaptation of the Last Aid Course?—A Mixed-Methods Study across the Danish-German Border. *Healthcare* **2022**, *10*, 658. [CrossRef]
45. Zelko, E.; Vrbek, L.; Koletnik, M. Last Aid Course—The Slovenian Experience. *Healthcare* **2022**, *10*, 1154. [CrossRef]
46. MacAden, L.; Broadfoot, K.; Carolan, C.; Muirhead, K.; Neylon, S.; Keen, J. Last Aid Training Online: Participants' and Facilitators' Perceptions from a Mixed-Methods Study in Rural Scotland. *Healthcare* **2022**, *10*, 918. [CrossRef]
47. Giehl, C.; Chikradze, N.; Bollig, G.; Vollmer, H.C.; Otte, I. "I Needed to Know, No Matter What I Do, I Won't Make It Worse"—Expectations and Experiences of Last Aid Course Participants in Germany—A Qualitative Pilot Study. *Healthcare* **2023**, *11*, 592. [CrossRef] [PubMed]
48. Woodworth, J. Building Death Literacy Through Last Aid: An Examination of Agency, Ambivalence and Gendered Informal Caregiving Within the Swedish Welfare State. *NORA-Nord. J. Fem. Gend. Res.* **2023**, *32*, 76–90. [CrossRef]

https://doi.org/10.3390/healthcare14010096

49. Bollig, G.; Gräf, K.; Gruna, H.; Drexler, D.; Pothmann, R. "We Want to Talk about Death, Dying and Grief and to Learn about End-of-Life Care"—Lessons Learned from a Multi-Center Mixed-Methods Study on Last Aid Courses for Kids and Teens. *Children* **2024**, *11*, 224. [CrossRef] [PubMed]
50. Bollig, G.; Mueller-Koch, S.; Zelko, E. Instructors' Views on and Experiences with Last Aid Courses as a Means for Public Palliative Care Education—A Longitudinal Mixed-Methods Study. *Int. J. Environ. Res. Public Health* **2025**, *22*, 1117. [CrossRef]
51. Bollig, G.; Heller, A. The last aid course—A simple and effective concept to teach the public about palliative care and to enhance the public discussion about death and dying. *Austin J. Palliat. Care* **2016**, *1*, 1010.
52. Bollig, G.; Brandt, F.; Ciurlionis, M.; Knopf, B. Last Aid Course. An Education For All Citizens and an Ingredient of Compassionate Communities. *Healthcare* **2019**, *7*, 19. [CrossRef]
53. Elder, A.B. A Narrative Review—Characterizing Palliative Care Curriculum Aimed at High School Adolescents and Young Adults. *Illn. Crisis Loss*, 2025; *online first*.
54. Seckin, M.; Tiwana, R.; Fry, D.; Bailey, C. Key themes and approaches in palliative and end-of-life care education for the general public: A systematic review. *BMC Palliat. Care* **2025**, *24*, 219. [CrossRef]
55. Last Aid Publication List. Available online: https://www.letztehilfe.info/wp-content/uploads/2025/10/newList-of-publications-Last-Aid-Sep-202572.pdf (accessed on 16 October 2025).
56. Romão, D.; Walshe, C.; Bingley, A.; Grinyer, A. Death education in practice: A scoping review of interventions. *Omega* **2025**. [CrossRef]
57. Hooper, M.; Rehn, M. Beyond life extension—Is it time for 'Emergency Last Aid' training? *Scand. J. Trauma Resusc. Emerg. Med.* **2025**, *33*, 20. [CrossRef]
58. Hooper, M.; Rehn, M. Response to Bollig and Zelko. *Scand. J. Trauma Resusc. Emerg. Med.* **2025**, *33*, 73. [CrossRef]
59. Phan, H.P.; Ngu, B.H.; Chen, S.C.; Hsu, C.S. How cultural beliefs and rituals may help alleviate grief and despair: A four-dimensional framework. *Front. Sociol.* **2025**, *10*, 1620016. [CrossRef]
60. Lenson, S.; Mills, J. First aid knowledge retention in school children: A review of the literature. *Australas. J. Paramed.* **2016**, *13*, 4. [CrossRef]
61. Ticozzi, E.M.; Fagoni, N.; Kacerik, E.; Bodina, A.; Perotti, G.; Lombardo, M.; Pregliasco, F.E.; Stirparo, G. Mandatory First-Aid Training in the Workplace: An Epidemiological Assessment of the Use of Acetylsalicylic Acid Therapy. *Epidemiologica* **2025**, *6*, 49. [CrossRef] [PubMed]
62. Rahim, A.; Asadollahi, A.; Mojadam, M.; Šparovec, E.D.; Kashfi, M.; Nazari, M. Effectiveness of First Aid Training at Home for Grandparents Caring Grandchildren Under 5 Years Old: A Randomized Controlled Trial. *Sci. World J.* **2025**, *2025*, 7457823. [CrossRef] [PubMed]
63. Kendall, I.; Laermans, J.; Daes, T.; Borra, V.; McCaul, M.; Aertgeerts, B.; De Buck, E. First aid training for laypeople. *Cochrane Database Syst. Rev.* **2025**, *8*, CD015538.
64. Da Cruz, K.B.; Cesario, E.S.; Gomes, J.L.; da Cunha, P.H.B.; Galvão, R.G.; Couto, S.B.; Luchesi, B.M.; Martins, T.C.R. Educational intervention in first aid for early childhood education professional: A quasi-experimental study. *Rev. Gasucha Enferm.* **2024**, *45*, e20240040. [CrossRef]
65. Abdelrahman, D.; Aleyeidi, N.A.; Alqahtani, H.T.; Aldosari, F.N.; Al Shammari, T.G.; Alrusaini, N.K.; Almahfouz, R.F.; Altamimi, S.A.; Alshehri, S.A.; Alsubaie, R.M.; et al. Assessment of knowledge, attitude, and practice toward first aid among female school educators in Riyadh, Saudi Arabia: A cross-sectional study. *Front. Public Health* **2024**, *12*, 1482181. [CrossRef]
66. Batzler, Y.N.; Schallenburger, M.; Schwartz, J.; Marazia, C.; Neukirchen, M. The General Public and Young Adults' Knowledge and Perception of Palliative Care: A Systematic Review. *Healthcare* **2024**, *12*, 957. [CrossRef]
67. Shahriah, S.; Dwivedi, S.; Amornmahaphun, S.; Seshkar, S.; Pouy, S.; Puri, S.; Kaur, H.; Aye, S.M.; Sangma, R.V.N.; Teo, S.P. Awareness building and improving participation of local communities in palliative care. *Palliat. Med. Pract.* **2024**, *18*, 3. [CrossRef]
68. Bylund-Grenklo, T.; Birgisdottir, D.; Beenaert, K.; Nyberg, T.; Skokic, V.; Kristensson, J.; Steineck, G.; Fürst, C.J.; Kreicbergs, U. Acute and long-term grief reactions and experiences in parentally cancer-bereaved teenagers. *BMC Palliat. Care* **2021**, *20*, 75. [CrossRef]
69. Dewhurst, F.; Turner, R.; Barett, L.; Westhead, E.; Wakefield, D.; Hanratty, B. Bereavement Training in the Workplace, Can it Help Bridge the Grief Support Gap? A Qualitative Evaluation of Employers' and Employees' Views. *Omega* **2025**. [CrossRef]
70. Lee, M.M.S.; Yeoh, E.K.; Wong, E.L.Y. Employers' Perspectives of Caregiver-Friendly Workplace Policies for Caregiver-Employees Caring for Older Adults in Hong Kong: Thematic Analysis. *JMIR Aging* **2025**, *8*, e68061. [CrossRef]
71. Matzinger, M.; Baum, E.; Bernhardsgrütter, D.; Kesseli, M.; Michelak, G.; Orosaj, F.; Kobleder, A.; Vetsch, J. Relevance and consequence of economic and social resources of severely ill persons and their informal caregivers at the end-of-life: A systematic review of qualitative studies. *BMC Palliat. Care* **2025**. [CrossRef]
72. Meunier, S.; De Montigny, F.; Zeghiche, S.; Lalande, D.; Verdon, C.; Da Costa, D.; Feeley, N. Workplace experience of parents coping with perinatal loss: A scoping review. *Work* **2021**, *69*, 411–421. [CrossRef]

https://doi.org/10.3390/healthcare14010096

73. Vanderstichelen, S.; De Moortel, D.; Nielsen, K.; Wegleitner, K.; Eneslätt, M.; Sardiello, T.; Martos, D.; Webster, J.; Nikandrou, I.; Delvaux, E.; et al. Developing and evaluating Compassionate Workplace Programs to promote health and wellbeing around serious illness, dying and loss in the workplace (EU-CoWork): A transdisciplinary, cross-national research project. *Palliat. Care Soc. Pract.* **2024**, *18*, 26323524241281070. [CrossRef] [PubMed]
74. Letzthelfer: Innen am Arbeitsplatz. Available online: https://letzthelferamarbeitsplatz.com (accessed on 6 December 2025).
75. Pyszczynski, T.; Greenberg, J.; Solomon, S. A dual-process model of defense against conscious and unconscious death-related thoughts: An extension of terror management theory. *Psychol. Rev.* **1999**, *106*, 835–845. [CrossRef]
76. Argyris, C. Double Loop Learning in Organisations. *Harv. Bus. Rev.* **1977**, *55*, 115–125.

https://doi.org/10.3390/healthcare14010096

MDPI AG
Grosspeteranlage 5
4052 Basel
Switzerland
Tel.: +41 61 683 77 34

Healthcare Editorial Office
E-mail: healthcare@mdpi.com
www.mdpi.com/journal/healthcare

www.ingramcontent.com/pod-product-compliance
Lightning Source LLC
Chambersburg PA
CBHW040822250926
51850CB00007BA/1240
9783725869367